HORMONAL BALANCE

Understanding Hormones, Weight, and Your Metabolism

by Scott Isaacs, M.D., F.A.C.P., F.A.C.E.
with Todd Leopold

BULL PUBLISHING COMPANY
BOULDER, COLORADO

Published by Bull Publishing Company,
Post Office Box 1377,
Boulder, Colorado 80306
(www.bullpub.com)

Library of Congress Cataloging-in-Publication Data

Isaacs, Scott, 1967-
Hormonal balance: understanding hormones, weight,
and your metabolism / by Scott Isaacs, with Todd Leopold
p. cm.
Includes bibliographical references and index.
ISBN 0-923521-69-0
1. Hormones—Popular works. 2. Weight loss—Endocrine aspects—
Popular works. 3. Endocrine glands—Diseases—Popular works.
4. Metabolism—Popular works. I. Leopold, Todd. II. Title.
QP571 .I833 2002
612.4'05—dc21
2002003824

INTERIOR DESIGN AND TOPOGRAPHY BY DIANNE NELSON,
SHADOW CANYON GRAPHICS

COVER DESIGN BY LIGHTBOURNE IMAGES

Second Printing, October 2003

CONTENTS

FOREWORD

BY NEIL SHULMAN, M.D.

HORMONAL BALANCE IS THE ESSENTIAL MANUAL FOR KEEPING YOUR BODY HEALTHY. It gives you the most up-to-date, cutting-edge facts about hormones and how they may be contributing to obesity. This book is a first. The hormone factor has been ignored, but may be critical. Before embarking on a series of diets, alterations in lifestyle, and pill taking, you should determine whether hormones are contributing to your problem.

Only after ruling out hormone problems can you make a rational decision about treatment. If you make a commitment to losing weight, you want to make all your agony worthwhile. For every minute and every dollar you put into losing weight, you want a payoff.

Finally, a physician expert in obesity and hormones is willing to reveal the secrets and intricacies of the hormone-obesity connection in an excellent, comprehensive, easy-to-read format.

Scott Isaacs, M.D., F.A.C.P., F.A.C.E., is board-certified in endocrinology, diabetes, and metabolism and has been treating patients, training doctors, and conducting research on hormones, stress, and obesity his entire career. Dr. Isaacs is a caring doctor who listens to his patients and explains things in easy to understand language. This book reflects that philosophy.

INTRODUCTION

IN MY CAREER AS AN ENDOCRINOLOGIST, I'VE ROUTINELY DEALT WITH PEOPLE WHO HAVE TROUBLE LOSING WEIGHT. An overweight patient will come to my office and tell me his or her story. "I've tried everything, doc," the patient will say. "I've followed diet books, I've taken diet pills, I exercise regularly. But nothing works. I'm really not eating that much, but I'm still fat. I can't lose the weight. What's wrong with me?"

What's wrong, I tell these patients, is not simply their diet or exercise regimen—at least, not at the root. The problem, I suggest, may be with their very body chemistry—their hormones.

Sometimes the patients believe me and we get right to work. Sometimes they thank me, leave the office, and go see another doctor —or two, or three—and take diet pills or try yet another diet plan. I wish them well. They may just be treating the symptoms, but not the disease.

You can do all the dieting, exercise, medicating, and thinking you want, but you're not going to lose the weight, keep it off, and live a healthy life unless you address the real problem: hormones.

Hormones are the misunderstood part of our whole weight-obsessed culture. Yes, you can lose weight on a diet — but you might not be healthy, and you'll probably put it all back. This book doesn't exist to give you a new diet. There are plenty of diets out there already, and several of them work just fine. I'll even include variations of some of them in this book.

And this book isn't going to give you great buns in 30 days. It may give you great buns in a few months, or a flat stomach in a year, but that won't be because of me. *That will be largely because you learned to understand your hormones.*

Diet and exercise are important, but they aren't the whole story. Underneath all the meal suggestions, exercise programs, and everything else in the dietary lexicon are little messengers within your body, your hormones. Your hormones—and there are hundreds of them—carry messages from your brain to your body and from your body to your brain. When you eat certain foods, some hormones kick in telling you whether you want more food, where that food will go, what effect it will have on the body and on the brain. When you exercise, hormones go to work, directing the body to move energy stores here, consume energy stores there, boost this part of the body, shut down that part. It's a very delicate dance.

And it's very easy to throw off. If one of your glands—the places in your body that produce hormones—shuts down, becomes overactive, or develops a tumor; if your consumption of a particular food throws off your body chemistry; if depression, pregnancy, any kind of emotional, psychological, or physical turmoil occurs—the body goes a little haywire.

Sometimes, it's self-correcting. It might be off for a few minutes or a few days, but pretty soon things return to normal. But sometimes it's a "new normal." The body has gotten used to its condition and you eat more, or metabolize less, or vary between those two extremes. That's when you start to gain weight.

And, lest we think that "new normal" can be caused only by an "extreme" situation—like tumors or gland failure—consider the aging process. If you could consume pizza and beer every night during your college years without gaining an ounce, you've probably found you can't do that any more.

What's the reason? Hormones. The production of many hormones declines with age, slowing metabolism. It's a fact of nature. But that doesn't mean we have to be captive to weight gain.

The hormonal changes that cause weight gain and occur because of weight gain are complex. The myriad of diet books and hormone books that are currently available are incomplete. Most of these books focus on the hormone *insulin* as the major hormone that makes you fat. Books on other hormones, such as *estrogen, thyroid,* and *growth hormone,* are also available, but none of these really get to the heart of the matter. All of your hormones work in concert to control your metabolism, body composition, and body weight. I wrote this book because I became frustrated with the incomplete messages these other books provided.

The information contained in this book is not a bunch of theories I invented myself. This book contains the most up-to-date scientific information about your body's hormones. Most of the topics in this book have been the major focus at national and international medical meetings. There are hundreds of scientific studies to back up this information; many of these are listed in the Bibliography at the end of this book. Some of the information I present in this book is pretty technical, but I have made every effort to walk you through the concepts step by step so that you understand all the variables involved.

My intention with *Hormonal Balance* is to bring hope and some new solutions to overweight people who suffer needlessly because of hormonal imbalance.

This book is dedicated to my mother,
Sheryle Isaacs,
my first (and best) teacher
on healthy eating and nutrition.

ACKNOWLEDGMENTS

I AM GRATEFUL TO EVERYONE WHO HAS HELPED MAKE THIS BOOK POSSIBLE. Thank you to Fiona Farrelly, Holyn Ivy, and Cindy DeWitt, R.N., M.S.N., who helped with the preparation of this manuscript. Thank you to my family, Howard Isaacs, Sheryle Isaacs, Lori Johns, and Chase Johns. Thank you to Sarah Gardner. I would also like to thank and acknowledge the following people who have been my mentors: Neil Shulman, M.D., Coach Phil Hayford, David Edwards, Ph.D., Janet Rubin, M.D., Guillermo Umpierrez, M.D., and Rabbi David Silverman.

I would also like to give special acknowledgement to Valerie Young, R.D., L.D., Ph.D., for her assistance with preparation of the Hormonal Health Diet, as well as with nutritional guidance throughout this book.

Many, many thanks to my mother, Sheryle Isaacs, for her healthy recipes that have been incorporated into the Hormonal Health Diet.

HORMONES AND METABOLISM

WE ARE FAT.

Americans are fatter than ever. Our comfortable couches, our reliance on fast food, our speedy cars and road systems and spread-out cities that mean you never have to touch a foot to the ground—they help make us fat. We spend billions of dollars on diet books; we throw fifty-dollar bills at jars of diet pills; we scarf up diet supplements, diet magazines, and turbo-quick diet weight-loss plans; we sign up for subscriptions at health clubs that we never use, book appointments at diet doctors whom we ignore, and we make half-hearted attempts at starting exercise programs that we never finish.

And still we are fat.

Why is this? Why can we not lose the weight? Why can we not be the thin, svelte, sexy, beautiful human beings we picture ourselves to be?

Well, part of it is in our minds. Until we can separate ourselves from images of what a sexy, beautiful human being *appears* to be (thin, svelte, rapturously muscled, and sleek), we have no chance of getting there. That ideal version of a human being—those actors, athletes, and supermodels we see on television and in magazines—is a trick of the photographer's light, a creation of the makeup artist's pencil. That ideal version of a human being is an impossibility.

But part of it, a large part of it, is in our bodies. The human body is a terrifically complex machine. Each piece of the machine has an impact on every other piece of the machine, and the machine is constantly analyzing input from inside and outside and adjusting itself accordingly. If one part of the machine goes "off," other parts can follow.

Obesity can be a result of the human machine getting off track. And one reason for this book is to help you understand *why* it gets off track and *how* it gets off track—reasons that are greatly influenced by our hormones. And, finally, it will tell you how to maintain your body so that it doesn't get off track at all, and so that your weight is under safe and healthy control.

A NEW WAY OF THINKING ABOUT YOUR WEIGHT

The statistics are staggering: According to the National Heart, Lung and Blood Institute, 55 percent of Americans are now overweight or obese. Thirty years ago, the figure was 43 percent. Twenty-five percent of children under the age of 19 are at risk for becoming overweight. Ninety-eight percent of people who lose weight on a diet gain it all back within 5 years. Some gain more than that.

Science has yearned to discover the cause of obesity. People try diet after diet, losing some weight only to gain back more, desperately trying any solution they see. But there is no magic cure. There won't be in this book either, so if you're expecting one, put it down now and blow $50 on those "diet pills" over there. If there were a magic cure, you'd know about it. It would not be a secret.

Fortunately, the last few years has brought a change in the way doctors and scientists view obesity. Most thought of obesity, except in the rarest of patients, as a question of willpower. Obese people ate too much. They didn't exercise. They didn't have a balanced diet or a regular workout program. They could lose the weight if only they'd have some guts and determination.

Obesity is no longer considered a problem of willpower. It's a lot more complicated than that.

Obesity used to be considered almost a problem in itself. Now doctors realize it's more a part of a syndrome. Obesity is the *number-two* preventable killer, second only to smoking, because it's connected with a host of medical problems ranging from heart disease and high blood pressure to diabetes, arthritis, gallbladder problems, and even certain types of cancer. The thing about many of these medical problems is that they cause other medical problems. Obesity is merely a part of the whole thing.

But think of how we treat these medical problems: individually. Pharmaceutical companies get rich making the vast array of medications needed to treat these conditions. I'm not putting down medical science; these medications have extended our lives and prevented certain death for many people. But it's a sign of the times that we treat so many individual diseases with drugs—and not the root causes of our problems.

In fact, these diseases—which are known as "diseases of civilization"—were almost unheard-of generations ago among our lesser-weight ancestors. And doctors have discovered that even a miniscule amount of weight loss—say, 5 or 10 pounds—can reduce our risk for many of these diseases.

The key to that weight loss? Hormonal balance. Hormonal balance can help you lose the weight you need to prevent or alleviate, or even cure many of these "diseases of civilization."

YOUR HORMONES CONTROL YOUR WEIGHT

Whether you are lean or overweight, your hormones regulate your fat cells or fat tissue. This is a simple fact, one many women already know to be true. For example, when some women gain weight, their menstrual cycles go out of whack.

But the hormones that control the menstrual cycle are only some of the many hormones that regulate your weight. And hormones don't go out of whack in a vacuum. Many overweight people have an intuitive sense that something's wrong in their bodies. Hormones regulate not only weight, but mood and emotion as well, and the desire for food (or lack of desire for food) and ability to process that food is intimately related to hormone levels in the body. Again, it has nothing to do with willpower.

Listen to Dr. Björntorp of the University of Göteburg, Sweden:

With visceral fat accumulation multiple endocrine perturbations are found, including elevated cortisol and androgens in women, as well as low growth hormone and, in men, testosterone secretion. These hormonal changes exert profound effects on adipose tissue metabolism and distribution. At the adipocyte (fat cell) level, cortisol and insulin promote lipid accumulation by expressing lipoprotein lipase (fat cell enzyme) activity, while testosterone and growth hormone and probably estrogens exert opposite effects.

What does this mean? Hormones have powerful interactions with your fat cells and have a major influence on your weight. And insulin, notwithstanding the good doctor, is only one of many hormones involved.

And what are hormones?

Hormones are as fundamental as life itself. All living creatures, as a matter of fact, have hormones. They are powerful molecules that control your metabolism. Hormones regulate how much fat you have and where you have it; they control your appetite; they affect your energy level; they influence your mood, your emotions, even your desire to exercise. Hormones determine the size and strength of your muscles. And hormones help determine your body weight.

This book will show you that by balancing your hormones, you will improve your metabolism, increase your energy level, lower your appetite, and quite possibly correct your body weight.

DON'T BLAME ME; IT'S ALL IN MY GENES

There have been great strides made in determining the genetics of obesity, and many genetic links to obesity will be discussed in this book. To date, more than 48 genes have been linked to obesity; however, this number may soon grow to 250. Because of our genes, our hormonal systems are almost identical to those of our ancient ancestors. Very little has changed over the generations.

Unfortunately for us, our environment has changed even if our hormone systems have not. No longer do we need to forage for nuts and berries; no longer do we need to kill our dinner or go without. There are McDonald's, Snickers bars, bags of Doritos, Ben and Jerry's, and cars to get us to the restaurant or grocery store. "Becoming obese," says obesity expert Dr. James Hill of the University of Colorado, "is a normal response to the American environment."

It's an environment created by the industrial revolution. Before the industrial revolution and all its advances in agriculture, transportation, and processing, granulated sugar was an extravagance. Ice cream was a delicacy. Anything requiring refrigeration existed only for the wealthy (or those in very cold climates). It all changed almost overnight, given the context of human history: suddenly, high-calorie, high-fat, high-refined sugar foods were inexpensive and readily available.

And we *like* those foods. We want more; we want more for our money. Think of "super-sizing." A double cheeseburger for 99 cents! A 48-oz Coke for only a dime more than a 32-oz Coke!

Seems like a bargain, right? But does "more" mean "better"? We are paying a price for all that "free" extra food. Sugars and fats bombard our delicate hormone systems. Our genes can't keep up with the changes.

Many nutrition experts today recommend that we eat the way our ancestors did thousands of years ago. Dean Ornish, creator of the diet that bears his name, has said that thousands of years ago "it was survival of the fattest."

But things have changed. Back then the problem was finding enough food to avoid starvation. And different cultures had different diets. The Inuits of northern Canada had (and have) a high-protein, high-fat diet, the better to insulate their bodies during the long, hard winter (the body burns that fat for heat and keeps itself alive). The ancient tribes of Africa, Mexico, and India adhered to a whole-grain, high-carbohydrate diet. Either way, the bottom line was the same: Different diets resulted in hormonal balance and lean bodies.

Today, we look for a "one-size-fits-all" solution. That's why so many diet books contradict each other. Different authors select the diet of a particular ancient culture to match the diet they're writing about. This anthropological basis for dieting falls short in the fact that it does not take hormones into consideration at all. *Obesity today is caused because the food of our civilization disrupts the delicate hormonal balance we are genetically programmed to have.*

"Genetics loads the gun. Environment pulls the trigger," says obesity guru George Bray.

Well, we can't change our genetics (not yet, anyway). But we can change our hormones. And you can change your hormones without eating like our Stone Age ancestors. This book will show you how.

HORMONES REGULATE YOUR METABOLISM

Metabolism (n.)—The sum of all the chemical and physical changes that take place within the body and enable its continued growth and functioning.

Metabolism is a critical determinant of your weight. Why is it that two people can eat the same amount of food and one will gain weight while the other does not? It's metabolism. A fast metabolism will burn off the weight, while a slow metabolism applies the food directly to your hips.

And what regulates metabolism? Hormones.

Hormones and metabolic rate help explain the paradox that exists between those who pig out and never gain weight and the calorie counters who gain weight even when they only smell doughnuts.

Think of your body as an engine. Metabolism is the rate at which the engine runs. Hormones are the push on the accelerator. Step on the gas and raise your metabolism.

Most of us have a very efficient metabolism. This means that the food—the fuel—you eat is efficiently burned, conserving as much as possible. But unlike cars, where the more efficient the better, an efficient metabolism means you need less food to maintain your metabolism. So the more efficient your metabolism, the less food you need to consume.

And what happens to that extra food? It's stored as fat.

Why do most of us have such an efficient metabolism? The answer is *genetics*. We have been genetically selected for our efficient metabolism. Keep in mind that, until very recently, food was scarce. Many people died of starvation. There was no such thing as a fat caveman or fat cavewoman. The key to survival was a slow metabolism: Save every excess calorie as fat, because you'll need it during the famine.

And times of famine were plentiful. The world revolved around agriculture, and agriculture was far less refined in those days. Any natural event—and, of course, there were no weather forecasts—could wipe out a year's crops and influence the crops for years to come.

So only those with an efficient, slow metabolism survived. Those people who would be considered naturally thin in today's environment died in famines.

There are some who have inefficient metabolisms who have survived the centuries. You know these people. These are the ones who eat and eat and never get fat. Their internal processes are so inefficient that they need to take in as much fuel/food as possible just to keep their body going. There is never enough left over to be stored as fat. At one time this was a survival disadvantage, but times have changed. Metabolically inefficient people are able to eat large quantities of food and never get fat.

But what about the rest of us? Are we doomed to keep piling fat on until the next famine? Of course not. There is a lot you can do to change your metabolism, and changing your metabolism will improve your health.

If your metabolism is efficient and slow, you are sluggish and tired all the time. When you speed up your metabolism, you burn calories quicker. Your energy levels are raised and you feel great.

Unfortunately, there is no perfect medication to make this happen. Medications that do exist have side effects: They'll make your heart beat faster or your mind to race, both of which put psychological and physiological stress on the body.

Maybe you're thinking you can do the job with exercise alone; after all, if you burn the calories, you'll lose weight, right? Well, you will. But there are limits. Most people exercise one, or a maximum of two, hours each day. But a revved-up metabolism works 24/7. Take jogging: You'll need to jog about 35 miles to lose just 1 pound. But boost your metabolism via your hormones and your weight will come off consistently, and stay off the right way.

As you read this book, you'll learn about the various hormone systems in the body—and the hormones specific to each one. You'll also learn how the systems work together, how one hormone can influence another (or several), and how the most efficient system for losing weight is the one in balance. Throughout the book and at the end, I'll supply eating suggestions to help you on your way to losing weight—and keeping it off.

BEYOND INSULIN

You may be familiar with the hormone *insulin* and its links to body weight. You also may have heard that too much insulin makes you fat.

That's what the experts say, anyway. (They are only partially right.) Dozens of books offer solutions on how to lower your insulin levels and ultimately lose weight.

This book goes beyond insulin. This book explains many more of your body's hormones and their relation to metabolism, hunger, body weight, and body composition. There are many medical conditions that can cause you to be overweight. We will discuss conditions such as Cushing's syndrome, the polycystic ovary syndrome (PCOS), male and female menopause, aging, growth hormone deficiency, insulin resistance, and even stress and depression. **All** of these conditions can slow your metabolism and make you gain weight.

Insulin is important. I don't mean to question that. But it is not the only hormone that affects your weight.

Human beings can have countless hormonal problems. These can bring about a variety of symptoms, physical attributes, moods, and emotions. And by identifying specific hormonal deficiencies or excesses, you can alter your diet, add certain nutraceutical or herbal products, or even go on medications to help balance your hormones.

Recent medical breakthroughs have revealed that insulin is only a small part of the complete hormonal picture. Dozens if not hundreds of hormones are involved in the regulation of your body weight. Glands like the adrenal gland, the thyroid gland, the pituitary gland, the ovary, and the testicle all make hormones that influence your body weight and body composition.

Hormones contribute to obesity, and obesity creates a hormonal imbalance that slows metabolism and perpetuates the obese state.

Now, insulin does have an effect. Improper insulin action leads to high insulin levels resulting in hunger and weight gain.

But there's also the thyroid. Low thyroid hormone or inefficient processing of thyroid hormone slows metabolism and causes weight gain.

Also, low androgen and growth hormone levels cause reduction in muscle mass and increased fat mass.

In women, low estrogen levels increase fat in the belly, but high estrogen levels increase fat in the hips and buttocks.

High cortisol levels increase fat in the belly and cause tremendous weight gain.

And leptin, a newly discovered hormone, is produced by the fat cell itself. Leptin has powerful actions on the hunger centers in the brain.

Various genetically controlled "hunger hormones" affect your appetite, metabolism, and body weight.

Also, food affects your hormones. Food is a powerful drug that triggers a vast array of hormonal, chemical, and brain effects.

But you're not hostage to your hormones. You can alter them and achieve hormonal balance. With hormonal balance you will experience weight loss and increased energy, but the benefits do not stop there.

Hormonal balance can dramatically reduce your susceptibility to the medical problems we discussed above and can improve a wide variety of complaints. Hormones also have powerful effects on the immune system.

Put simply, hormonal balance can save your life.

The eating principles in this book are not designed specifically for weight loss; they are designed to help you achieve hormonal balance. With hormonal balance, you will optimize your metabolism and you will lose weight. And by learning the principles of your body's hormones, you can tailor the optimal diet and vitamin/mineral/supplement program for yourself and your family members.

This book explains how.

YOUR HORMONAL IDENTITY

You are an individual. Your fingerprints are not like anyone else's fingerprints; your sense of humor is not like anyone else's sense of humor; your taste in music, in clothing, in colors or animals or people is not like anyone else's tastes in those things or most any other thing.

So, of course, your hormones are not the same as anyone else's hormones.

But keep in mind that hormones control all facets of life. In addition to body weight and metabolism, hormones control mood, the menstrual cycle, and your biological clock.

Hormones are also the key that unlocks the door to a healthy body weight.

Hormonal balance will help you achieve health, wellness, physical and mental well-being, and optimal metabolism. *The answer to achieving a healthy body weight is in your hormones.*

And *your* hormones, in particular, reflect your internal chemistry. Hormones are the reason some people remain youthful and vital later in life and others quickly deteriorate both mentally and physically.

You may not know what your hormonal identity is, but this book will help you find it. Subtle clues—from physical symptoms to physical traits—help us find our hormonal identity. In addition, hormonal testing, *when done properly*, may also help us to discover our hormonal identity.

Each chapter in this book will offer methods of determining your hormonal status for a particular hormone. Your levels may be too high, too low, or right where you want them—but you can have them right where you want them all of the time.

HORMONES CHANGE WITH AGE

Want to know why we get fatter when we age? Want to know why our muscles start to droop, our sex drive diminishes, our sleep gets a little harder to come by?

The answer: our hormones.

Many of our vital hormones are at a fraction of what they were when we were young. These low levels, once considered a normal part of aging, are now considered by many physicians to be abnormal.

Aging will be a major focus of this book, because hormones, aging, and metabolism are so closely related. We become older; our metabolism slows; we gain weight. But that need not be the end of the story. This book will show you how you can reverse some of the hormonal changes that occur with aging.

Much of that is due to modern medicine. We no longer accept anymore that aging means falling apart and crawling into that long goodnight. Doctors are now treating hormonal deficiencies, and a new branch of medicine, called *anti-aging medicine*, has evolved. Anti-aging physicians routinely prescribe hormones as a way of reversing some of the effects of aging. It's a whole new paradigm for medicine.

This may sound like science fiction, but you see it every day. You might be familiar with estrogen replacement therapy in menopausal women; this was almost unheard-of until a few years ago. Back then, it was reserved for only the most stricken of women. Now, doctors agree that most menopausal women should take estrogen replacement.

And what is estrogen? A hormone. What brings on estrogen deficiency? Aging.

Estrogen isn't the only hormone that declines with age. Thyroid hormone, growth hormone, and androgens also reach lower levels. But I believe that many people can benefit from increasing their hormone levels to where they were when they were younger (and leaner). This book will discuss not only methods of hormone replacement but also alternative ways to raise hormone levels using diet and specific vitamins and herbal remedies.

FOOD AND YOUR HORMONES

What's the most powerful drug you take on a regular basis? You might think it's some sort of high-tech medication, and there are many such medications that have profound effects on the body. But on a day-in, day-out regimen, that most powerful drug is **food**. Food can create or cure illness; every bite you take affects your hormones. Hormones can even be affected by the *sight or smell* of food.

Powerful stuff, indeed.

Every time you eat, a chemical reaction takes place between your hormones and the food. Hormones control your digestive system, and, in turn, your digestive system produces its own set of hormones. Hormones control your appetite and hormones control your cravings. Carbohydrate cravings, for example, are closely linked to several hormones. (You chocolate lovers will find out there's a reason for craving chocolate the way you do.)

The hormone most closely linked to food is insulin. But insulin isn't the only hormone affected by food, nor is it necessarily the most important.

And sometimes *hormones in food* can affect us without our even knowing about it. Hormone use in the livestock industry is commonplace, and those hormones are ingested by us when we eat the cows, pigs, sheep, and chickens that have ingested them. The toxins and chemicals that get into our foods frequently contain substances that mimic hormones.

There is a positive side to this: Some foods and many common herbs contain natural substances that mimic hormones. These can sometimes be used as an alternative form of hormone replacement.

In this book, we will discuss food—carbohydrates, proteins, and fats—and how each of these affects your hormones. We will also discuss food cravings, how hormones control your cravings, and how you can eliminate your cravings by controlling your hormones.

But we'll also go beyond that. Specific foods affect specific hormones. Foods contain micronutrients that control the production and processing of hormones. Today's processed foods lack many of the vital nutrients that your body requires for proper hormone production and efficient hormone action.

The eating suggestions in this book are not an attempt to force a rigid system into your life. Rather, we offer simple eating guidelines as a way to help you achieve hormonal balance.

THE ENDOCRINE SYSTEM: YOUR BODY'S HORMONES

Hormone has an interesting etymological root: The word comes from the Greek, meaning "to stir up" or "to urge on." Classically, a hormone is a substance produced by a gland, and secreted into the bloodstream, that has its action at a distant location in the body.

We now know that almost every organ, not just glands, makes hormones. Nerve cells, fat cells, intestinal cells, even heart cells all make hormones. Most of the "classic" hormones are controlled by the *pituitary gland*—referred to as the "master gland"—in the brain (see Figure 1.1). These include thyroid hormone, androgens, estrogens, cortisol, and growth hormone. The pituitary gland makes yet another set of hormones that control these glands. The pituitary gland is actually controlled by a portion of the brain known as the *hypothalamus*. Higher centers in the brain, influenced by your thoughts, moods, emotions, and other hormones, control the hypothalamus.

Ultimately, then, your brain controls your hormones.
But: Your hormones also control your brain.

Your hormones are constantly in a state of flux. They are never steady; they are always going up or down. Your brain "listens" to your hormones to figure out what to do. High hormone levels feed back to the brain telling it to shut down production of a particular hormone level. Low hormone levels do the opposite, making brain hormone levels surge.

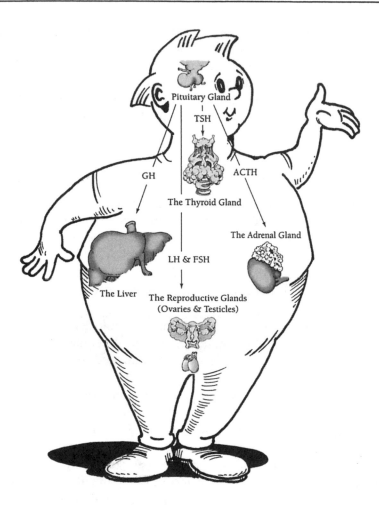

Figure 1.1
THE ENDOCRINE SYSTEM I: Control by the "Master Gland"

The pituitary gland, also known as the master gland, produces hormones that regulate other glands in the body. Thyroid-stimulating hormone (TSH) regulates hormone production from the thyroid gland. Adrenocorticotrophic hormone (ACTH) regulates adrenal gland hormone production including cortisol and dehydroepiandrosterone (DHEA). Luteinizing hormone (LH) and follicle-stimulating hormone (FSH) regulate gonadal (ovaries or testicles) hormone production including estrogen, progesterone, testosterone, and androstenedione. Growth hormone (GH) regulates the production of insulin-like growth factor-1 (IGF-1) in the liver. Hormones made by the target glands send signals back to the pituitary gland.

The rhythms are not always predictable, either. Some hormones follow a regular 24-hour cycle, known as a circadian rhythm. But those rhythms aren't in sync. Cortisol, for example, peaks at 7–8 A.M. Growth hormone, on the other hand, peaks about 3 A.M.

Many other hormones are not under the control of the pituitary gland (see Figure 1.2). Insulin is not officially controlled by the pituitary gland, but imbalances of thyroid, growth hormone, cortisol, estrogen, or testosterone can affect insulin. Various other hormones are not regulated by the pituitary gland, such as gut hormones, leptin, and other brain hormones.

Many things can go wrong with hormones. There can be too much or not enough; the receptors might not work, there might be proteins in the blood binding up specific hormones . . . the possibilities are endless.

HOW DO HORMONES WORK?

Think of a lock and a key. The key (hormone) unlocks the lock (receptor), "directing" it to open or close, as the case may be. The key changes the lock's status from locked to unlocked, or vice versa (see Figure 1.3).

Hormones, in the great scheme of things, are tiny. A single drop of blood contains literally thousands of hormones. The hormones travel through the blood and other bodily fluids, serving as chemical messengers. The message directs the organism at the receiving end— known, likely enough, as a "receptor"—to do something. *Receptors* are special proteins that can recognize and bind a particular hormone, and when hormone and receptor merge in a cell, a chain of events begins. Hormones cause specific genes in the cell to turn on and off.

Because hormones work by turning on and off genes, you can fight against your genetic predisposition to being overweight by changing your hormones!

The keys—the hormones—are made by glands. The pituitary gland (the "master gland") makes special hormones that control many of the glands (think of the pituitary gland as the CEO of the key company). And the brain makes other hormones that control the pituitary gland (like the chairman of the board). So, ultimately, everything is controlled by the brain. But in nature's delicate balance, a system known as *feedback* exists. Hormones made by the glands have reciprocal influences on the brain

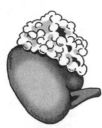

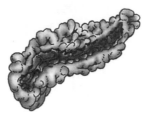

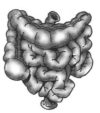

The Adrenal Gland
↓
Epinephrine
Norepinephrine
Aldosterone

The Pancreas
↓
Insulin
Glucagon
Somatostatin
Amylin

The Intestines
↓
Cholecystokinin
Glucagon-like peptide-1

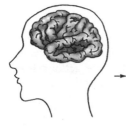

Neuropeptide Y
Pro-opiomelanocortin
Melanocyte Stimulating Hormone
→ Agouti-Related Protein
Melanin Concentrating Hormone
Serotonin
Urocortin
Melatonin

The Human Brain

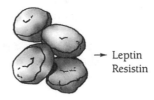

→ Leptin
Resistin

Fat Cells

Figure 1.2
THE ENDOCRINE SYSTEM II: Hormones that Function
Independent of the Pituitary Gland.

Many hormones are not under the control of the pituitary gland. The adrenal gland produces the stress hormones epinephrine and norepinephrine as well as aldosterone (a steroid hormone that regulates blood pressure). The pancreas makes several important hormones including insulin, glucagon, somatostatin, and amylin. The intestines make cholecystokinin (CCK) and glucagon-like peptide-1 (GLP-1). Fat cells make a newly discovered hormone, known as leptin. The brain makes many hormones including neuropeptide Y (NPY), pro-opiomelanocortin (POMC), melanocyte-stimulating hormone (MSH), agouti-related protein (AgRP), melanin-concentrating hormone (MCH), serotonin, urocortin, and melatonin.

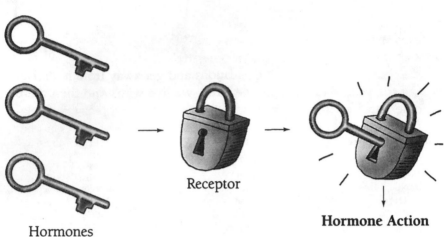

Receptor

Hormone Action

Hormones

Figure 1.3
HORMONES AND RECEPTORS: How Hormones Work
The specific hormone molecules are like specific "keys." Only the appropriate hormone corresponds to a receptor (lock). When a hormone and a receptor interact, it sets forth a chain of events that ultimately lead to the actions associated with each specific hormone.

and pituitary gland. In other words, your brain controls your hormones, and hormones control your brain. The situation works both ways because, as messengers, hormones can tell parts of the body what to do— and then they have to obey a part of the body telling *them* what to do.

After all, every living cell has hormone receptors, and hormones control every living cell. They do so by working through the most fundamental component of living beings: DNA. Glands "secrete" hormones into the bloodstream. There they travel to every nook and cranny of your body until they locate their specific receptor. Virtually every cell in the body has receptors for a wide variety of hormones.

STRESS DISRUPTS HORMONAL BALANCE

We are living in stressful times. Certainly many generations have uttered those words, but think of what our generation faces: instantaneous communication, constant availability, "just-in-time" production methods. Even our children, once largely free of the stresses of adult life, now make "play dates." Our lives have been sped up in ways previous generations never could have imagined.

We cope, or try to. We take vacations and get away from it all. But most of the year, there it is, all the stress we live with. And then there are other stresses: the death of loved ones, the heartbreak of a relationship that ends, even the "good-for-you" hunger of a crash diet (which, of course, isn't really good for you at all).

Usually, two things happen. The first is that our body goes into conservation mode. Metabolism slows and even the normal diet we were adhering to makes us put on weight. The second thing is that we look to one of the most familiar items in our lives for consolation: food. And often not just food, but chocolate bars, sugary sodas, and super-size containers of french fries. "Comfort food," it's sometimes called.

Why do we do this? Because of our hormones. Any kind of stress—whether mental, physical, or emotional—can disrupt hormonal balance in our bodies in ways that make us gain weight.

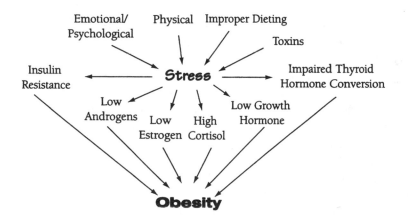

Figure 1.4
HORMONAL CHANGES THAT OCCUR WITH STRESS
Stress disrupts the body's hormonal system by creating insulin resistance, lowering sex hormones (estrogen and testosterone), lowering growth hormone, and increasing cortisol levels. Stress also reduces the body's ability to convert thyroid hormone to an active form. Each one of these hormonal changes slows metabolism and causes weight gain.

Stress causes the brain, pituitary gland, and adrenal glands to pump out *stress hormones* (see Figure 1.4). These hormones cause the biological reactions we associate with stress, from rapid heartbeat to a rise in blood sugar to slowed digestion. They prepare us for the "fight or flight" response.

Now, all of us experience stress. Furthermore, our bodies have adapted to handle the normal hormonal surges that occur with stress. This acute, short-term stress does not cause us to gain weight.

Chronic, long-term stress, however, is something else entirely. Too much stress causes longer-term elevations of stress hormones which result in weight gain.

Many diets make you lose weight in such a way that it becomes a tremendous stress on your body. This is why most diets ultimately fail. Chronic stress also causes the body to shift its focus away from its normal activity. Stress causes the immune system to wane, muscles to shrink, and, in general, a lousy feeling throughout your body.

We'll discuss the hormonal effects of stress further in each chapter.

DIETS CAN WRECK YOUR METABOLISM

When you go on a diet, your metabolism is dramatically altered. When your body is losing weight, it can be "stressed"—causing all the hormonal disruptions that make you stop losing weight.

Dieting, ironically, slows your metabolism. This is why 98 percent of diets ultimately fail.

How does this happen? Think of a famine. When you go on a diet, your body doesn't realize that you are doing this for its own good. Your body thinks it is starving. It cannot tell the difference between a diet and a famine. It is all about survival.

Your body slows its metabolism, making it even more efficient. After all, it has no idea when the famine will end. And how is metabolism slowed? Through your hormones, of course.

During dieting, thyroid and androgen levels plunge and cortisol (a hormone that makes you gain weight) surges. Eventually your body succumbs to this hormonal pressure and your diet ultimately fails.

This book will show you how to prevent this from happening. We will show you how to lose weight consistently—and you will *keep the weight off*. In fact, it is possible to lose weight and maintain—or even increase—your metabolism. It all relies on hormonal balance.

HORMONES REGULATE BODY COMPOSITION

The amount of muscle you have is perhaps the most important determinant of your metabolism. Your hormones, most notably androgens and growth hormone, control your muscle mass.

Think of the bodybuilder on steroids. He eats all day and puts on more and more muscle. Without the boost of "'roids," all that food would become fat. As the old saying has it, "muscle burns fat"—and it's true. If you want to boost your metabolism, a surefire way is to increase the amount of muscle mass you have.

Now, many of us actually have a normal body weight but have a very high percentage of body fat. This condition has been described by Dr. Neil Ruderman as the "metabolically obese, normal weight individual," or MONW. But obese or not obese, if you have a high percentage of body fat, you are likely to have hormonal problems.

This book explains how hormones affect your body composition and how your body composition affects your hormones. For example, as we age, our levels of growth hormone and testosterone plunge. Once considered a normal part of aging, doctors have been treating these low levels back to the level of a 30- or 40-year-old. Why? Growth hormone and testosterone both have an effect of building muscle mass. In this book, we will go over the effects of growth hormone, testosterone, and other androgens (testosterone-like hormones).

HORMONAL DISORDERS IGNORED BY MANY DOCTORS

Doctors learn about hormonal disorders in medical school, as they learn about so many other things. But the medical school curriculum stresses that hormonal disorders are usually rare. Not only is this not true, but it does a disservice to endocrinologists, who study hormones and hormonal disorders, and patients, who are told that the problem lies elsewhere. Medical schools will teach about hormonal disorders in their extreme cases but fail to teach about less severe cases of the same disorders.

In real life, hormonal disorders can occur in many ranges and be due to many things. Some hormonal disorders are caused by tumors (sometimes cancer, sometimes not cancer) of glands—the glands pump out tons and tons of a particular hormone. Other hormonal disorders are caused by complete failure of a gland.

The flaws of medical education don't stop there. In med school, the blood test is emphasized as the be-all and end-all. Symptoms are brushed aside; other tests aren't considered as seriously. But tests can be wrong. Many people with hormonal problems can have normal blood test results.

Medical schools don't teach much about the hormonal disorders caused by a mild overproduction or a mild deficiency of a hormone. They also don't teach much about receptor problems or other ways that a hormone could go haywire. The result: Over the years, many doctors forget to look for any type of hormonal disorder. Why should they? They've been practically trained to ignore them.

But that can have costly effects for patients in more ways than one. Many overweight patients seek advice from their physicians. They are usually told their hormones are normal. "It's not your hormones," they say. "Just eat less and exercise more."

Meanwhile, the doctor may think to herself, "This poor obese patient. I know that the odds are less than 2 percent that he will ever lose weight, so why even bother to try." This attitude has become so prevalent that doctors now openly debate the utility of trying to have their patients lose weight at all.

Sometimes doctors miss extreme hormone problems because they are not in the frame of mind of looking for hormonal disorders. I have seen many of these cases myself. These doctors ignore subtle complaints and attribute your problems to your weight. They forget to consider that perhaps your symptoms may be clues to the *cause* of your weight gain, not *because* of it.

And though our hormones are affected by food, dieting, stress, and the other factors listed earlier, sometimes hormone problems go beyond these issues. Many things can go wrong, causing hormone levels to be too high or too low or, simply, to not work properly.

Many hormonal disorders will make you gain weight, and all the dieting in the world will not help until the hormonal disorder is corrected. Maybe a simple blood test won't find them, but other testing methods can—and hormonal testing techniques continue to improve. We can detect hormones in blood, urine, and even saliva. But even there, a well-trained doctor will know what else to ask for, because tests can only go so far: They should be given at certain points of the day, test certain parts of the body, and follow other guidelines that many doctors aren't aware of.

This book will discuss symptoms of various hormonal disorders. Your symptoms will help you determine if you may have a hormonal disorder. This book will also explain various tests and help you to interpret the results.

This book is not meant to be a substitute for your physician. It is simply a guide to help answer questions. It is also intended to bring about your awareness of symptoms so that you can make your physician aware of them.

HORMONE PROBLEMS CAN BE TREATED

Hormone treatments cover a wide range. For some people, dietary recommendations are enough. For others, specific vitamin and/or minerals may also be helpful. For yet others, medications may be required.

Fortunately, hormones and hormone treatments come in many forms: pills, patches, shots, gels, and creams. And they work in many ways. Some boost the body's natural supply of certain hormones, such as estrogen, while others work by stimulating a particular gland to make more of its own hormone.

Treatment with hormones goes back to the 19th century, when French physician Charles Edouard Brown-Sequard injected himself with an extract of crushed dog and guinea pig testicles in order to test its efficacy. At the time, the good doctor was 72 years old, and, as in many 72-year-olds, aging had taken a toll on his appetite and sex drive. However, after the injection—and to the amazement of his colleagues—the extract had the same effect as modern-day testosterone.

While testosterone medications are derived from different sources nowadays, not all hormone medications have strayed from an animal form processed for human consumption. For example, a popular thyroid hormone medication, Armour Thyroid, consists of ground pig thyroid glands. And a popular estrogen medication is made from the urine of pregnant mares.

But hormones come from a variety of sources, and natural does not always mean better than synthetic. Moreover, some hormones work better when taken by mouth; others get digested in the stomach and work only if taken by injection, patch, cream, gel, or other creative delivery device.

In today's managed care environment, the average doctor has only about 10 minutes to spend with each patient. He or she simply doesn't have enough time to go into as much detail as this book. So this book is written as a guide for you and your doctor. It will explain your treatment options in some detail.

This book is also recommended for doctors and other health care providers as a guide to up-to-date treatments for hormonal problems. One of my goals is to help demystify hormone treatments for both patients and professionals. Whether you're already taking hormones—or merely considering it—I believe this book will still be very helpful to you.

HORMONE WEIGHT-LOSS PRODUCTS
AND HORMONE PREPARATIONS

Health-food store shelves are filled with herbal products that make claims to affect your hormones and/or your weight. In a clever bit of marketing, herbal products are now referred to as *nutraceuticals*—"functional foods," including vitamins and minerals, which are available from health-food stores and drug stores without a prescription.

Nutraceuticals are not under as strict regulation as prescription medications. The quality control is highly variable. Many of them have not been properly tested. Prescription medications are held to a much higher standard. This is not to put down nutraceuticals completely; many of them show great promise.

But **know what you're getting**. Many nutraceuticals are derived from plants, but some are hormone preparations *made from ground animal glands or brains*. The labels can be disguised ("bovine" means cow, "porcine" means pig), and consumers may end up buying something that, at worst, can hurt, not heal.

Think of this: Many nutraceutical products make weight-loss claims. And many of these products claim to affect your metabolism and/or your hormones. **The important point is that these products, although considered "natural," can be just as potent as prescription medications and should be treated as such.**

In this book, I will explain many nutraceutical products. Moreover, this book will help you put things into perspective. It will tell you what products are worthwhile, what products are garbage … and what products are dangerous.

This book will also point out specific instances where a common vitamin or mineral affects your hormones. Many of us eat too much processed food, lacking in vitamins and minerals vital for proper hormonal balance. In addition, many crops are grown in nutrient-poor soil, so that even fresh fruits and vegetables may be lacking in specific vital nutrients. Hormones require specific vitamins and minerals in order to be made or processed efficiently.

This book will show you simple dietary changes you can make to increase the nutrients you need to achieve hormonal balance. Vitamins and minerals can come from the foods you eat. You don't always have to "pop a pill."

HORMONAL BALANCE: YOUR GUIDE TO A HEALTHY LIFE

It all comes down to *hormonal balance*. Whether you want to lose a significant amount of weight, get in shape, or even want to reverse the effects of aging, hormonal balance is critical.

How can this be done? It starts with diet. You can tailor your diet to achieve a perfect equilibrium of hormones. The hormones themselves will do the rest of the work.

We've come to assume that once out of control, hormones are always out of control – that we are powerless to these messengers circulating throughout our body. That isn't true, even if you've already suffered from a hormonal ailment. You *can* control your hormones. You *can* control your metabolism. Follow the lessons in this book, and you will be on your way to a *healthier, thinner, well-tuned* version of **you**.

CHAPTER TWO

FOOD AND INSULIN

UNDERSTANDING INSULIN

EVERY BITE OF FOOD THAT YOU PUT IN YOUR MOUTH AFFECTS YOUR HORMONES. Whether you eat junk food, healthy food, large quantities or small quantities, even if you starve yourself, your hormones are affected. When it comes to hormones and food, one hormone stands out above all the rest: insulin.

You've probably heard of insulin, but you may not have realized that insulin is a hormone. It's the hormone that diabetics take to regulate their blood sugar. If we're not diabetic, we seldom think of our own bodies' insulin production. But we should, because when it comes to food, insulin is critical.

Insulin is one of several hormones made by the pancreas. The pancreas is really two separate organs in one. The **endocrine pancreas**, also known as the islets of Langerhans, consists of hormone-producing cells that make hormones responsible for the *metabolism* of food. Special cells, known as beta-cells, make insulin. Other cells in the endocrine pancreas synthesize the important hormones glucagon and somatostatin. Hormones produced in the endocrine pancreas are secreted into the blood and act on tissues throughout the body. The **exocrine pancreas** makes enzymes needed for the *digestion* of food. These enzymes are secreted into the intestines. Damage or injury to the pancreas can cause problems with both hormones and enzymes.

25

All the pancreatic hormones work together to help control your metabolism and body weight. Insulin regulates the metabolism of food—carbohydrates, proteins, and fats. Insulin promotes weight gain by increasing appetite as well as promoting *storage* of nutrients as fat. When insulin levels are high, weight loss is very difficult. Glucagon and somatostatin also affect body weight and appetite and are discussed in more detail in Chapter 10.

Later in this chapter, I will focus on how you can keep your insulin levels low. Also in this chapter, I'll discuss dietary carbohydrates such as starches and sugars and their effects on insulin, showing how the shorthand many diet books are using—proteins "good," carbohydrates "bad"—paints an incomplete picture.

I'll give you dietary suggestions to help regulate your insulin levels, emphasizing not only types of foods but also total amount of food, portion size, and frequency of meals. I'll explain the **glycemic index**, a system that rates how fast a carbohydrate enters the bloodstream. I'll discuss the hormonal value of beneficial foods and how the wrong types of carbohydrates can cause rapid fluctuations in blood sugar, giving rise to problems such as hypoglycemia, fatigue, and extreme hunger. (Think of how sleepy you feel after eating a big meal . . . and yet your hunger returns quickly.) I'll also talk about **carbohydrate cravings** and ways to counter them.

In Chapter 3, I'll address the problem of **insulin resistance**. This is one of the most common hormonal imbalances in overweight people. Insulin resistance causes very high insulin levels because receptors for insulin do not work efficiently, a condition caused by a combination of your genes and your environment. If you have insulin resistance, you require higher insulin levels to maintain your metabolism. When insulin does not function properly, a vicious cycle ensues. Fat cells release toxic chemicals known as free fatty acids into the blood. These "toxic blood fats" poison insulin receptors, further worsening insulin resistance. Much attention has been given to a disease of insulin resistance known as **"The Metabolic Syndrome" or Syndrome X,** whose features include obesity, diabetes, high blood pressure, high cholesterol and triglycerides, Polycystic ovary syndrome (PCOS), gout, and heart disease. I will also discuss a variety of new treatments for insulin resistance.

THE TRUTH ABOUT CARBOHYDRATES

Scientifically, carbohydrates are simply any compound that features hydrogen and oxygen—the elements of water—combined with carbon. They are the most common organic compounds found in nature, and are the substances produced by green plants during photosynthesis. Your body requires insulin to properly metabolize carbohydrates.

Carbohydrates have received a bad rap lately. Books like *Dr. Atkins' New Diet Revolution, Protein Power,* and *The Carbohydrate Addict's Diet* place the brunt of the blame for obesity on carbohydrates and their effects on insulin. For most of these plans, breads, pasta, sugary foods, and grains are off limits; the idea is to keep insulin production low. The upshot is that high insulin levels will make you fat. These "low-carb" or "no-carb" diets have helped people shed pounds. Unfortunately for most, once the diet is stopped, the excess weight returns with a vengeance.

Why? All foods affect insulin, not just carbohydrates. Carbohydrates, however, have received too much of the attention when it comes to insulin. The pancreas also produces insulin when you eat proteins and fats. Ironically, books like the ones mentioned above don't touch on the effects of other hormones. Low thyroid, androgen, estrogen, and growth hormone levels can be as dangerous as high insulin levels; all can lead to heart disease, blood pressure problems, and all the accompanying ailments of obesity.

CARBOHYDRATES: A QUICK GUIDE

Carbohydrates are often referred to as coming in two kinds: simple and complex. Simple carbohydrates are usually sugars; complex carbohydrates are usually starches. Regardless of what kind they are, carbohydrates—in the form of sugar, wheat, rice, grains, fruit, and vegetables—are the principal components of almost every human's diet and are the primary source of energy in our diet.

Although the recent trend in diet books has been to emphasize low- or no-carbohydrate intakes (Atkins recommends just 20 grams a day), carbohydrates are a necessary part of the diet. Your brain requires the basic building block of carbohydrate, glucose—the most simple sugar—in order to function properly.

The liver can store about 18 hours' worth of carbohydrate. After this point, however, to provide energy, the liver must make new sugar (glucose). This process, known as *gluconeogenesis*, literally means "the birth of new glucose." The body must break down muscle and fat to provide the liver with the building blocks needed for gluconeogenesis. This may sound attractive to overweight people; who wouldn't want to start getting rid of some of that excess chubbiness? And, indeed, that's part of the point of low-carbohydrate diets.

But this diet change comes at a price. After a while, the body breaks down its own tissue for food in its desperate need for more glucose. Metabolism slows down, so if your carbohydrate intake increases, you'll gain the weight back faster than you took it off. And, if the body doesn't get the carbohydrate and glucose it needs, your muscles will break down and weaken. *It is essential that your body get ample supplies of carbohydrate in order to prevent muscle breakdown.*

There is a happy medium, of course. Too much carbohydrate can cause problems, such as insulin spiking after meals. This spiking causes rapid blood sugar drops, also known as *hypoglycemia*, and since insulin makes you hungry, you get hungrier and eat more. Moreover, this constant "pounding" on the insulin receptors leads to insulin resistance. Finally, high insulin levels lead to storage of nutrients as fat. Given Americans' sedentary nature and love of sweets and fast food, we tend to get far too much in the way of carbohydrate—and a quick look down any city street shows what dietitians already know: We are the fattest country on earth.

The terms *sugar* and *starch* are very nonspecific. I'd like to provide a more detailed, scientific description of carbohydrates, to help you understand exactly what a carbohydrate is, and how sugars and starches are all made up of the same building blocks. Those of you who got an "A" in high school science can skip to the next section.

- **Monosaccharides** are the building blocks of all carbohydrates, just as amino acids are the building blocks of protein. All carbohydrates are made up of these three simple sugars:

    Glucose: The most abundant monosaccharide. It has the strongest effect in stimulating production of insulin. Most of the time the terms *blood sugar* and *blood glucose* are interchangeable.

Fructose: Half of what makes up table sugar; fructose is best known as the primary sugar found in fruit. Fruit provides only mild insulin stimulation, which is why it's an essential element to hormonal balance. I recommend that you consume at least 5 servings of fruit every day (see Chapter 11).

Galactose: No, not the kind of sugar they use on *Star Trek*, but a form of sugar found only in milk and milk products.

- **Disaccharides** are created when two monosaccharides come together to form a simple sugar. During digestion, the disaccharides are broken down into monosaccharides by special enzymes in the intestine. There are two primary disaccharides:

  Sucrose: Made of equal parts glucose and fructose. Sucrose is found in fruits and table sugar.

  Lactose: Made of equal parts galactose and glucose. Lactose is found only in milk and milk products. It is digested by the enzyme *lactase*. People with lactase deficiency have problems digesting milk (see below).

- **Polysaccharides** are created by many monosaccharides linked together in very complex arrays. However, they're still nothing more than a string of monosaccharides. Polysaccharides are also known as **starch** or **complex carbohydrate**.

CARBOHYDRATES AND INSULIN

What actually happens when you eat carbohydrates? It's a seemingly complex process, but it takes only a matter of hours to occur—sometimes less. Let's run through it step by step.

Carbohydrates are broken down to their most basic form, monosaccharides, by digestive enzymes in your intestines. Most of the enzymes needed to digest carbohydrates come from the pancreas (the same organ that makes insulin). Monosaccharides are transported through the intestinal lining into the bloodstream. Carbohydrate-rich blood is brought straight to the liver through a vein known as the portal vein. Here, the liver does not treat all monosaccharides the same. Glucose zips straight through the liver; however, fructose and galactose are slowly converted to glucose before they move on. Glucose ultimately fuels the body. This is why fruits which are high in fructose cause less insulin spiking than other carbohydrates.

Glucose is also sensed by the beta-cells of the pancreas. The pancreas responds by pumping out insulin. There are two phases of insulin release (see Figure 2.1). The immediate (first phase) is a release of pre-made insulin and is always a set quantity. The later (second phase) insulin release comes as new insulin is synthesized and is a variable amount depending on the body's needs.

Insulin itself is one of the body's most important hormones, if not *the* most important. It affects every cell and every organ. Insulin instructs the liver to stop making glucose. This prevents the breakdown of muscle and fat. Insulin also causes these tissues to transport glucose out of the blood into the cell, a process known as *glucose uptake*. Together, these actions of insulin result in lowering blood glucose and the buildup of muscle and fat. Insulin also acts to turn on hunger centers in the brain.

Once carbohydrates hit the bloodstream, blood glucose rises and insulin responds. This glucose rise and subsequent insulin response after a meal can be measured and even predicted. In response to the insulin surge, several **counter-insulin hormones** (glucagon, growth hormone, cortisol, and epinephrine) are released. These hormones

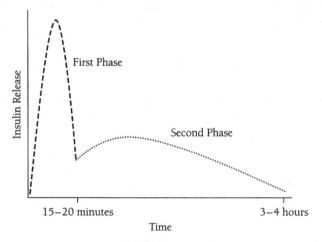

Figure 2.1
THE TWO PHASES OF INSULIN RELEASE
Insulin is released in two phases. The first phase occurs in the first 30 minutes and represents pre-made insulin that is stored in the pancreas. The second phase of insulin release occurs over the next 3 hours and represents the production of new insulin.

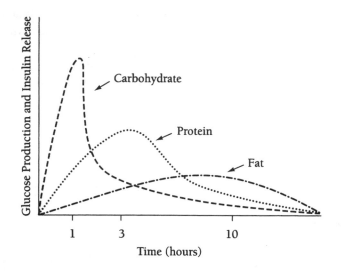

Figure 2.2
GLUCOSE AND INSULIN RELEASE WITH
CARBOHYDRATES, PROTEIN, AND FAT
Various nutrients have different effects on glucose production and insulin release. Carbohydrates cause rapid spiking of insulin. Protein and fat also cause insulin release that is longer lasting but has less spiking.

have activities in direct opposition to insulin. Counter-insulin hormones can disrupt hormonal balance and cause insulin resistance. Remember, carbohydrates are not the only nutrient that affects insulin—proteins and fats also stimulate insulin release (see Figure 2.2).

Here are some ways you can have too much insulin:

* *Overeating any type of food.* Overeating starts the body on a vicious cycle: production of insulin, intense hunger, more overeating, and more production of insulin, ad infinitum. Eventually, insulin receptors shut down, creating insulin resistance and even higher insulin levels.
* *Too much of the wrong type of carbohydrate.* Not all carbohydrates are created equal. Different carbohydrates affect your blood sugar and insulin differently.

- *Medications.* Certain medications, including some diabetes medications, raise insulin levels. This is why many people with diabetes have such a hard time losing weight.
- *Tumors.* A tumor called an *insulinoma* produces huge amounts of insulin. People with insulinomas are invariably obese due to very high insulin levels.

DO CARBOHYDRATES CAUSE OBESITY?

Recently, there has been great public interest in the composition of the American diet. The high fat content of the typical diet has been linked to a wide variety of diseases including coronary heart disease, diabetes, and cancer. In the fervor to cut back on fats, we have increased our consumption of carbohydrates. Diet experts continue to debate the perfect balance of carbohydrates, protein, and fat.

Americans eat too many carbohydrates. Amazingly, several health organizations—including the American Diabetes Association, the American Heart Association, and even those affiliated with the U.S. government—have recommended that we further increase the carbohydrate content of our diet. I don't think that's appropriate. Forty to 50 percent carbohydrate is plenty for most people. If you eat good carbohydrates—ones with a low glycemic index—all the better. My belief—and the belief of many other physicians and dietary experts—is that a diet should feature a healthy balance of carbohydrates, protein and fat. Keep in mind that exact percentages aren't critical. As long as you're in the ballpark, you'll be eating a proper, balanced diet and one that should help you stay healthy and be at your proper weight. Just don't overeat: Calories *do* count.

The average American now consumes over 20 teaspoons of sugar every day. Sweeteners make up as much as *one-third* of the carbohydrate content of the typical American diet. Think about that: *thirty-three percent* of everything the average American consumes is simply sugar. Thirty-three percent! That's the cup of sugar you add to a Kool-Aid packet to make a pitcher. That's the sugar applied to your Frosted Flakes. That's the sugar in soft drinks, ketchup, snack cakes, and your morning coffee. And if you don't think you're eating so much sugar, check the labels of some of your favorite products.

Low-carbohydrate diets are the biggest diet fad in America. People are passing on the baked potato but loading up on steak. The fad is actually a re-emergence of an early-'70s trend begun by Dr. Robert Atkins, author of the 1972 best-seller *Dr. Atkins' Diet Revolution* and the more recent *Dr. Atkins' New Diet Revolution*. Other low-carbohydrate diet books have arrived in his wake, including *The Zone, Sugar Busters!, The Carbohydrate Addict's Diet,* and *Protein Power*. Recently, the top four best-selling advice/how-to books on the *New York Times* best-seller list were all low-carbohydrate diet books.

Yet controversy remains. There are still many unanswered questions. Some doctors are skeptical of the claims of the low-carbohydrate diets. The American Heart Association recently advised against high-protein, low carbohydrate diets. The authors of these diet books themselves argue over the proper proportions of carbohydrate in the diet and what form that carbohydrate should take. Many don't address the subject of calorie counting, as if merely watching the serving size takes care of that need. And most offer "one-size-fits-all" diets, relatively generic recommendations expected to work equally well for everyone.

Meanwhile, as I noted, several health groups are pushing diets in a different direction, increasing the amount of carbohydrate intake to as high as 60 percent of the diet. Their versions stress starch in the diet but do not differentiate between high- and low-glycemic index starches. They also emphasize monosaccharides, particularly glucose and fructose. I certainly agree with the latter determination—fructose, since it comes from eating fruit, is the best monosaccharide you can eat.

Even some diet books buck the trend. The highly regarded Dr. Dean Ornish poses a more traditional diet, heavy on fruits and vegetables and low on fat, in his 1993 book *Eat More, Weigh Less*. The Ornish diet contains up to 80 percent carbohydrates, but almost no fat. This diet does work, but because of our craving for fat, it can be a difficult diet to adhere to. The high-carbohydrate diet has another problem: detrimental effects on glucose, insulin, and triglycerides that may, paradoxically, increase the risk for heart disease.

Ornish's book inadvertently suggests the reason low-carbohydrate diets have taken off. For years, diet experts and health agencies have been encouraging us to cut fat, cut fat, cut fat. Well, there's a reason we like to eat fat: It's comforting. (Think of that bagel slathered with cream cheese, or vegetables simmering in butter, or that rich chocolate cake at dinner.) Through hormones, dietary fat helps us feel full and satisfied. If you cut fat, there are only two places to go: protein or carbohydrates. Carbohydrates tend to be more accessible than proteins—after all, we're dealing with sugar—so people started eating more carbohydrates without paying attention to calories.

And American food producers responded. Think of all the low-fat or no-fat products that have hit the shelves in recent years: low-fat cheese, low-fat chips, fat-free ice cream, and even fat-free chocolate cookies. But these foods aren't calorie-free; just because you substitute applesauce for vegetable shortening doesn't mean the food suddenly has the same calorie count as water. In fact, some fat-free or low-fat foods have a higher caloric content than their fat-full counterparts. Americans are deceived by "fat-free" and are getting fatter because of it (see Table 2.1). So much for trying to lose weight.

Thus, the backlash. Still, most of the current low-carbohydrate diets frown on fat; so lower carbohydrates mean higher protein.

Carbohydrates need not be all evil, however. I've already noted that fruit is good for you *and* contains "good" carbohydrate in the form of fructose. There are many "good" carbohydrates. Each one is unique, and each has its own special properties.

VEGETABLES AND FRUITS

Vegetables and fruits are by far the best carbohydrates that you can eat. If there is such a thing as a "miracle food" for weight loss, vegetables and fruits are just that. The meal plan at the end of this book allows you to have unlimited amounts of most fruits and vegetables. Why? Pound for pound, vegetables, and to a lesser extent, fruits are extremely low in calories. Fresh vegetables and fruits are high in fiber and health-promoting nutrients called *phytonutrients*. In fact, many studies have been published proving the effect of consuming vegetables and fruits on the reduction of cancer, heart disease and strokes, among other ailments. These benefits have not been replicated by taking vitamin pills.

I strongly encourage you to consume at least 5 servings of vegetables and 5 servings of fruits every day. I consider these numbers minimums. As far as vegetables and fruits go, more is better! If you are

Table 2.1
FAT-FREE VERSUS REGULAR FOOD CALORIE COMPARISON

Whether it comes from carbohydrate or fat, a calorie is still a calorie. Any food eaten in excess can cause insulin surges and can lead to weight gain.

Fat-Free or Reduced Fat	Calories	Regular	Calories
Reduced-fat peanut butter (2 Tbsp)	190	Regular peanut butter	190
Reduced-fat cookie	128	Regular cookie	136
Fat-free fig cookie	70	Fig cookie	50
Nonfat frozen yogurt (½ cup)	190	Ice cream (½ cup)	180
Fat-free caramel topping (2 Tbsp)	130	Caramel topping (½ Tbsp)	130
Reduced-fat granola cereal (¼ cup)	110	Granola cereal (¼ cup)	130
Reduced-fat croissant roll	110	Regular croissant roll	130
Baked tortilla chips (1 oz)	110	Regular tortilla chips (1 oz)	130
Reduced-fat breakfast bar	140	Regular breakfast bar	130

Source: *The Practical Guide to the Identification, Evaluation, and Treatment of Overweight and Obesity in Adults.* National Institutes of Health, September 1998, p. 31.

hungry, vegetables and fruits are the first thing you should eat. It is important that you have only fresh vegetables and fruits (although frozen is also acceptable). Dried fruits, canned fruits, and fruit juices are high in calories and should be consumed only in very limited quantities. Grapes, bananas, and watermelon can also lead to problems with insulin spiking if overeaten and should not exceed 5 servings total in a given day.

Many people who are not used to eating vegetables and fruits have trouble eating 5 servings of each on a daily basis. I encourage you to stick with it. Eventually you will begin to feel bad if you do not get all your servings of vegetables and fruits each day. When you fill your belly with these healthy foods, you will feel less hungry for the bad foods. See Chapter 11 for more information on vegetables and fruits.

COMPLEX CARBOHYDRATES

Complex carbohydrates, also known as starches, are incredibly variable in regard to their effects on insulin. Some starches barely nudge insulin; others make it shoot up out of control. Regardless of the starch, the body treats it the same: All starches—complex carbohydrates—are converted to simple sugars. But good carbohydrates are digested and broken down slowly, providing a more gradual release of sugar into the body. Bad carbohydrates, on the other hand, cause huge sugar and insulin spikes. The former is what you want, because if the sugar is released gradually into the body, less insulin is produced—and so is less fat.

Starch, as a chemical compound, exists in very specific structures. Scientists can look into a microscope and use special light settings—polarization—to identify different starches. Some starch granules are encased in a "lattice" of protein or a different carbohydrate molecule. In order to digest a starch, your body must first disrupt this latticework. The more lattice present, the more difficult a starch is to digest (and easier for your hormones to process).

As noted earlier, starch is made up of a combination of monosaccharide molecules that form polysaccharides. Two of the polysaccharides in starch found in varying ratios are **amylose** and **amylopectin**. The ratio of amylose to amylopectin is what determines how digestible the starch is: Amylose is a dense polysaccharide which stays together in tight clumps, whereas amylopectin is loosely stacked, like a group of coat racks that have been put together. So amylopectin molecules can be incredibly complex, with a fine, intricate branching structure of glucose molecule chains. Because amylopectin molecules are not stacked as tightly as are amylose molecules, enzymes can break in easier, digesting the glucose more rapidly and causing a sudden rise in blood sugar levels. With the insulin spike, your appetite returns quickly—and you want more food. Foods high in amylopectin, such as potatoes and bananas, produce the same effect as sugary foods.

Ideally, you want foods with a higher percentage of amylose, because they'll be harder to digest, provide longer lasting energy, provoke less insulin release, and satisfy appetite better.

GOOD CARBOHYDRATES ARE HARD TO DIGEST

It's not only the amylose-amylopectin ratio that affects digestibility. How the starch is packaged in its specific plant sources—the latticework—also has an influence.

Let's use the humble bean as an example. In a bean, the latticework is difficult to penetrate because beans have a lot of this lattice protein encasing the starch. So beans are an excellent part of any diet: They're a source of both protein and carbohydrate, but have little fat. The protein protects the carbohydrate from digestion, resulting in lower insulin release and an overall better effect on the body.

Of course, beans do have one notable side effect: gas. In addition to not being fully digested because of the protective latticework, they contain a carbohydrate that is not digestible by our enzymes, as well as a lot of fiber. For these three reasons, undigested bean particles are passed from our small intestine—where digestion occurs—to the colon. Here, the "colonic flora," some healthy bacteria that live in our colon, work hard to digest the beans for us. The by-product of this colonic fermentation process is gas. A similar process produces gas in lactose-intolerant people.

Other factors that affect digestibility are cooking, processing, chewing, and digestive enzymes.

- **Cooking**. The more a carbohydrate is cooked—heated—the more its chemical bonds are broken down and the higher its glycemic index becomes. The upshot is the food becomes much easier to digest. Interestingly, however, there's a flip side to cooking called *retrogradation*: When food is heated and then cooled, then heated again, the process can actually modify starches and make them harder to digest. So, if you bake a potato, place it in the refrigerator overnight, then reheat it the next day, it will become harder to digest than it was after first baking. Leftovers, in other words, are a *good* thing.

- **Processing**. Grinding of grains raises the glycemic index, so finely milled flour is digested more quickly than whole-wheat flour or simple cracked wheat. In general, the more something is processed, the higher the glycemic index.
- **Chewing**. Back in the 1800s, many families followed the teachings of clergyman Sylvester Graham. Today, Graham would be considered prescient in many ways: a vegetarian, he encouraged his followers to eat fruits and vegetables and avoid fried foods, and he invented an unsifted wheat flour that has taken his name (as has a cracker made from that flour). But one of his pronouncements was dead wrong. He believed, probably rightly so, that Americans ate too fast. His answer, however, was that one should chew food at least 32 times (one chew for each tooth) before swallowing, and many more times if possible. This process, and some of the philosophy behind it, became known as "fletcherism," after one of Graham's followers.

  Unfortunately, excessive chewing liquefies and almost completely digests the food in your mouth. The saliva contains an enzyme, amylase, which breaks down amylose, so we actually start to digest sugars and starches before we swallow. By the time the overchewed food hits the stomach and intestines, it's ready to be instantly absorbed into the bloodstream—creating a huge insulin surge. (And, as 19th-century Americans found out, excessive chewing also leads to colossally boring meals. When do you get a chance to talk?)
- **Enzymes**. Many of the enzymes needed to digest types of carbohydrates come from the pancreas, as do enzymes that digest proteins and fats. The main enzyme for starches, pancreatic amylase, is essentially the same one found in saliva, in fact.

  The thing is, it doesn't matter how many enzymes you have participating in the process. Our bodies come equipped with these enzymes far in excess of what we need; if you ate three-quarters of a pound of pure starch, you'd still have plenty of enzymes to digest the starch. Moreover, nothing can change the digestibility of the starch you just ate. You can down a half-gallon of water after that serving of pure starch; you can chow down on other food groups; you can even throw some enzyme supplements into your system. It doesn't matter. The enzymes are going to do their job at their own pace.

So it's too late once you've eaten the starch. The key is to watch what you eat in the first place. *Any diet that combines specific foods for the purposes of enhancing digestion is, at its heart, fundamentally flawed.* Slower digestion is beneficial. It produces a more gradual source of energy to the body. If digestion of starches is speeded up, the energy load comes hard and strong and all at once and you get an insulin surge. The insulin surge causes energy to be converted into fat, instead of being burned as fuel, and results in a rapid lowering of blood sugar, causing symptoms of hypoglycemia. So beware of diets that base their food combinations on "enhancing digestion": All they're doing is enlarging your waistline.

THE GLYCEMIC INDEX

The concept of the glycemic index dates back to 1981, when Dr. David Jenkins and Dr. Thomas M. S. Wolever published a paper detailing the concept that not all carbohydrate foods break down at the same rate. As noted in the popular book *The Glucose Revolution* (co-authored by Dr. Wolever), the ones that break down quickly during digestion produce a fast and high blood sugar response; these foods have high glycemic indices. The ones that break down slowly and release glucose gradually into the bloodstream have lower glycemic indices. Examples of the former group are potatoes, bagels, corn chips, and jellybeans; the latter group includes most fruit, milk, yogurt, and beans. (Chocolate, incidentally, has a glycemic index of 49. Not bad. Unfortunately, it's loaded with fat.)

Unlike the concept of the calorie, the glycemic index is measured using real people and real food. Calories are measured in a laboratory, using a device called a *bomb calorimeter*. A food is placed in the bomb calorimeter and literally burned to a crisp. The amount of heat produced by the food is measured. A true calorie is the amount of heat required to raise the temperature of 1 cubic centimeter of water by 1 degree Celsius; the calories we're familiar with—the ones noted on the nutrition information boxes listed on every supermarket food product—are actually kilocalories (1 kilocalorie is 1000 calories). Either way, what's being determined is simply a measure of energy—not the effect a food has on the body.

Enter the glycemic index. Instead of calculating measurements in test tubes or bomb calorimeters, the glycemic index is determined using real people. Several volunteers, usually eight to ten, are tested on two or three separate occasions. Each volunteer is fed a serving of food containing 50 grams of carbohydrate. (Obviously, because some foods are denser with carbohydrates than others, serving sizes differ from food to food.) The volunteers are then checked continuously to see what effect that food has on their blood sugar: Their blood glucose is measured every 15 minutes over the course of about 3 hours. When the testing is concluded, all the values are averaged and a food is given a glycemic index number. The reference food, a portion of white bread containing the equivalent of 50 grams of carbohydrate, equals 100, so each food's glycemic index is compared to white bread. In general, foods with a glycemic index of more than 70 are considered high-glycemic-index foods. Those less than 55 are low-glycemic-index foods. Table 2.2 gives the glycemic index of selected foods.

The glycemic index measures glucose in the blood, but what we are really interested in is insulin. Scientists make a giant leap of faith and assume that the response of insulin parallels the response of blood glucose. Some have suggested the formation of an "insulinemic index" as a true measure of the body's insulin response to food.

The glycemic index can be affected by a number of variables. Acidity lowers the glycemic index; so does a high degree of fiber. And foods eaten in conjunction with each other—as we would in real life—must be averaged to compute their glycemic index, according to some theories. In this way, some foods can slow down the digestion (and thus the insulin spike) of others.

Measuring blood glucose is not the same thing as measuring insulin response. However, the two are closely related, so it can be assumed they work in conjunction. The body requires less insulin to process low-glycemic-index foods. In general, less glucose means less insulin, which means less fat.

Interestingly, the American Diabetes Association does not support the glycemic index. The reason is that there is such variability in the testing as well as the fact that we have no idea what these foods do in combination. As noted earlier, you can arrive at a rough estimate of the glycemic index of a meal by averaging the indices of each item based on the serving size you're eating, but this hasn't been determined to be reliable as of yet. Furthermore, the insulin response to proteins and fats in combination with various carbohydrates is totally unpredictable—and insulin is really what we're concerned about, not the glycemic index.

The experts do agree on some things. Slowly digested carbohydrates are more beneficial than quickly digested carbohydrates: Beans and lentils are better than baked potatoes, for example. In fact, vegetables that grow above the ground are generally better than those that grow below the ground (onions are an exception). Fruits are also an excellent carbohydrate because they're high in fiber and have fructose as their source of sugar.

In addition, studies have shown that glycemic index diets improve diabetes and reduce the risk of getting diabetes, improve cholesterol, and increase "fecal bulk"—the size of the stool, a factor known to reduce the risk of colon cancer. And fiber, which plays a role in lowering the glycemic index, keeps the colon healthy.

But the glycemic index isn't everything. Diets that rely heavily on the glycemic index are missing the point as much as diets that stress low levels of carbohydrate. The body requires balance. The glycemic index is only one of the factors to be considered in a weight-loss program.

SUGARS

The three principal sugars consumed by people are sucrose, fructose, and lactose.

Sucrose is better known as simple table sugar. After starch, it's the second most common carbohydrate in our diet. On the glycemic index, it rates about a 65—considered intermediate on the scale.

Interestingly, table sugar enters the bloodstream slower than breakfast cereals—considered a model of dietary goodness—do. The reason for this is that table sugar is actually made of two simple sugars—glucose *and* fructose. While the glucose half enters the bloodstream quickly (after all, it's in the basic form the body uses), the fructose portion must be processed by the liver. So the overall rise in blood sugar is hindered.

Table 2.2
THE GLYCEMIC INDEX OF SELECTED FOODS

The glycemic index represents the impact that various carbohydrates have on blood sugar levels and insulin response. The higher the glycemic index, the greater the glucose and insulin response. Foods with a glycemic index greater than 70 are considered high, 55–70 is considered intermediate, and less than 55 is considered low.

Low Glycemic Index

14 Yogurt, nonfat, plain
14 Peanuts
22 Cherries
25 Barley, boiled
25 Grapefruit, fresh
26 Lentils, red
27 Whole milk
32 Fettucini
33 Yogurt, nonfat, flavored
37 Spaghetti, whole wheat
38 Pear, fresh
38 Apple, fresh
39 Plums, fresh
40 Apple juice
41 Spaghetti, white
42 Peach, fresh
44 Orange, fresh
46 Grapes, green
46 Orange juice
46 Pineapple juice
46 Linguine pasta, thick
48 Grapefruit juice
49 Oatmeal, old fashioned
49 Carrots
49 Chocolate
50 Ice milk
52 Soudough bread
52 Kiwi, frsh
54 Pound cake
54 Sweet potato
54 Potato chips
55 Banana

Low Glycemic Index (cont'd)

55 Corn, canned
55 Brown rice
55 Oatmeal cookie
55 Linguine pasta, thin
55 Popcorn

Intermediate Glycemic Index

56 White rice
57 Apricots, frsh
58 Basmati white rice
58 Peach, canned in syrup
58 Honey
59 Blueberry muffin
60 Oat bran muffin
60 Pizza, cheese
61 Ice cream
63 Coca-Cola™
64 Beets, canned
64 Raisins
65 Rye bread
65 Cantaloupe
66 Pineapple, fresh
67 Croissant

Table 2.2
THE GLYCEMIC INDEX OF SELECTED FOODS (cont'd)

High Glycemic Index

70 White bread	77 Vanilla wafers
72 Bagel	78 Gatorade™
72 Corn chips	80 Jelly beans
72 Watermelon	86 Mashed potatoes, instant
74 Graham crackers	87 Instant rice
74 Soda crackers	88 Potatoes, red skin, boiled
74 Saltine crackers	93 Potatoes, red skin, mashed
75 French fries	95 French baguette
75 Pumpkin, boiled	103 Dates, dried

Sucrose actually has less glucose than refined flours, potatoes, or white rice, and its glycemic index is less than that of white bread. Its bad name is purely because we've demonized sugar in our society. Our bodies need some sugar; sure, we overdo it with the chocolate bars and the Twinkies, but without sugar, we wouldn't be able to survive. There are very few sources of pure glucose in our diet, even though glucose is the most important carbohydrate we talk about. Of course, glucose—as noted previously—is contained in all other carbohydrates.

When sucrose goes into the digestive system, an enzyme called *sucrase*, present in the small intestine, breaks it down. This enzyme is available in amounts far exceeding that which we need. It breaks sucrose into its two component parts, glucose and fructose. Glucose is quickly run through the liver and put into general circulation.

Fructose, the other half of the sucrose molecule, is also run through the liver, but it's not released into the bloodstream. Instead, the liver uses the fructose to make glycogen. *Glycogen*, you'll recall, is one of the principal polysaccharides. It's the body's way of storing carbohydrate; we can store about an 18-hour supply of carbohydrate in the liver in the form of glycogen.

Fructose is found primarily in fruits, but not in the same proportions, as you might expect. Oranges and orange juice are about half fructose, half glucose; apples and apple juice are about two-thirds fructose, one-third glucose. Apple juice, therefore, has a lower glycemic index and a slower blood glucose peak than orange juice. So, when people with diabetes have low blood sugar, they'll drink orange juice to get their blood sugar up quickly. Unprocessed fresh fruits are very healthy and should be a major component of your diet. For more information on fruits, see Chapter 11.

Lactose, a disaccharide, is the other sugar important to human nutrition. Made of equal parts glucose and galactose, the only source of this sugar is milk. Like fructose, the liver must process galactose before it goes into the general circulation.

You might be familiar with a condition known as **lactose intolerance.** This condition is caused by a deficiency of *lactase*, the enzyme needed to break down lactose. When a lactose-intolerant person consumes milk products, lactose cannot be digested and absorbed into the bloodstream. The milk products then pass through the small intestines into the large intestine where they are then "fermented" by coliform (bacteria that inhabit stool). The by-product of this fermentation is gas and other toxins, and people who experience lactose intolerance frequently suffer from bloating, flatulence, or diarrhea when they consume milk products.

There are enzyme supplements available to combat this condition—but I recommend against them. Basically, if you are lactose intolerant, it's because your body does not want dairy products. It rejects the dairy, sending it to the scavenger bacteria in your colon. If you take lactase enzyme tablets, you are forcing your body to accept a nutrient it has chosen to reject. Many people have allergies to milk proteins. Lactase enzyme tablets can overcome your body's defense against milk. This can have serious consequences, including disrupting hormonal balance and altering metabolism. Because milk and dairy products are a prime source of calcium, people suffering from lactose intolerance should seek out other sources of this key nutrient (see Chapter 6 for more information on calcium).

SPREAD YOUR CARBOHYDRATES THROUGHOUT THE DAY

The glycemic index, by noting which foods are high in easily digested sugars and which are low, encourages the consumption of certain foods with low glycemic indices. But it's not always easy to follow the glycemic index: Few people carry a list of every food's G.I. around, and even fewer commit it to memory.

One alternative is nibbling. All glycemic index measurements are done with a 50-gram portion of carbohydrate. But quantity matters: You eat more, your glucose and insulin levels go even higher. Eating a huge portion of a so-called "healthy" food, such as beans or lentils, can prompt an insulin surge as easily as a fistful of Twinkies. But the opposite is also true: Eating a small portion of a "bad" food, such as white bread or potatoes, will induce a low glucose and insulin response.

So, if you nibble tiny portions of high- or low-glycemic index foods throughout the day, you will provide a constant low-level source of glucose (energy) to your body, and your body will not respond with a huge insulin surge. The body becomes *accustomed* to receiving a constant supply of energy. On the other hand, if you starve the body by skipping meals, then gorging on a huge meal once or twice a day, the body freaks out. It thinks it's starving and does everything it can to store the food.

What happens then? Metabolism is slowed, you get sleepy after the meal, and the huge insulin surge created by the huge meal allows the meal to be stored as fat instead of burned as energy. Big meals make you sleepy *because* your metabolic rate is slowed. The body is conserving energy because even though it just got a huge meal, it is still in starvation mode and doesn't know when the next meal is coming. When you provide a continuous source of calories to the body in the form of nibbling, the body relaxes: It goes out of starvation mode and starts using the calories instead of storing them. The result is less hunger, more energy, and weight loss.

Faith's Story
Faith didn't like diets. A New York attorney with a large firm, she couldn't stick to them: too much to remember, too many schedules to keep. Besides, she usually worked right through lunch anyway, and dinner had to wait until she could take the subway to Grand Central Terminal, catch a 6:32 to Westchester, and get home from the local train station. She usually didn't eat until 7:30 at the earliest, weary and cranky. She was also carrying 160 pounds on her 5-foot-5-inch frame, at least 30 pounds too much.

Ironically, considering her work habits, Faith would have been a good subject for a nibbling diet. She could have kept carrot sticks and fruit in the office refrigerator, or even taken a bagel from the snack cart in the morning, eating half then and half in the afternoon. Exercise could have been easy, too: Instead of the elevator, she could have taken the stairs to her seventh-floor office, or she could have walked 11 blocks from Grand Central to her Midtown Manhattan office instead of taking the subway.

Faith decided, however, that she was just going to skip meals. No lunch, no mid-morning or mid-afternoon snacks, no protein bar at the newsstand before boarding the commuter train. Her food intake would consist solely of a light breakfast, usually coffee and cereal, and a dinner of high-protein, low-carbohydrate foods, such as chicken and fish.

This worked well in the beginning. Faith dropped 5 pounds the first week; she attributed her fatigue and short temper to the diet, and told people that. But after a few more weeks, the weight wasn't coming off anymore, yet Faith remained tired and irritated. She snapped at co-workers, her memory was foggy, and her work suffered.

Her body had fallen into starvation mode. Even though Faith still weighed over 150 pounds, her body was trying to conserve energy, not use it.

Faith eventually figured out that her starvation diet wasn't doing the trick. She started following the meal plan in Chapter 11, with six small meals each day, and adding exercise to the mix, and the pounds gradually came off. More importantly, Faith felt better.

Studies show that nibbling results in a lesser glucose surge than gorging. Nibbling reduces high insulin levels and prevents the "undershoot" of glucose that is seen when high-glycemic foods are consumed. After all, because food is introduced to the body gradually, the insulin surge is less and the glucose response of rapid decline is less as well.

Nibbling has proven to be an accepted treatment for hypoglycemia. Hypoglycemic patients are told to eat six small meals a day. Doing so has some positive side effects: Nibbling prevents the insulin surge that comes with wolfing down big meals or high-glycemic foods, which in turn stops calories from being stored as fat.

When you think about our evolution, this all makes sense. Our ancient hunter-gatherer ancestors lived from moment to moment, often off whatever nuts and berries they came across in their daily search for food. A big meal was a treat! It's only in modern times, when even our agriculture workers are governed by the time clock, that we've focused on eating three big meals a day—giving us the morning and afternoon to work. Not that we stick to that, of course . . . our three big meals are usually augmented by countless snacks.

The bottom line is that nibbling is good. By nibbling, you are supplying the body with its nutrients in a gradual fashion, in the way it handles them best. The concept matches that of the glycemic index: With low-glycemic foods, the natural digestive process allows for the gradual release of glucose into the bloodstream; with nibbling, the small portions allow for the gradual release of glucose into the bloodstream. Either way, no foods are forbidden. If you eat high-glycemic foods, simply eat them in small quantities. Calories do count. *The amount of carbohydrate consumed is much more important than the type of carbohydrate.*

THE PROBLEM WITH SKIPPING BREAKFAST

Have you ever seen a sumo wrestler? These Japanese titans often weigh well over 400 pounds, a handy size to be when you're trying to force your opponent out of the ring—or simply knock him down.

But do you know how a sumo wrestler gains all that weight? Sumo wrestlers don't eat breakfast. They wake up, exercise and practice their technique all morning (for big men, sumo wrestlers can be quite nimble), and have a big lunch. It's a healthy lunch—the Japanese have notably healthy diets, high in protein from seafood and low in fat—but it's also loaded with starch in the form of white rice, a high-glycemic food. After that lunch, they sleep for several hours. As I've noted, metabolism slows after a big meal, and sleep slows metabolism (and digestion) even more. Sumo wrestlers become very fat.

Interestingly, at least during their careers, they're not in terrible shape. They exercise frequently, so the fat tends to form under the skin (subcutaneously) and not in the stomach (visceral fat). Incidence of diabetes and cholesterol is very low among sumo wrestlers.

But once they retire, all those problems hit with a vengeance. Suddenly fat shifts to the belly; incidence of high cholesterol and diabetes shoots way up. All the weight they carry around becomes a burden, not an advantage.

Several studies have linked obesity to skipping breakfast. In fact, the *more* meals you have per day, the *less* likely you are to be overweight.

Many of my patients have told me that they simply aren't hungry for breakfast. I have found that the most common reason for not being hungry for breakfast is overeating the night before. It is a vicious cycle. Skip breakfast and get too hungry for lunch and dinner. Overeat at night and feel full the next morning. The cycle repeats itself. If you follow the eating suggestions in this book, you will become hungry for breakfast.

Breakfast is a critical element to hormonal balance. Breakfast prevents insulin surges that occur if you feast and then starve yourself.

You should also try to incorporate protein with breakfast. Protein at breakfast has been shown to reduce hunger and cravings throughout the day. In fact, if you have protein with your breakfast, you will be less likely to overeat at both lunch and dinner. There are many ways to enjoy protein in the morning. My personal favorite is an egg white omelet packed with fresh vegetables and a slice of fat-free cheese. For more suggestions on healthy breakfasts, see Chapter 11.

FIBER KEEPS INSULIN LOW

If you want to lower your insulin levels, fiber is the way to go. Like starch, fiber is a polysaccharide, with one major difference: The body cannot digest fiber. That's bad, right? Nope. It's a good thing. Fiber lowers the glycemic index of food by delaying digestion. This, in turn, lowers insulin levels. It also plays a major role in maintaining good health in a variety of other ways:

- Fiber makes you feel full. Soluble fibers swell in the stomach and bowels, reducing feelings of hunger and making you feel full.

Soluble fibers also slow gastric emptying, keeping other food in the stomach longer. And since the body cannot digest fiber, the fiber harmlessly makes its way through the digestive system, eventually passed out into the stool.

- Fiber nourishes your *colonic mucosa*, the innermost layer of the large intestine, by helping in the production of a substance called *butyrate*. Butyrate is thought to have a role in the prevention of colon cancer and other colonic diseases.
- A high-fiber diet reduces LDL (or "bad") cholesterol by as much as 10 percent.
- Although it has little effect on blood glucose overall, fiber does lower the glycemic index of foods.
- Fiber prevents constipation.

A 1999 study published in the *Journal of the American Medical Association* concluded that fiber lowers insulin levels and helps people lose weight. There have been many other studies published on this subject. Most, but not all, have agreed that fiber helps you lose weight.

Not all fiber is created equal, however. *Soluble* fibers, referred to above, are foods such as legumes, oats, and psyllium, as well as pectin, found in apples; *insoluble* fibers are foods like whole wheat or bran, foods often found in certain cereal grains. Insoluble fiber may actually raise cholesterol, so it's best not to eat too much. Even soluble fiber won't benefit you much unless it has been mixed well with other foods, which—for lack of a better term—improves the viscosity (thickness of flow) of the food in the stomach. And fiber also causes gas, for similar reasons as beans and lactose: The body can't digest it, so the colonic bacteria ferment the material and produce gas as a by-product.

That said, fiber is still an overall positive. You need 25 to 35 grams a day of fiber each day, minimum, in your diet. At the least, it keeps you regular, reduces the risk of colon cancer, and promotes good digestion; at best, it can also help you lose weight, partly because it helps you feel "full," partly because of its glycemic-index-lowering and insulin-lowering properties.

The best way to get fiber in your diet is to eat lots of fresh vegetables and fruits. And more is better when it comes to vegetables and fruits. Yes, vegetables and fruits have calories, but it is difficult to overeat these items. For more information, see Chapter 11.

PROTEIN IS UNPREDICTABLE

Once again, you've heard the dietary litany: protein good, fat bad. The fact is that our bodies need both protein and fat in order to function—just as our bodies also require carbohydrate.

Proteins, you may recall from high school biology, are made up of molecules called *amino acids*. Amino acids can be easily converted by the body into glucose and fat. The body can also use amino acids as the building blocks for potent hormones and neurotransmitters. (Neurotransmitters are the chemical signals the nervous system's cells, neurons, use to communicate with one another. There are three major chemical families of neurotransmitters; one family is made out of amines, the same carbon-hydrogen-nitrogen compounds that make up amino acids.)

High-protein diets are currently all the rage; they're the flip side of low-carbohydrate diets. (Proponents of low-carbohydrate diets require that you eat lots of protein to make up for the lack of carbo-hydrates.) One reason to consume lots of protein, the proponents argue, is that—because of lowered carbohydrate consumption—it's a diet that promotes less insulin release. Protein also tells the body to release cholecystokinin, a hormone that reduces appetite and makes you feel satisfied.

However, that's not always true. Protein turns out to be a potent insulin stimulator in its own right. Protein enthusiasts have based their dieting principles on a theory but not fact. They only look at the effects of individual nutrients—carbohydrates, proteins, and fats—on the body's production of insulin. They rarely actually measure (instead of predicting) the body's response to combining nutrients. Research com-bining carbohydrate and protein has been done, however. Dr. Rabinowitz, at Johns Hopkins School of Medicine, studied the effects of carbohydrate alone, protein alone, and carbohydrate combined with protein on a group of healthy women. To the amazement of the med-ical community, the insulin response to the mixed carbohydrate-protein meal was *not predictable* from the responses seen from consuming each alone (see Figure 2.3). This study and others have shown that when carbohydrates and protein are consumed together (like most of our meals), insulin levels soar.

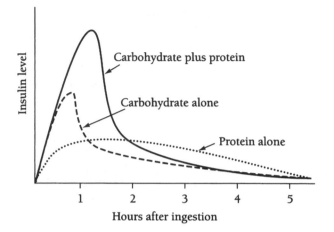

Adapted from Rabinowitz, et al. Patterns of Hormonal Release After Glucose, Protein and Glucose Plus Protein, *Lancet*. Vol 2(7461), 1966, 454-456.

Figure 2.3
INSULIN RESPONSE TO CARBOHYDRATE, TO PROTEIN, AND TO CARBOHYDRATE PLUS PROTEIN

When protein is ingested alone, the insulin response is less than that to carbohydrate. However, the effects of a mixed carbohydrate-protein meal cannot be predicted from the response seen from consuming each alone. The insulin response to carbohydrate plus protein is higher than what would be predicted.

For protein to be effective in lowering insulin levels, you must, as much as possible, eat it in a meal separate from carbohydrates. In the long run, this type of eating pattern will lower your insulin levels. This is a very difficult way to eat in real life. Michel Montignac, in his French cuisine best-seller, *Dine Out and Lose Weight*, promotes this eating principle. Montignac goes off base, however, by claiming that if you follow this principle, you can eat as much as you want and not gain weight or actually *lose* weight.

I recommend that you eat about 0.4 grams of protein each day for every pound you weigh. So, a 150-pound person should consume about 55 to 60 grams of protein each day. However, this formula isn't perfect, since it doesn't take into account body composition. Remember, protein, especially when combined with carbohydrate, can cause insulin spiking. The diet at the end of this book provides for unlimited quantities of egg whites. In theory, this could lead to eating too much protein; however, most people find it difficult to eat too many egg whites. If you have kidney problems, you should consume much less protein. So it pays to be careful and be cautious. If you have any doubts, see your doctor.

You should spread your protein throughout the day, but in particular, **you need protein at breakfast.** Many people are accustomed to all (or mostly) carbohydrate breakfasts such as juice and toast, cereal and skim milk (has minimal protein), pancakes or waffles and syrup. High-carbohydrate breakfasts cause glucose and insulin spiking and result in hunger, sleepiness, and carbohydrate cravings (usually in that order) later in the day. In fact, these symptoms are so common that many people skip breakfast. The problem is that skipping breakfast causes other problems with insulin (see earlier discussions). The answer: **protein at breakfast.** Protein at breakfast will help control hunger and cravings for the entire day. You will eat less at lunch and dinner. Protein at breakfast will also supply your body with a source of long-lasting glucose that will give you energy and prevent fatigue associated with glucose crashing (hypoglycemia). See Chapter 11 for more information.

FAT

Fat has become the most discriminated of the nutrients. Many diets encourage people to cut their fat consumption way, way back; the thought is, the less fat, the better. But fat is an essential part of our diet, and an essential cog in body function. A good diet has about 30 percent fat.

Like protein, fat has a number of benefits. It slows down the rate of carbohydrates entering the bloodstream. It has little effect on insulin response. And, perhaps most importantly, it produces a hormone—cholecystokinin—that tells your brain that it's time to stop eating. It's the fat that makes you feel full. Besides, even if you think you're completely addicted to fat, you aren't. When was the last time you ate a

stick of butter or a tub of shortening? Even if the butter had been flavored with chocolate, you wouldn't have gotten very far until your
brain said, "No more."

There are different types of fat. *Saturated* fats are substances like
butter; their chemical bonds, between carbon atoms, are already full of
hydrogen atoms. Almost all saturated fats have an animal origin and are
usually solid at room temperature. *Unsaturated* fats, which include
cooking oils, are usually liquid at room temperature; their chemical
bonds have room for more hydrogen atoms. Within the unsaturated-fat
category, there are monounsaturated fats and polyunsaturated fats; the
former include olive, peanut, and canola oils, while the latter include
vegetable oils and the fat in fish.

Most fats are a combination of saturated and unsaturated fats, and
unsaturated fats can be turned into saturated fats by a process called
hydrogenation—literally adding hydrogen to the mix. All fats have the
same caloric content: 9 calories per gram. Proteins and carbohydrates
have about 4 calories per gram, so fat has more than twice the calories
as an equivalent amount of protein or carbohydrate.

Fats are known to have an effect on cholesterol. The best for your
cholesterol is monounsaturated fat; the worst, saturated fat. Most kinds
of unsaturated fats have a lesser effect on cholesterol than saturated fat,
but there is one kind of unsaturated fat—trans-unsaturated fat—that is
as bad as saturated fat. When manufacturers hydrogenate fats, they will
add hydrogen atoms in no particular order—unlike nature, which adds
hydrogen atoms in a very precise way. If the process is stopped in the
middle, as it is with many brands of margarine (the idea being to add
hydrogen until the fat becomes solid), it's called *partial hydrogenation*.
The result is a product containing "trans-fatty acids"—transformed,
toxic substances that can be detrimental to our health. What's worse is
that this trans-unsaturated fat is listed on packages as being simply
unsaturated. Technically it is, but only because there are hydrogen
atoms floating around, unsure of where to bond.

Cholesterol-lowering margarines and salad dressings (Benechol
and Take Control) are now sold in the United States. These products
contain compounds known as *hydrogenated sterols*, which help lower
cholesterol. Although effective for cholesterol, these products have the
same number of calories as regular margarine and do not help you
lose weight.

Though most diets try to cut fat, one in particular—the Atkins diet—proposes eating *more* fat. The theory behind this is that by replacing carbohydrate with fat, insulin levels go down and, as we've seen, it's the spike in insulin which can lead to weight gain because the body is both storing more calories and, when the spike ends, slowing metabolism. Also, as previously noted, fat supplies the brain with the "off" switch when it comes to appetite. Eat more fat, the theory goes, and the off switch clicks sooner; don't eat enough, and we'll remain hungry.

Certain fats are, indeed, vital to our well-being. These are known as *essential fatty acids* (EFAs). Two EFAs, linoleic acid and lenolenic acid, are chief among the body's requirements. The former is an omega-3 fatty acid, the latter an omega-6 fatty acid. Linoleic acid has been shown to prevent diabetes in laboratory animals. Without EFAs, we fall victim to a variety of symptoms, including dry flaking skin, hair loss, arthritis, weakness, incoordination of muscles, and numbness and tingling of the hands and feet.

Ironically, despite all the fat we get from our modern diets, we seldom get the right kind of fat. Most of our dietary fat consists of processed oils and meat fat. Manufacturers process oil to prevent it from becoming rancid. This processing removes many of the vital nutrients. Meat fat is full of saturated fat and, in today's society, filled with hormones. In the name of building a bigger, leaner, better-producing cow, agribusinesses shoot cattle up with growth hormone, testosterone, and hormones to stimulate milk production, and with high-potency antibiotics and vaccines. Moreover, think of what cattle eat: grass and hay that has probably been treated with herbicides, pesticides, and other chemicals to eliminate pests and bugs. Unfortunately, those chemicals never go away; they are stored in the fat of the animal. The cow eats them on the feed, and we eat them from the cow (or sheep, or goat, or whatever meat is at hand).

The bottom line is that we're not getting enough natural vegetable fat and fat from sources besides processed oils and meat. We're surrounded by sources, too: fish, nuts, sunflower seeds, olives, and avocados. Unrefined oils, extracted from an old-fashioned screw press, are available in some health-food stores; however, they tend to become rancid quite easily. Fish, especially fish that live in cold water (sardines, herring, lake trout, and salmon) are very high in omega-3 fatty acids. Flax, soybeans, sunflower seeds, sesame seeds, peanuts, and walnuts are also good sources of this beneficial fat. Omega-3 enriched eggs, laid

by hens fed a diet of flaxseed meal, fish meal, or algae, are an interesting new product on the market (the omega-3 fatty acids are only in
the yolk). Omega-3 fatty acids play a role in lowering insulin levels and
reducing insulin resistance (see Chapter 3). By lowering blood triglycerides, these beneficial fats have also been found to reduce your risk
of heart disease.

The heart-healthy benefits of omega-3 fatty acids have prompted
the American Heart Association to recommend that everyone eat two
3-ounce servings of fish each week. But the fish oils sold in capsules
deserve caution. Overdoses have been linked to impaired immune
function, elevations of vitamins A and D to toxic levels, and a worsening of diabetes.

Fat Substitutes

In the midst of escaping from fat, we have created fat replacers, the two
primary brands being Simplesse and Olestra. Simplesse is a protein-
based substance. It carries as many calories as a carbohydrate, but
that's still only half as much as the equivalent amount of fat. Besides its
caloric content, there has been little problem with Simplesse.

Olestra, also marketed under the name Olean, is another matter. It's
essentially a fat the body cannot absorb, so it's passed through the
digestive system without entering the body. In large amounts, it has
been shown to prompt diarrhea and gastrointestinal pain. On the plus
side, it adds virtually no calories to products and is said to have a better texture than Simplesse. There is a concern that these fat replacers
can leach your body of vital nutrients. In order to prevent vitamin deficiencies, the Food and Drug Administration has mandated that the fat-
soluble vitamins A, D, E, and K be added to these products.
Replacement of these four vitamins may not be enough. In general, I
recommend using these products sparingly.

Fat Blockers

With obesity and its treatment a major industry in this country—from fat-
free products to the extreme of stomach-stapling operations—there is
now a medication for the treatment of obesity. Called orlistat, marketed

under the brand name Xenical, it works by blocking the digestion and absorption of some of the fat you eat. This medication does work; however, orlistat coupled with too much fat consumption can overload your intestinal tract with fat and cause gastrointestinal problems, including diarrhea and leakage of oily stool.

Natural-foods partisans also have an obesity product, chitosan. Chitosan is made from crustacean shells and is supposed to block fat absorption. However, a 2001 study in the journal *Obesity Research* found that chitosan blocks *zero* of the fat in your diet. The next time you see one of those infomercials for chitosan, don't be tempted. It's just a come-on and a rip-off. A newer product, nopal cactus, claims to have the same effect as chitosan. At this time, it is not known whether or not nopal cactus actually works.

HYPOGLYCEMIA

Glucose is the body's main fuel. In a good diet, the idea is to keep the level of glucose more or less constant, increasing it at times when you need more energy and letting it wane when you need less—but usually not to the point where it causes a negative reaction.

Of course, almost none of us do that. Think about it: have you ever eaten a huge meal? Have you ever consumed a rich dessert, often in an oversized serving, in a fine restaurant? Have you ever gotten home late at night, tired but not sleepy, and had a comforting bowl of ice cream? Have you ever quenched your afternoon carb craving with a bag of potato chips or a candy bar?

All of these actions spiked your blood sugar. That in itself isn't terrible; our bodies are well equipped to deal with spikes in blood sugar, and the worst thing that usually happens is we gain weight.

But some people are afflicted with a condition called *hypoglycemia*. Literally, hypoglycemia is simply "low blood sugar." The glucose level in the blood drops below the point where it can fuel the body's activity. This form of hypoglycemia usually occurs after eating large meals or high-glycemic index foods: The blood sugar rises, the insulin surges, and then—very rapidly—blood sugar levels decline. The hypoglycemia is caused by an "undershoot" whereby blood sugar levels fall below the level that existed *before* you ate. This type of hypoglycemia, known as "reactive hypoglycemia," invariably occurs as a reaction to food.

When blood sugar drops rapidly, symptoms of hypoglycemia set in. You feel hungry (already!), sleepy, tired, fatigued; your heart rate picks up and your sweating increases. All you want to do is take a nap, which is the worst thing you can do—your metabolism slows to a crawl. But you probably can't sleep anyway, even though you feel sleepy; with your heart pounding and the extra sweating, you feel irritated, jazzed, and annoyed. Eating carbohydrates makes brain serotonin levels surge (see Chapter 10). Serotonin calms you and makes you sleepy, slowing your metabolism. This, of course, leads to weight gain and creates a vicious circle.

As I've noted earlier, we've all probably had these symptoms periodically. We all like to eat, and we don't always eat what's good for us. What we can do is fight the appetite and the urge to sleep: We can take a walk or engage in some other physical activity. We can do something to maintain or raise our metabolism and level out our blood sugar. Endocrinologists treat people with reactive hypoglycemia by having them eat low-glycemic-index carbohydrates spread out in multiple small meals throughout the day. This type of eating reduces blood glucose surges and the insulin spikes that follow.

Brooke's Story

Brooke, a 47-year-old financial analyst, came to me with what she thought was a strange collection of symptoms. She'd been gaining weight, she told me, even though she believed her diet hadn't changed much in many years. She also had periods of confusion. She'd forget where she was when out for a walk, or couldn't keep a list of numbers straight—a disastrous condition to have, considering her job. She noted that the symptoms came on anytime she went more than 2 to 3 hours without eating. She became accustomed to the problem, eating more and more.

Her symptom of mental confusion was disconcerting, as was the weight gain. We performed some tests and determined that she had hypoglycemia. Brooke's hypoglycemia was not in response to eating the wrong types of carbohydrates, though. The cause of her hypoglycemia was an insulinoma—a tumor that produces far more insulin than is needed. Fortunately, the tumor was found on an MRI scan and Brooke was scheduled for surgery. A tumor about the size of a marble was

*removed from Brooke's pancreas. After the surgery, her prob-
lems with hypoglycemia were gone. More importantly, with
lower insulin levels, Brooke was finally able to lose some
weight.*

ABOUT INSULINOMAS

Sometimes hypoglycemia can be a life-threatening condition. Very high
insulin levels produced by a small tumor in the pancreas can cause
severe low blood sugar levels. Unlike reactive hypoglycemia, the hypoglycemia caused by an insulinoma almost never occurs after a meal.
Instead, this type of hypoglycemia occurs when you have not been eating. Without a constant source of food, blood sugar levels can drop
dangerously. Low blood sugar can affect the brain, a condition known
as *neuroglycopenia*, causing symptoms such as personality changes,
confusion, and seizures or passing out. Once food is consumed, blood
sugar rises and the symptoms disappear. The symptoms of an insulinoma can be subtle. Many patients are not diagnosed for 10 years or
more, and keep getting fat because of the high insulin levels and
because they keep eating, trying to fight low blood sugar. They learn
that if they do not eat large amounts of food all the time, they pass out.
If you have symptoms of this disorder, you should see an endocrinologist to make sure you're not suffering from this potentially fatal, if
rare, problem.

Miriam's Story

*Miriam was a 42-year-old woman with a loving husband, two
children, and a secret: a constantly replenished chocolate-bar
stash, which she kept in a cabinet above the vent for her stove.
Miriam wasn't overindulgent with her chocolate craving, at
least not at first: in the afternoons, usually after finishing
some housework, she would dip into a bag of Hershey Kisses or
a similar sweet and eat about 2 ounces' worth. She wasn't ter-
ribly overweight, maybe 15 pounds.*

*But Miriam was extremely conscious of her extra weight,
and since she didn't exercise much, she frequently tried diets.
Most of these were faddish and lasted only a couple of weeks.
With the recent trend in low-carbohydrate diets, however,*

Miriam decided to go that route. That, of course, would mean cutting the chocolate bars almost entirely out of her life.

It didn't work. The late-afternoon cravings for sweets and other carbohydrates not only killed the diet but also ended up making Miriam gain even more weight. (With few carbohydrates in her new diet, her blood sugar levels would spike higher every time she consumed some carbo-heavy food, and the fat of the chocolate bars didn't help.) She was hungry all the time, particularly a couple hours after a meal, and generally sleepy in the late afternoon, her craving time. She started going through bags of Hershey Kisses, not just a couple ounces. Miriam needed help.

Miriam started a meal plan similar to the one at the end of this book—eating protein and low-glycemic-index carbohydrates, spread out throughout the day. She started snacking on lean protein snacks like turkey and tuna. Most importantly, she started having protein with her breakfast. She stopped tempting herself with bags of chocolate. At first the cravings continued on with a vengeance, but this time Miriam did not give up. When her body said, "Eat chocolate," she ate a chocolate protein bar. Within a couple of weeks, the cravings subsided. She still ate chocolate, but her cravings were controllable. Before she knew it, Miriam had dropped two dress sizes and felt better than ever.

CARBOHYDRATE CRAVINGS

Typical symptoms of carbohydrate cravings are

- Feeling hungry all the time, especially 2 to 3 hours after a meal
- Feeling sleepy and sluggish in the afternoons
- Feeling anxious
- Feeling calm and satiated when eating sugars, candy, chips, pretzels, and other heavy-carbohydrate foods

Carbohydrate cravings are caused by insulin and serotonin. As insulin falls after its normal post-meal rise, a brain chemical known as *serotonin* is released. You may have heard of serotonin; it's the neurotransmitter whose quantities are increased after taking anti-depressant drugs, such as Prozac, Celexa, Zoloft, or Paxil. Serotonin makes you feel better and also provides a key signal to the brain: I am satisfied. I don't need to eat anymore right now.

If insulin goes too high, serotonin is not released in the brain. When this happens, people become anxious, easily irritated, and generally out of sorts. Moreover, the brain hasn't received that key message to stop eating. So people continue stuffing themselves, often with carbohydrate-laden comfort foods, in an effort to finally get that calm, satisfied feeling. Interestingly, several weight-loss medications work by increasing serotonin levels. See Chapter 10 for more information on serotonin.

How do you avoid carbohydrate cravings? Keep your insulin low. Eat protein with breakfast. Eat small frequent meals. Eat lots of fruits and vegetables. The diet principles discussed in this book and the meal plans in Chapter 11 offer the ultimate solution for completely eliminating carbohydrate cravings.

DIET GUIDELINES

- Eat the correct number of calories. The amount of calories you consume each day depends on your body weight and activity level. In general, men and women should eat 10 to 12 calories per pound per day. Read food labels. Look for hidden sources of sugar and fat.
- Eat at least 5 servings of fruits and 5 servings of vegetables every day. Fruits and vegetables are key to hormonal balance. If you are hungry, eat more vegetables and fruits instead of snacking on more fattening foods. As far as vegetables and fruits go, more is better! It's tough to overeat vegetables and fruits.
- Maintain a healthy balance of carbohydrates, proteins, and fat. Exact percentages aren't important, as long as you satisfy your protein requirements and do not eat too much fat.
- Eat low-glycemic-index carbohydrates. If you eat high-glycemic carbohydrates, do not eat them alone; instead, incorporate them into a meal. Alternatively, nibble on high-glycemic carbohydrates slowly, over several hours. This diminishes the impact on your blood sugar and insulin levels.

- Don't give in to carbohydrate cravings. Eat vegetables and fruits or a protein snack instead.
- Eat multiple small meals each day. Your goal should be 5 or 6 meals per day.
- Do not skip meals, especially breakfast.
- Make sure you get enough protein. The minimum protein requirement for healthy adults is 0.4 grams of protein per pound of body weight each day (roughly 55 to 60 grams of protein per day for a 150-pound adult).
- Eat protein (egg whites, lean meat, turkey, chicken, fish, or tofu) at breakfast. This will help you eat less at lunch and dinner.
- Don't eat too much protein. Remember, protein, especially when combined with carbohydrate, can cause insulin spiking. The diet at the end of this book provides for unlimited quantities of egg whites because most people find it very difficult to eat huge quantities of this food.
- Eat low-fat foods. I recommend that your diet be no more than 30 percent fat. Despite the benefits of healthy fats, remember that fat is high in calories and calories still count.
- Eat healthy fats. Replace saturated and trans-unsaturated fats in your diet with monounsaturated and polyunsaturated fats. Good sources of healthy fat include olive oil, avocados, nuts, and fish.
- Avoid fat substitutes.
- Drink at least eight 8-ounce glasses of water each day.
- Do *not* attempt to speed digestion with enzyme supplements or special food combinations. The slower your digestion, the better.

CHAPTER THREE

INSULIN RESISTANCE

THE PIMA INDIANS

THE PIMA INDIANS LIVE JUST SOUTH OF PHOENIX IN SOUTHERN ARIZONA'S GILA RIVER INDIAN COMMUNITY. Their North American ancestry goes back countless generations; indeed, they are believed to have been among the first settlers of North America, first moving here 30,000 years ago.

For 2,000 years, the Pimas were a subsistence agricultural people. They grew wheat, beans, squash, and cotton, and were well known for their generosity. But in the late 19th century, their water supply was diverted by Western settlers and the Pimas suffered from famine and poverty. To maintain their survival, they began eating foodstuffs given them by the U.S. government: lard, white flour, and sugar.

When the United States entered World War II, many Pimas left the reservation and joined the thriving wartime industry in Phoenix and other southwestern cities. Others joined the U.S. military. Both provided the Pimas with greater prosperity; both also prompted a further change in their diet to one similar to that of most Americans.

And, like many Americans, the Pimas started growing fat. But their obesity was on a scale far different from that of people in the rest of the country: By some indications, the majority of all Pima adults were well overweight.

In 1963, the National Institute of Diabetes and Digestive and Kidney Diseases (NIDDK) did a survey of rheumatoid arthritis among the Pimas and another tribe, the Blackfoot tribe of Montana. What they found was that the Pima Indians had an extremely high rate of diabetes, far beyond that which was considered normal for the general population. Two years later, the NIDDK and several other organizations, including the Pima community itself, began another study to explain this phenomenon. By figuring out the secret of the Pimas' affliction, the researchers hoped to shine a light on the underlying causes of diabetes, particularly reasons why diabetes affects Native Americans, Hispanics, and other nonwhite North American peoples at a rate 10 times that of Caucasians.

The Pimas provided an excellent scientific sampling, and continue to do so. They have lived in the Gila River region for hundreds of years, and members of the tribe usually marry other members of the tribe and stay in the area. Families thus have intermingling lineages, and it's easy to trace the transfer of key genetic characteristics. The Pimas have also maintained their agricultural roots, so to speak, for centuries. Even today they are a farming people, cultivating orange groves, pistachios, and olives.

So, why the high rate of diabetes? The researching organizations turned up a number of causes and indicators:

- **History**. Until the late 19th century, the Pima diet contained about 15 percent fat and was high in starch and fiber. Today the Pimas consume about 40 percent fat. Moreover, like most of us, the Pimas don't exercise much. One hundred years ago, their agriculture required more physical labor; today, machines do a lot of the work, and leisure time is spent in sedentary activities. Interestingly, a community of Pima Indians in Mexico—which still adheres to the ancient traditions and diet—has a much lower rate of diabetes and obesity. Diabetes and obesity are, of course, closely related.
- **Genetics**. The Pimas have several genetic "markers" that occur less often in the white population. One gene, known as FABP2, is found more regularly in Pimas than in the general population; it makes an intestinal fatty-acid-binding protein using one of two amino acids. In turn, the National Institutes of Health scientists who discovered the gene believe it could lead to a higher level of fats in the blood, contributing to insulin resistance. Pimas also seem to have a genetic tendency to maintain fat.

The "thrifty gene" theory plays a role here. Geneticists believe that populations that underwent continuous cycles of feast and famine developed a gene that conserves energy (that is, fat) during the fallow times. Today's cornucopia of foods—particularly high-fat foods—makes this gene superfluous, but it's still there, doing its job. In the Pima, it does its job all too well.

Children stand a strong chance of inheriting insulin resistance from their parents. In a population like the Pimas, it's almost a certainty that the children will be at high risk. Given the Pima diet, many of these children develop diabetes before they reach adulthood—and then they, too, risk passing insulin resistance and diabetes along to *their* children.

- **Metabolism**. Studies on the Pima Indians have shown that overweight people, before they gain weight, have a slower metabolic rate compared to that of people of the same weight. Coupled with the Pimas' high-fat diet, the body cannot burn fat fast enough, and weight gain is inevitable.

However, the story doesn't necessarily have an unhappy ending. Both genetics *and* environment play a role in perpetuating insulin resistance, and health workers have worked with the Pimas to change their diet and their degree of physical activity. The Pimas have cooperated closely with health authorities; in physical and mortal cost, they've seen what diabetes can do. The Pima Indians aren't genetically doomed—and neither are the rest of us.

What Is Insulin Resistance?

Insulin resistance has become a buzzword in the dietary community. Insulin, of course, is a powerful hormone that stimulates storage of nutrients as fat. We saw in Chapter 2 the problems of insulin spikes: fatigue, tiredness, and a desire to eat more to pump the blood sugar level back up—a process which eventually makes you fat.

The idea of insulin resistance starts with the concept that routinely high insulin levels cause fat cells to gradually malfunction. Fat cells have insulin receptors; as the cells have to cope with more and more insulin—in amounts beyond that which they were programmed to handle—they shut down those receptors. What finally emerges is a classic vicious cycle: The more the receptors are shut down, the more insulin is required to make them work properly.

The problem is that the body starves without insulin acting as the transporter for glucose to get into the cells. The body produces more and more insulin to achieve this natural process. Eventually, the pancreas, which produces the body's insulin, is unable to keep up with the demand and runs out of the hormone. Once that happens, diabetes has set in.

Diabetes Is a Disease of Insulin Resistance

It is estimated that as many as 75 percent of obese people have some form of insulin resistance. Many have no signs of diabetes. Others, however, do have undiagnosed diabetes, or at least a reduced ability of the body to process carbohydrates, known as *impaired glucose tolerance.*

Moreover, there is a relationship between weight and diabetes. The heavier you are, the more intense the level of insulin resistance. Your risk for insulin resistance—as for diabetes—is as much genetic as anything else, so being overweight coupled with a family history of obesity or diabetes puts you at greater risk. The bottom line: Genetics will determine at what body weight you *will* get insulin resistance—not *if* you will get insulin resistance. It's the classic case of genetics and environment working together to cause disease.

Most people start to develop insulin resistance when they become 35 to 40 percent above their ideal body weight. "When a nondiabetic person consumes excessive calories and gains weight," notes Dr. Ralph DeFronzo of the University of Texas Health Science Center, "the body becomes markedly resistant to the action of insulin." Insulin resistance is not something just seen in diabetics, though that remains a common belief in the medical community. The fact is that most overweight individuals have some level of insulin resistance, and for many it *makes them* diabetic.

Here's how it works. In the beginning, the body is able to meet its own demands by increasing insulin production. "The net result," says Dr. DeFronzo, "is a well-compensated metabolic state in which the insulin resistance is closely counterbalanced by an increase in insulin secretion such that glucose tolerance remains normal or only slightly impaired. The trade-off is hyperinsulinemia [excessive insulin production]. With advancing duration of obesity or with further weight gain, the excessive rates of insulin secretion cannot be maintained."

Diets high in sugar not only boost this need for insulin, but also cause the body to lose excessive amounts of chromium. Chromium deficiency worsens insulin resistance. At this point, it takes only the slightest decline in insulin secretion to set off diabetes.

Dr. DeFronzo calls insulin resistance "a multi-faceted syndrome responsible for diabetes, obesity, hypertension, dyslipidemia [high cholesterol] and atherosclerotic cardiovascular disease." He notes the incidence of these problems has reached "epidemic proportions."

So insulin resistance isn't some rare disease you'll find only in a medical textbook. This is everyday stuff. *This is what the majority of people die from in this country.* Think about that before having that extra helping of mashed potatoes.

TOXIC FAT

Your fat is a toxin. It causes insulin resistance and many other hormonal problems as well, which I will get to in future chapters.

Insulin is a "fat-storage" hormone. It stops the breakdown of fat, a process known as *lipolysis*. So low insulin levels mean you can burn fat (instead of the alternative—storing fat). Under normal circumstances, insulin helps maintain the body's metabolism by regulating the flux of nutrients into and out of fat cells.

Because metabolism and insulin are so critically connected, insulin resistance is associated with a state of abnormal metabolism. In short, insulin resistance makes fat cells freak out, causing them to release toxic fat (known as free fatty acids) into the blood.

According to Debra Waterhouse, a nutritionist and the author of *Outsmarting the Female Fat Cell*, lipolysis is always a good thing. Waterhouse suggests that the reason women have a difficult time losing weight is because they don't have enough enzymes for lipolysis. As usual, hormonal balance is critical. Too much lipolysis makes blood fats soar. A healthy weight-loss program mandates the breakdown of fat; however, too much lipolysis and you're in trouble.

Blood fats released from the breakdown of fat cells which are known as *free fatty acids*, poison the insulin receptor, turning a bad situation to worse. What occurs is **lipotoxicity**—literally, the toxic effect of fat.

The free fatty acids cause the liver to make more glucose and to stop muscle from converting glucose into energy. Both of these events lead to high blood glucose levels, which is the last thing you need if you already have high insulin levels. And a vicious cycle is being kick-started, as the high glucose level tells the body to make even more insulin. (Remember, the body is a constant source of and listener to its own feedback.)

Both glucose and free fatty acids are major sources of energy. They're also competitors: Glucose and free fatty acids compete to get inside of cells, a process known as the *Randle fatty acid cycle*. Given the high levels of both at this time of insulin resistance, the competition is particularly intense.

Who's the winner?

Insulin resistance creates an environment that allows the free fatty acids to triumph. They're the substances that get pumped into cells by the insulin, instead of the glucose. The result is even *higher* blood glucose levels (after all, the glucose is still floating around), which further stimulate higher insulin levels, which lead to more weight gain. It's the beginning of yet another vicious cycle: As the glucose rises, the body tries to compensate by raising insulin levels even more.

A toxic hormone, **resistin,** has recently been linked to fat cells and insulin resistance. Resistin, made by white adipose tissue (WAT—see Chapter 10 for more information) makes other tissues, such as muscle and liver, less sensitive to insulin. Scientists have proposed using medications to neutralize resistin (known as *resistin antagonists*) as a treatment for insulin resistance and diabetes. Many questions remain unanswered about this newly discovered fat-cell hormone.

Insulin resistance can lead to a condition known as *impaired glucose tolerance*. This, the final step before developing diabetes, begins with the body being unable to process the carbohydrate load after a meal properly. (It's also referred to as "borderline diabetes," a term I mistrust—to me, a person either has diabetes or doesn't have it, so this remains one step short of the disease.) At some point, the pancreas gives up and can no longer keep up with the demand for insulin. Blood sugar levels now rise unchecked by further insulin increases, and the person now has diabetes.

Impaired glucose tolerance can be checked with the common OGTT, the oral glucose tolerance test. In this test, a patient's blood sugar is tested, then the patient drinks a pure-glucose beverage and receives periodic blood tests. The blood-sugar response to the sugar drink gives doctors information about how well the patient's body handles sugar. Because pregnancy-induced diabetes is so common, all pregnant women receive a modified version of this test.

Fat-Cell Mutations

Now, it's easy to blame obesity on overeating and eventual destruction of insulin receptors. But researchers have recently been determining that genetics may have a lot to do with it.

In 1999, researchers at the Joslin Diabetes Center in Boston found that 3.3 percent of the subjects in a study they were performing on obese persons had a mutation in a gene known as the PPAR (pronounced "pee-par," peroxisome-proliferator activated receptor). PPAR-gamma protein is thought to be involved in the body's mechanisms to make fat cells. The defect interferes with the body's mechanisms to switch off the PPAR-gamma protein, so it is always turned on. Thus the body makes bigger fat cells, but there's a catch: it also allows insulin to function more efficiently. So these people are insulin resistant, but much less than would be expected, considering their body weight.

(Incidentally, two diabetes medications—rosiglitazone and pioglitazone—work by stimulating the same receptor. These medications improve insulin resistance, but they also make you gain weight.)

The upshot is that people with PPAR-gamma mutations tend to be very heavy but have less insulin resistance, lower insulin levels, and a lower frequency of diabetes.

Syndrome X (the Metabolic Syndrome)

There are several medical problems that have been linked to insulin resistance. Given that they're all related, both to insulin resistance and each other, they're placed under the umbrella term Syndrome X (or the "metabolic syndrome"). Improving your insulin resistance, for which I shall offer tips at the end of this chapter, should have a positive effect on these medical problems and will prevent you from getting them if you're not already afflicted.

These problems include:

- *Central obesity.* This is apple-shaped obesity: big belly, small arms, and small legs. However, any type of obesity may be associated with insulin resistance.
- *Diabetes (or impaired glucose tolerance).*
- *High blood pressure.*
- *Unfavorable cholesterol profile (dyslipidemia).* This refers to low levels of HDL (good cholesterol) and high levels of LDL (bad cholesterol) and triglycerides (another "blood fat" other than cholesterol—commonly treated if high).
- *Heart disease and heart attacks.*
- *Circulation problems (peripheral vascular disease).*
- *Strokes.*
- *Gout.*

I shall go into more detail about each of these in a minute.

Floyd's Story

He came into my office one day, a large man with his shirttail untucked, his tie loosened, and his face red from overexertion, even though he had spent some time waiting in the waiting room. He stood 5-foot-10 and weighed 320 pounds. His chart told the story: Hypertension. High cholesterol. Diabetes. He also had a touch of angina—no surprise, given his age (46) and his condition.

Floyd knew he had to lose weight. His diabetes was of the late-onset variety; with a poor, sugar-filled diet and the excess weight, he had simply pushed his pancreas past its breaking point and it had stopped doing its job. The diabetes wasn't going to go away with weight loss, but at least he could get into condition to live a longer, fuller life. The way things were now, he wasn't going to have many years left, and what time he did was going to be increasingly uncomfortable.

THE PRICE OF INSULIN RESISTANCE

Let me explain what each of the problems of Syndrome X means in real terms:

Diabetes

There are two types of diabetes, conveniently named "type 1" and "type 2." In type 1 diabetes, previously known as insulin-dependent diabetes mellitus (IDDM) or juvenile-onset diabetes, the body does not produce insulin. It usually (but not always) occurs in persons 35 years of age or younger. Type 1 diabetes is an autoimmune disease—the immune system attacks cells in the pancreas that produce insulin.

Type 2 diabetes is what we're talking about here. In **type 2 diabetes**, previously known as non-insulin-dependent diabetes mellitus (NIDDM) or adult-onset diabetes, the body makes tons of insulin but because of the insulin resistance, it can't use the insulin it makes. Somewhere around 90 to 95 percent of the diagnosed diabetes cases in the United States are type 2 diabetes. And 80 percent of those are people who suffer from obesity. As Dr. DeFronzo stated earlier, the insulin resistance suffered by people with advancing obesity eventually becomes diabetes; the pancreas simply can't keep up with the growing need for insulin.

There's another entity related to all of this, known as *glucose toxicity*. After an individual develops diabetes, elevated blood sugar levels act as a toxin to the pancreas, further shutting down insulin secretion—thus worsening the diabetes. The entire process is a tale of mounting woe: First insulin resistance creates lipotoxicity, the lipotoxicity worsens insulin resistance and puts a strain on the pancreas, and then high blood sugars and glucose toxicity provide the final blow.

But, in its early stages, glucose toxicity is reversible. Good blood sugar control, whether by diet, exercise, pills, or insulin, will take the stress off the pancreas and glucose toxicity can be alleviated. It's only when the blood sugar levels become *chronically elevated* that the problem becomes impossible to stop; by then, the pancreas is permanently damaged. (Lipotoxicity causes insulin resistance; glucose toxicity causes insulin deficiency. Both worsen diabetes.)

How is all of this related to weight loss? Weight loss alleviates insulin resistance so you need less insulin to do the job it has to do. The same amount of insulin once considered deficient is now sufficient if the insulin resistance is lessened.

High Blood Pressure

People with insulin resistance have many reasons to have high blood pressure. Consider these:

• Obesity, on its own, causes high blood pressure.
• Insulin resistance only makes matters worse. Insulin resistance causes "fluid overload" because of effects on the kidney. Too much fluid means bloating and high blood pressure.
• High blood pressure caused by fluid overload can be treated by avoiding salt and taking diuretics. However, these diuretic medications also worsen insulin resistance.
• Insulin resistance causes the heart to pump too strongly: high blood pressure.

Interestingly, one of the primary ways doctors treat high blood pressure is with medications known as *beta-blockers*. However, beta-blockers solve one problem—high blood pressure—and cause another: They slow the body's metabolic rate, leading to weight gain. Moreover, they make you feel tired, so it is harder to exercise. And they turn off a sure-fire stress reliever by making some men impotent.

Experts estimate that patients on beta-blockers convert an extra 100 to 200 calories into fat every day, just due to the reduced metabolism. So it's a catch-22: Treating one offshoot of obesity, high blood pressure, with beta-blockers may actually cause patients to become *more* obese, worsening the overall problem.

Unfavorable Lipid Profile

Cholesterol comes in two basic kinds: **HDL**, high-density lipoproteins or "good cholesterol"; and **LDL**, low-density lipoproteins or "bad cholesterol." An unfavorable lipid profile features a high count of LDL and a low count of HDL.

Women are somewhat protected from a poor lipid profile because of the estrogen in their bodies. *Estrogen* is a hormone that maintains HDL levels and helps keep LDL levels low.

But if a woman has reduced estrogen levels—such as what happens after her childbearing years have ended—coupled with insulin resistance, the combination can be a double whammy. The lipid profile changes, with HDL levels lowering and LDL levels getting higher. It puts a woman at risk for heart disease, and also ends up increasing insulin resistance because of a cycle started by an increased appetite and weight gain.

Elevated triglycerides, also part of an unfavorable lipid profile, are blood fats linked to heart disease. A very low-fat, high-carbohydrate diet—such as the Ornish or Pritikin plans—can raise your triglycerides.

Heart Disease

According to some controversial hypotheses, insulin itself may cause coronary artery disease and heart attacks. Critics say it's not the insulin; they say that high insulin levels merely correlate with—but do not cause—heart disease.

However, recent evidence asserts that's not true. Insulin acts as an "anabolic hormone" and a growth factor, and both aspects have powerful effects on blood vessels, particularly the heart's coronary arteries. Insulin increases the formation of cholesterol plaques—fatty deposits— inside blood vessel walls, and this effect is compounded by other related diseases, such as diabetes, high blood pressure, and high cholesterol. (Remember: The point of Syndrome X is you seldom find one ailment without finding others.) Throw in obesity and you have a very dangerous mix.

Moreover, in a 1998 study published by the *Journal of the American Medical Association* (JAMA), it was determined that insulin resistance increases cardiovascular risk by a variety of mechanisms, including facilitation of blood clotting and atherosclerosis. This doesn't even take into account what happens in the insulin resistance cycle: the decrease in good cholesterol, the increase in bad cholesterol and triglycerides.

Interestingly, there have been a number of long-term studies that have looked at intensive control of diabetes using high doses of insulin.

Although these studies have shown a reduction in most diabetes complications, none have ever shown a reduction in the rate of heart attacks. In fact, heart attack is the number one killer of people with insulin resistance.

Polycystic Ovary Syndrome

Polycystic ovary syndrome, or PCOS, is a condition in which the ovary and adrenal gland make too much male hormone. This disorder has its roots in insulin resistance, although this type of insulin resistance is closely linked with overproduction of male hormones. When insulin resistance is relieved, testosterone levels plummet.

PCOS is commonly treated with special diets or diabetes medications that improve insulin resistance. I'll talk more about PCOS in Chapter 5.

WHAT CAUSES INSULIN RESISTANCE?

So far, we know that obesity, overeating, and diets too high in carbohydrates work together with your genes to cause insulin resistance. But there are several other factors that contribute to this condition, not all of them physiological:

Stress

- First of all, *elevations in cortisol and epinephrine*—two hormones secreted when the body is under stress—promote insulin resistance.
- The stress of *poor health* also jacks up insulin levels. A diabetic with a cold, for example, has a rise in blood sugar levels because his insulin resistance is worse. This is true for any number of ailments, from infections to mental illness. Indeed, depression and insulin resistance are closely related.
- *Extreme physical exercise*, such as marathon running, can cause insulin resistance. Interestingly, milder forms of exercise have the opposite effect.

- There is even an entity known as *stress hyperglycemia*. The stress of a severe illness can cause such acute insulin resistance that very ill patients will often have high blood sugar levels—even if they've never been diagnosed with diabetes. To put it simply, the sicker you are, the higher your blood sugar. Though this isn't a hard-and-fast rule, it's true in a majority of situations.
- Finally, I've talked about *subclinical disease*—disease that exists at such low levels that it's difficult to pick up medically. If a person is overweight and can't figure out exactly why, it may be due to a subclinical insulin resistance caused by a great deal of stress in his or her life. Avoidance of stress lowers insulin levels and helps you lose weight.

Laura's Story

Laura, a law professor, was living a stress-filled life. She and her husband had recently purchased a large house that cost a little more than Laura had been willing to spend. Her two children were approaching college age, and Laura wondered how she was going to be able to afford their educations. And she had a punishing workload of classes, committees, and consulting.

One day, it all came crashing down. Laura suffered a heart attack during class and was rushed to the hospital. It was touch-and-go for a while, but Laura was in reasonably good shape for a woman of 49—she didn't smoke and she was only a few pounds overweight—and she pulled through.

While she was in the hospital, physicians performed several tests. One of them determined that Laura's blood sugar was exceptionally high. This surprised Laura, who had never known she was diabetic.

Perhaps, it turns out, it's because she wasn't diabetic. Laura's recovery was slow and arduous: exercise, an improved diet, and—above all—a cutting back on her previous responsibilities. Six months later, she submitted to a new round of tests. This time, her blood sugar level was fine and she had no signs of diabetes. The hyperglycemia may have been caused entirely by excessive stress.

Dieting

There are two types of diets that increase insulin resistance: ketogenic diets and low-fat/high-carbohydrate diets.

- A *ketogenic diet* is one in which the body gets little or no carbohydrate. Ketones are a by-product of the breakdown of fat, which is supposed to happen if the consumption of carbohydrates is cut. (The Atkins diet, if followed properly, is a ketogenic diet.) Ketogenic diet proponents claim that these diets lower insulin levels, but they may actually make the situation worse. Consider this: Without carbohydrates, the body thinks it's starving.
- *Low-fat/high-carbohydrate diets*, such as the Pritikin plan and the Dean Ornish diet, take the opposite tack from Atkins. But carbohydrates are sugars, and a gain of sugars tends to produce more insulin to cope with the increase. Low-fat/high-carbohydrate diets are well known to cause insulin resistance, high triglyceride levels, and—in some cases—full-fledged diabetes.

Smoking

For decades, smoking has been a way for some people to keep their weight down. Nicotine acts as a stimulant, after all, and the buzz of a nicotine high can keep thoughts of eating more food away. (Many smokers suffer a great gain in weight when they quit smoking or even try to quit; the desire to put something, anything, in one's mouth is overwhelming.) But smoking is also a known cause of insulin resistance. For this reason—as well as many others—it should be avoided.

Menopause

Decreased *estradiol* (healthy estrogen; see Chapter 6) levels in menopausal women can promote insulin resistance. In fact, there's a whole condition that revolves around high insulin levels at this age: Syndrome W.

Syndrome W—so called because it involves *w*omen, *w*eight gain, *w*aist size increase, and *w*hite-coat hypertension (situational or occasional high blood pressure, such as during visits to doctors' offices)—was first proposed by Dr. Harriet Mogul in 1999. As reported in *Internal Medicine News* (July 1, 1999), Dr. Mogul and her colleagues studied 278 women who came to the Menopausal Health Program at their suburban New York City institution over a 2½-year period. Of the 278 subjects, 67 had body mass indices between 25 and 32 and also reported having gained 20 pounds or more since their 20s (you are overweight if your body mass index is greater than 25). More than half of the 67 had hyperinsulinemia. These were all healthy women, around age 40, who led active lives with no history of insulin-related problems.

If they had stayed on their current trend, many of the women would have developed full-blown Syndrome X sometime in their lives. But given a low-glycemic-index diet, the women were treated successfully.

Other therapies can also work on Syndrome W. Estrogen has a protective effect on body composition, preventing the accumulation of abdominal body fat. (Many of the women in the study had gained fat around the abdomen and hips.) So hormone-replacement therapy, in particular, will help bring insulin levels back into line and cut down on insulin resistance and Syndrome W. Estrogen also lowers bad cholesterol and raises good cholesterol. (See Chapter 6 for more information on estrogen, weight gain, and insulin resistance.)

Other Physiological Factors That Contribute to Insulin Resistance

- *Aging* makes people more insulin resistant. In some respects, changing your diet to improve (i.e., lower) insulin resistance is like giving yourself anti-aging medicine. There's some controversy about aging, actually: Some experts say it's not aging itself as it is our decreased physical activity that makes us overweight and insulin resistant; others maintain aging itself can have these effects. More research needs to be done, and the conclusion may very well turn out to be a combination of those factors and many others.
- *Puberty* gives adolescents low levels of insulin resistance, but obese adolescents going through puberty have very high levels of insulin resistance. This would seem to correlate with other effects

of puberty: Some children lose their baby fat and become strapping young adults, whereas for others their weight problems just get worse. We are now seeing an alarming increase in rates of type 2 diabetes (previously known as *adult-onset diabetes*) because of the epidemic of adolescent obesity.

- *Pregnancy* is the classic insulin-resistant state. The prototypical insulin-resistant person is apple-shaped: big stomach, thin arms. Sound familiar? With a pregnant woman, all the weight—in this case, the baby—is on the stomach, while the arms and legs stay thin. In fact, all pregnant women are tested for *gestational diabetes* because insulin resistance makes the condition so common.
- *Kidney or liver problems* may cause insulin resistance.
- *Hormonal excess* can promote insulin resistance. I'll deal with some of these hormones more extensively in later chapters, but cortisol, growth hormone, and glucagon, in atypical quantities, can make people insulin resistant. These hormones are considered "counter-insulin hormones" in that they provide checks and balances for insulin.

Of these, conditions with too much glucagon are the rarest to occur. There is a tumor of the pancreas called a *glucagonanoma* that manufactures too much glucagon. Patients afflicted with this condition develop a strange red rash over their entire body and usually have diabetes. I bring this up only because several popular diet books talk of glucagon as a wonder hormone—glucagon good, insulin bad. But too much of any hormone is bad—even glucagon.

DO YOU HAVE INSULIN RESISTANCE?

Measuring Insulin Levels

Insulin is measured from a blood sample and—when determining diabetes—is best done in the fasting state (on an empty stomach), usually first thing in the morning after an overnight fast. A high insulin level is considered to be greater than 10 to15 µU/mL. Some doctors will also measure insulin levels after ingestion of a pure-glucose beverage. This test, similar to a glucose tolerance test, can detect insulin resistance at very early stages.

However, overweight people are almost always insulin resistant, so I personally believe that *blood tests on overweight people to determine insulin resistance are usually not necessary*. Moreover, a person who has any of the medical problems detailed above (Syndrome X or Syndrome W) is at even a greater risk for having insulin resistance—and a severe case at that.

Glucose and Insulin Test, and Meal Tolerance Test

These are tests typically done in a physician's office. After the person consumes a pure-glucose beverage or a liquid meal replacement (with carbohydrate, protein, and fat), measurements are taken every hour or so. In general I find that these tests are a waste of time. If you are overweight or have excess fat in the middle, you have insulin resistance and probably do not need to be tested.

Fat in the Gut Is Worse Than Fat in the Butt

Obesity comes in many forms. A person with *android obesity* has fat in the middle section and skinny arms and legs—"apple-shaped" obesity. A person with *gynecoid obesity*, on the other hand, has a large rear end and hips—"pear-shaped" obesity. Think of the two kinds as "gut vs. butt."

As I've noted previously, people who fit into the former category are at great risk for insulin resistance and may already be afflicted with the condition. Men with a waistline of more than 40 inches and women with a waistline of more than 35 inches are likely to be insulin resistant. In the past, obesity experts have used a different measurement, the waist-to-hip ratio, to help determine insulin resistance. However, the waist-to-hip ratio isn't a very good guide. The simple waistline measurement is much more accurate.

The reason central obesity puts people at greater risk for insulin resistance is that the fat literally surrounds the organs. This fat is also known as *visceral* fat (*viscera* is a term for innards) because of its location. The other fat, the fat of love handles, large buttocks and big hips, is subcutaneous fat. Of the two, visceral fat is bad fat—I would even call it ***metabolically evil***.

Why? Because visceral *adipocytes*—the fat cells surrounding internal organs—are the bad boys of obesity and insulin resistance. This metabolically active adipose tissue is regulated by a number of hormones, and all you need is one hormone to go out of whack to make this tissue grow. Increased cortisol and decreased growth hormone can cause central obesity; so can decreased testosterone in men and increased testosterone and decreased estrogen in women. The combination of any of these hormonal problems, along with insulin resistance and high insulin levels, promotes the accumulation of fat in the abdomen.

In other words, if subcutaneous fat is merely a sign of overeating, then visceral fat is a sign of a hormonal imbalance. That's oversimplifying the situation—as we shall see in future chapters—but as a rule of thumb, just like the waistline guideline, it works.

Black Velvety Skin Rash

Acanthosis nigricans is a skin condition caused by excess insulin. It has a black velvety appearance. It's usually found on the neck, in the armpits, and on the knuckles and face. It looks dirty, but it won't come off when you try to wash it. As we have discussed, insulin is a growth factor—and insulin also makes skin grow. In the presence of abnormally high insulin levels, skin grows in very strange ways, making it turn dark.

If you have acanthosis nigricans, you are virtually guaranteed of having insulin resistance. But it's not an incurable condition: As you lose weight, the acanthosis nigricans disappears as well.

One word of warning, however: On rare occasions, acanthosis nigricans is not caused by insulin resistance; it is caused by cancer. If you have this condition under *any* circumstances, see your doctor.

TREATING INSULIN RESISTANCE

Insulin resistance is not incurable. At the beginning of this chapter, we saw how the Pima Indians, despite being genetically disposed to insulin resistance, still could avoid obesity, diabetes, and a host of other Syndrome X ailments that surround insulin resistance. The same is true for all of us, particularly because many people become insulin resistant through poor dietary choices—not through any genetic predisposition. The answer to insulin resistance is a healthy diet and lifestyle. A 2001 study published in the *New England Journal of Medicine* has even proven that modest diet and lifestyle improvements can prevent people from getting type 2 diabetes. The Nurses Health Study has also found that the majority of cases of insulin resistance and type 2 diabetes can be prevented by following a healthier diet and exercise.

Cut Down on Carbohydrates and Have a Little Extra Protein

To counter insulin resistance—and, by no coincidence, to promote balanced nutrition—I stress a high-protein diet consisting of about 40 percent carbohydrate, 30 percent protein, and 30 percent fat. This is a slight deviation from American Diabetic Association (ADA) guidelines, which support a diet containing 20 percent protein and 50 percent carbohydrates. Many other diet experts, most notably Barry Sears, also promote this ratio of carbohydrate, protein, and fat.

Critics of high-protein diets claim that improvement in insulin resistance occurs when you lose weight, regardless of how much protein is in your diet. This is true, as far as it goes: Weight loss *does* improve insulin resistance. However, a diet slightly higher in protein actually improves insulin resistance *beyond* what is seen with weight loss on a traditional ADA diet.

The diet I recommend to optimize insulin levels is found in Chapter 11.

Eat Fish High in Omega-3 Fatty Acids

Omega-3 fatty acids help to reduce insulin resistance. Moreover, fish is a terrific source of both protein and "healthy fat." Fish oil lowers bad cholesterol and raises good cholesterol, and diets high in fish improve insulin resistance beyond what is seen in diets without fish. If possible, feel free to add omega-3 fatty acid supplements; but follow the suggested dosage, and don't use the supplements as a substitute for fish. Table 3.1 lists the omega-3 fatty acid content of various fish.

Eat Low-Glycemic-Index Foods

As I noted in Chapter 2, experts have shown that low-glycemic-index foods have a variety of positive effects. The body breaks them down slowly, so there are fewer insulin spikes, and the body can absorb the energy from sugar gradually, which has a salutary influence on other body processes. High-glycemic-index foods are fine—but only in tiny amounts.

Eat Reasonable Portions at Proper Times

Nibbling, as I mentioned in Chapter 2, is an excellent way to eat. The reverse is also true: Don't eat too much at one time. No diet is effective if you overload your hormonal system with too many calories; calories *do* count.

Also, don't eat late at night. Our bodies secrete hormones cyclically. Growth hormone and cortisol, both counter-insulin hormones that create insulin resistance, are secreted mostly at night, usually during the peak time between 3 A.M. and 6 A.M. If you eat during your growth hormone and cortisol peaks, your body will have to pump out more insulin to process your meal to overcome the effects of these hormones.

Finally, as also noted in Chapter 2, don't eat just before bedtime. Sleep slows metabolism, so foods eaten during this time not only will take longer to break down, but also won't be burned up as energy.

Two quick notes: Avoid high-fat diets. They usually make you gain weight, and that will set you on the treadmill to insulin resistance. And sugar substitutes have absolutely no effect on insulin resistance. They don't cause it, and they don't cure it.

Alcohol, in Moderation

Moderate alcohol use—one or two drinks a day—can be good for your health. Alcohol decreases insulin resistance, a fact that doctors have known for years—but, with the fear of encouraging alcoholism, the information hasn't been well promoted. Beer, wine, and hard liquor—any alcoholic beverage—will lower insulin resistance, but **be aware of calories**. And remember moderation: When I say one or two drinks *a day*, I mean exactly that. You can't "save up" drinks for the weekend.

Table 3.1
OMEGA-3 FATTY ACID CONTENT OF FISH

Only certain fish, mainly those that live in cold water, contain meaningful amounts of omega-3 fish oils. Measurements are grams of omega-3 fatty acid per 100 grams of raw fish.

Sardines (in their own oil)	21.1 grams
Atlantic mackerel	2.5 grams
Lake trout	1.6 grams
Salmon	1.2 grams
Striped bass	0.8 grams
Tuna	0.5 grams
Pacific halibut	0.4 grams
Channel catfish	0.3 grams
Shrimp	0.3 grams
Dungeness crab	0.3 grams
Swordfish	0.2 grams
Red snapper	0.2 grams
Sole	0.1 gram

Source: Christine Gorman, "We Love Fish," *Time*, October 30, 2000.

EXERCISE AND STRESS REDUCTION

Along with these eating guidelines should come an appropriate exercise program. Part of what makes contemporary Americans so susceptible to diabetes and insulin resistance is our sedentary, comfortable lifestyle. We don't even get up to change the channel on the TV anymore—we simply click a button on a remote control.

Ironically, though, we're probably working harder than ever. In days past, we were allowed to take time to do our work, and if it didn't get done by the end of the day, we would always have tomorrow. Nowadays, with faxes, e-mail, and other forms of instant communication, not only do we not have to the end of the day, we don't even have to the end of the hour! No wonder we're so stressed: We don't exercise, we're trying to get things done yesterday, and there seems like there's more to do than ever.

Unfortunately, there's no magic pill, no as-seen-on-TV contraption that will take the place of a good solid workout. Imagine your body is an old-fashioned locomotive: It takes time to build up a head of steam; it takes time to get the heart pumping and the energy moving efficiently. If you exercise properly—if you take the 20 or 30 minutes a day to have a moderate aerobic workout, or an extra 10 or 15 minutes to add some weight training—that time will pay dividends in the long run.

Don't even think about an exercise regimen as a way to simply lose weight—and, by losing weight, improve your insulin resistance. Studies have shown that exercise improves insulin resistance even if you *don't* lose weight. Physical training allows your body to handle blood glucose better. Remember: Muscle needs glucose to function. When you exercise, the muscles are not only stronger, but *metabolically stronger*. Exercise allows your body to "dispose" of glucose more easily—it gets into the muscle more easily—and your insulin levels drop.

Simply put, if you have two people of identical body weight, and one exercises and the other doesn't, the one who exercises will have lower insulin levels and less insulin resistance.

Other facts about exercising and insulin:

- Weight training is critical. The more muscle you have, the more tissue you have to take up glucose, and the better your sensitivity to insulin. As the old saying goes, "Muscle burns fat."
    - Exercise increases the activity of a special enzyme in the cell known as *succinic oxidase*. This enzyme is located in the mitochondria of the cell, the part of the cell that produces energy (you may remember it from biology textbooks as "the powerhouse of the cell"). Increased mitochondria oxidative enzyme activity means the body can more effectively process nutrients into energy.
    - Exercise makes the insulin receptor more efficient.
    - Exercise improves blood flow to muscles, which also improves insulin resistance. People with diabetes are well aware of this phenomenon. If they exercise, they should reduce the dose of

insulin before the workout. Those who use insulin pumps have to shut them off when exercising, or the insulin dose will have more potency and their blood sugar will drop. Some diabetics who exercise regularly can often discontinue their insulin or other diabetic medications entirely.

One word of caution: Extreme exercise, such as marathon running, may temporarily worsen insulin resistance. And that gets us back to stress.

When your body is physically stressed, *cortisol*—the stress hormone—is released. Cortisol is a counter-insulin hormone and thus can undo much of the positive effects on blood sugar that exercise is having. Moreover, drinking high-glycemic-index beverages, such as Gatorade, before exercise can give you an insulin surge. The surge will soon make your blood sugar level *lower* than it was when you started exercising. Obviously, this isn't a good idea. Sports drinks are designed to refresh your body after (or during) a workout, not before.

I'll go into stress in much more detail in Chapter 8 (Cortisol), but let me leave you with two more words on the subject: hot tubs. Hot tubs have also been shown to improve insulin resistance. Why? We don't know. But consider: The fact is that hot tubs improve blood flow. Hot tubs relieve stress. Hot tubs improve sleep. Perhaps it's not so surprising that with all of these positives, they also improve insulin resistance.

NUTRACEUTICALS

Chromium

This element—yes, the same one from which "chrome" in automobiles is made—is essential to our health. Without chromium, insulin doesn't work properly. It is required only in trace amounts in the diet, but without those small amounts, people can suffer from a condition known simply as **chromium deficiency**, which can cause impaired glucose tolerance, hyper- and hypoglycemia, and insulin resistance.

A 1996 study indicated increased chromium intake could be beneficial for diabetics. Some of the study's subjects took 1,000 micrograms of chromium picolinate supplements a day. After 4 months, blood samples were taken, and these people's glycated hemoglobin levels had dropped—a significant indicator of diabetes control. While chromium

Table 3.2
FOODS HIGH IN CHROMIUM

Brewer's yeast

Organ meats

Mushrooms

Wheat germ

Broccoli

Chicken

Shellfish—especially clams

Corn oil

Whole grains

is not a cure for diabetes, it appears it can help diminish its effects. Chromium has also been shown to have no harmful effects on animals, even at extremely high dosages.

Maintaining chromium in the body is difficult. For one thing, we don't consume enough chromium-rich food; for another, chromium is easily passed out of the body in urine and sweat—even more easily if a person is diabetic or consumes a high-glycemic-index diet.

Foods high in chromium include brewer's yeast, organ meats, mushrooms, wheat germ, broccoli, processed meats, chicken, shellfish—especially clams—corn oil, and a variety of whole grains. I highly recommend incorporating these foods into a diet; if you are diabetic or suffer from insulin resistance, then a supplement may be beneficial as well.

Vanadium

Another periodic table element, vanadium—ironically—was mistaken for a form of chromium when discovered in the early 19th century. One of the hardest of all metals, it is never found in a pure state, but always in a compound form with other elements.

Scientists still aren't sure about the exact contribution of vanadium to our diet, but **vanadium deficiency** has been shown to cause decreased milk production, bone deformities, infertility, and increased infant mortality in some animals. Moreover, these defects were handed down to succeeding generations. Positive effects include improved glucose tolerance.

Although bodybuilders and diabetics have taken a form of vanadium, vanadyl sulfate, to improve insulin action, there is little proof it does this. What vanadium has been shown to do is mimic the action of insulin by turning on the insulin receptor. (Interestingly, vanadium consumption is recommended as a diabetes treatment in France.) Vanadium also improves cholesterol. However, another form of the

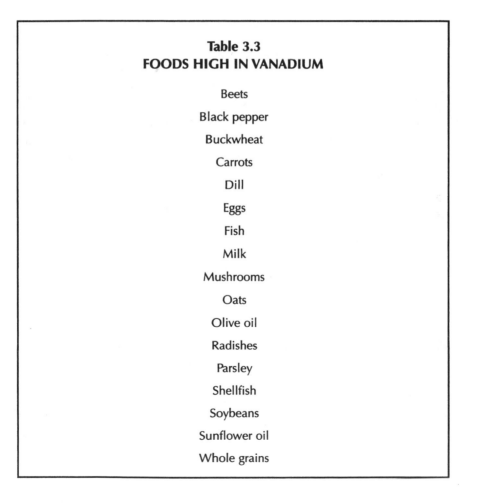

Table 3.3
FOODS HIGH IN VANADIUM

Beets

Black pepper

Buckwheat

Carrots

Dill

Eggs

Fish

Milk

Mushrooms

Oats

Olive oil

Radishes

Parsley

Shellfish

Soybeans

Sunflower oil

Whole grains

element, vanadate, is not recommended because of toxic effects, ranging from anemia and green tongue to cataracts and death. One recent development is a new compound called *peroxvanadium*. This substance is at least 50 times more powerful than vanadium. Reports indicate that it might normalize insulin resistance without as much toxicity as regular vanadium. Still, as with all forms of vanadium, more research is needed.

Although I don't approve of vanadium supplements, I staunchly support eating foods high in vanadium. These include beets, black pepper, buckwheat, carrots, dill, eggs, fish, milk, mushrooms, oats, olive oil, radishes, parsley, shellfish, soybeans, sunflower oil, and whole grains.

Biotin

This water-soluble B vitamin is essential for proper carbohydrate metabolism, as well as cell growth and replication. Eating foods high in biotin, or consuming biotin supplements, enhances insulin sensitivity and increases the activity of enzymes necessary for proper carbohydrate metabolism; conversely, a **biotin deficiency** can cause insulin resistance or diabetes.

Most of us have plenty of biotin in our diet, however. Among the foods that contain biotin are brewer's yeast, egg yolks, whole grains, breads, fish, nuts, beans, meat, dairy products, lentils, peas, peanuts, walnuts, and molasses. Moreover, biotin is a natural product of the bacteria in our intestines. The recommended daily allowance of biotin is 30 to 100 micrograms a day, a relatively miniscule amount.

However, other items in a diet can force a need for more biotin. Egg yolks, as I noted, contain biotin; however, raw egg whites inactivate the vitamin, so people who eat lots of raw egg whites can become biotin deficient. Alcohol raises the biotin requirement, as does estrogen. And food-processing techniques, such as canning and cooking, can destroy biotin.

Like the deficiency of any vitamin, a deficiency in biotin can cause a variety of ailments, not just insulin resistance. Symptoms include hair loss, scaly red rash around the nose and mouth, anemia, high cholesterol, loss of appetite, nausea, depression, sleeplessness, and hallucinations.

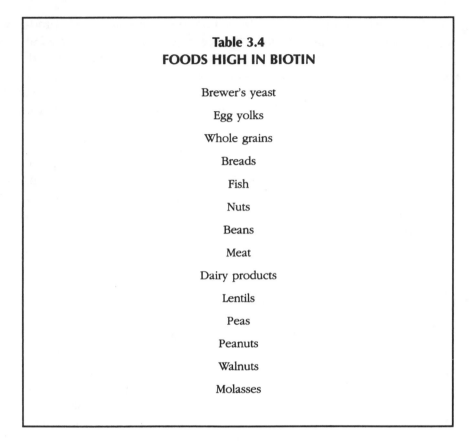

Table 3.4
FOODS HIGH IN BIOTIN

Brewer's yeast

Egg yolks

Whole grains

Breads

Fish

Nuts

Beans

Meat

Dairy products

Lentils

Peas

Peanuts

Walnuts

Molasses

Biotin is frequently a component of standard multivitamin tablets; however, if your diet includes at least some of the foods I'm recommending in this section, you shouldn't need to take special biotin supplements. But if you've had any of the above-listed symptoms, that might have been a source of your trouble.

Other Trace Minerals

Any diet should include a variety of vitamins and minerals, and one to improve insulin resistance—as well as overall health—is no exception. To protect against diabetes, I encourage a diet high in zinc, copper, and selenium, as well as vitamins A, C, and E.

- *Selenium.* Selenium-rich foods include meats, poultry, dairy products, and other animal foods. I'll discuss selenium in more detail in Chapter 7; selenium is key to healthy function of the thyroid gland.
- *Zinc.* Foods high in zinc include oysters, beef, wheat germ, lima beans, and dairy products. Zinc helps insulin work properly; in fact, certain types of insulin used by diabetics have zinc in the insulin, which helps the insulin last longer in the body.
- *Copper.* Copper-rich foods include oysters, shellfish, nuts, cherries, mushrooms, and beans. A high-fructose diet—that is, one high in fruit—can cause a copper deficiency. Copper is needed in exceptionally small quantities in the diet—about 1.5 to 3 micrograms, or about one-tenth the amount of zinc.
- *Vitamins A, C, and E.* These antioxidants may also be beneficial in lowering insulin resistance.

MEDICATIONS

Metformin (Glucophage)

Metformin is a diabetes medication that treats insulin resistance. The FDA has approved metformin for use in patients with diabetes, but it is increasingly being used to lower insulin resistance in nondiabetics. Metformin helps people lose weight. It has also been very effective for the treatment of PCOS (see Chapter 5). One of the most common side effects of metformin is nausea and diarrhea. In most people (but not all), this gets better with time. You can minimize the side effects by starting with a very low dose and increasing the dose slowly. Also, taking your pill with a meal helps alleviate the side effects. A new, long-acting version of metformin is now available, but the pills are very large and I see no advantage to these over the original formulation that is usually taken twice a day. People with liver or kidney problems should not take metformin.

Rosiglitazone (Avandia) and Pioglitazone (Actos)

These medications, known as *PPAR agonists* or *glitazones,* are also approved by the FDA for the treatment of diabetes. Unlike metformin, they cause weight gain.

You may wonder why one medication causes weight loss while another causes weight gain, even though both improve insulin resistance. Glitazones work at the level of the fat-cell DNA, making insulin work better. So insulin resistance is improved, but at the expense of making a bigger, healthier, and more efficient fat cell. These "super fat cells," which have a renewed ability to respond to insulin, get bigger and bigger. So improving insulin resistance does not always mean weight loss. Interestingly, the fat gain caused by these medications is mostly subcutaneous (under the skin) and not the metabolically evil visceral fat we discussed earlier.

Besides weight gain, the most common side effect of rosiglitazone and pioglitazone is fluid retention. This can cause or worsen medical conditions like edema and congestive heart failure. If you have these conditions, you probably should not take these medications. An earlier version of these medications was pulled from the market because of concerns of liver damage. So far, only very rare cases of liver problems have been seen with the newer medications. Nevertheless, if you take these medications, your doctor should periodically take blood work to monitor for liver problems.

Miglitol (Glyset) and Acarbose (Precose)

These diabetes medications work by blocking an enzyme in the intestine that breaks down carbohydrates, known as alpha-galactosidase. They slow, but do not prevent, the digestion of food and foster a mild decrease in the absorption of carbohydrates. Their effect on weight is minimal.

Orlistat (Xenical)

This medication, discussed in Chapter 2, works by preventing the digestion of about one third of the fat that is consumed. Orlistat is approved as a weight-loss medication; however, studies show that this medication also helps treat diabetes, high cholesterol, and insulin resistance.

CHAPTER FOUR

ANDROGENS

ANDROGENS, YOUR HEALTH, AND YOUR WEIGHT

NOWADAYS, TESTOSTERONE IS HIP.

The principle male hormone—or *androgen*, the term for any male sex hormone—has come to be associated with anything distinctly male. Hard-bodied weightlifters are fueled by testosterone. So are aggressive CEOs, deep-voiced baritones, and the raging members of the World Wrestling Federation. Testosterone helps men become strong, virile, and muscular; low testosterone levels can make men gain weight, or at least change body composition to less muscle and more fat.

What's not to like? No wonder men are bulking up on testosterone supplements and related boosters. Don't have enough? Don't worry—you can get it in a gel. Just apply to the skin and get ready to rrrrrrumble. It's good to have testosterone—it helps you keep up with our crazily competitive society.

But testosterone, naturally, isn't all good. First of all, it's not even all male—women have androgens too, just in far lesser amounts than men do. Second, testosterone is a steroid hormone, and steroids have their dangers. (Excesses of testosterone have been shown to cause cancerous tumors.) Finally, research continues to explore the links between testosterone, mood, aggression, and anger.

That's not to say testosterone isn't necessary—not at all. Testosterone in the womb is what makes a baby develop into a boy. A

93

spike in testosterone levels helps develop that boy into a man. Testosterone has important functions in many areas of the body including the brain, kidney, liver, and skin. Testosterone helps to maintain strong and healthy muscles and bones. Low testosterone has been linked to increased amounts of fat in the body. Recently, testosterone has been shown to have an effect on dilating the blood vessels of the heart. And there is a place for aggression, for anger, and even for machismo; in earlier civilizations, these traits almost certainly helped continue the survival of the human species.

But these days, testosterone is seen as just another supplement, something used to help mold soft bodies into well-muscled Adonises, something to give hard-driving business executives and athletes that extra "edge" in life. And it is from that perspective that testosterone needs to be better understood, because what you don't know about this hormone can be harmful to your health.

ANDROGENS INCREASE MUSCLE AND DECREASE FAT

A lot is made of the physical ideals we present to women in today's society: stunning models, many still in their teens, with large breasts and tiny waists—ideals that have prompted a generation of schoolgirls to go on crash diets just when their bodies are in desperate need of a stable diet. Even as women age they still have to face the perfection of the fashion models they see in magazines and on television, and that has led to a growth business in cosmetic surgery, health clubs, and books like this one.

And there have also been darker consequences of the model ideal, the desperation of eating disorders and depression that has overtaken many women who find it impossible to be happy with the way they look or what they weigh.

But what of men? The belief is that men aren't affected at all by the beefy, muscled representations of the ideal male. According to recent studies, however, that simply isn't true. First of all, those hard-body specimens have become even more pronounced: Harrison Pope, the co-author of *The Adonis Complex*, notes that Mr. America bodybuilding winners are much more developed than they were 50 years ago. And then there are the endless images of handsome celebrity males seen all over our culture. Perhaps there are more who look like Woody Allen than Mark McGwire, but the McGwire version—chiseled, muscular, *strong*—is the one that's now dominant. Besides, virtually nobody aspires to look like Woody Allen.

McGwire caught a lot of flak in 1998, during his chase of the home-run record, when it was revealed he took androstenedione. Androstenedione is a powerful steroid supplement that promotes muscle growth. McGwire has since stopped taking androstenedione and is, by many accounts, simply a terrific physical specimen who works hard to maintain his physique. However, many men prefer the shortcut that anabolic steroids provide. Some men, in fact, have a psychological condition called BDD—*body dysmorphic disorder*, in which they're convinced that their body is horribly unattractive. Their concerns can be focused on many parts of their body—from their hair to their legs—but, for many, it's the physique that's disappointing. They work out, and to help their workout along, they take steroids.

Women undergo plastic surgery and liposuction; men take steroids.

WHAT IS A STEROID?

In chemical terms, steroids are naturally occurring *lipids*, or fat-soluble substances. They all have similar chemical structures and are ultimately derived from cholesterol (see Figure 4.1). Yes, cholesterol: What you thought was bad can also be beneficial. (Not that you should start stuffing yourself with cholesterol-heavy foods. The body makes its own cholesterol from the fat in your diet.)

Steroid hormones, aside from the male sex hormones, include estrogen, aldosterone, progesterone, cortisol, and even vitamin D. Cholesterol is modified by special enzymes in a series of steps to become all of the various hormones.

The enzymes that make hormones are very different from the enzymes that digest food. The enzymes that make steroids are in your blood; enzymes for digestion are in your gut. You may have seen books that recommend certain diets based on their effects on enzymes. The enzymes in your blood can be affected by your diet, but many diet "experts" get confused and make recommendations that affect the wrong kind of enzymes.

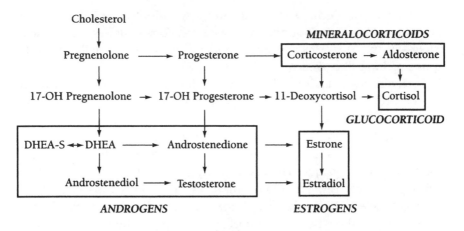

Figure 4.1
THE STEROID BIOSYNTHESIS PATHWAY
All steroid hormones are synthesized from a common precursor, cholesterol.
The enzymes present in each gland determine the final hormone produced.
Steroid hormones can be interconverted to one another.

All steroid hormones exert their action by controlling your genes.
Steroids act by literally turning "on" and "off" genes.

Anabolic steroids, the kind most closely associated with steroid
supplements, are derived specifically from testosterone and were originally developed for cancer patients and victims of starvation. Because
of their muscle- and strength-building qualities, athletes started to take
them for a competitive edge. The International Olympic Committee and
many American team sports for years have banned steroids, but secre-
tive use is widespread.

The positive effects of anabolic steroids are obvious: muscle
growth, enhanced physical performance, loss of fat—and through this,
enhanced metabolism. The effects of steroids are long lasting; the muscle gains can last for years.

Meanwhile, anabolic steroids boost testosterone levels, a key influence on increasing muscle mass and metabolism. Low testosterone levels
cause men (and sometimes women) to be tired and flabby. Men with low
testosterone put on weight in their bellies—the central obesity I talked
about in Chapter 3. This is the worst type of fat, increasing insulin resistance and causing further weight and fat gain from high insulin levels.

Many doctors prescribe steroids for their patients with low testosterone levels. A body requires decent testosterone levels to function properly, and for men with low levels of the hormone, the boost can be beneficial. It may even be life saving: Recently, AIDS patients have seen tremendous improvement from taking steroids at levels that might be considered high for a person in good health. Body weight and muscle mass predict how long someone with AIDS will survive. When AIDS patients start losing weight, it is likely that they will die within a year or two. Bulking up with steroids (and growth hormone; see Chapter 9) may prolong their lives.

But there's a thin line between using anabolic steroids to replace a deficiency and using high doses to bulk up. The latter is illegal and a doctor can lose his or her license for prescribing steroids for this purpose. More important, the effects of high steroid use can be emotionally and physically disastrous for the user. High steroid use has been associated with shrunken testicles, female breast characteristics, and even cancerous tumors.

TESTOSTERONE AFFECTS YOUR MOOD

Androgens affect the brain by controlling the "maleness" in our personalities. Even women's personalities are affected by androgens, a subject that I'll get to later.

Ironically, however, not only do androgens affect the brain, the brain affects androgens—by regulating the levels of these substances in our bodies. We have seen how the body is in a constant feedback loop and how much of the information in this loop comes from the glands. A gland produces a substance, the substance sends a message to the brain, the brain sends a message to a particular part of the body, action in that part of the body increases or decreases, the information gets back to the brain, which sends a message to the gland . . . and on and on and on.

In the case of androgens, the pituitary gland makes two hormones—*follicle stimulating hormone* (FSH) and *luteinizing hormone* (LH)—that turn androgen production on and off from the testicles or ovaries. In turn, FSH and LH are regulated by another hormone, called *gonadotropin-releasing hormone* (GnRH). GnRH comes from a higher level in the brain known as the *hypothalamus*. Figure 4.2 illustrates these hormone feedback loops.

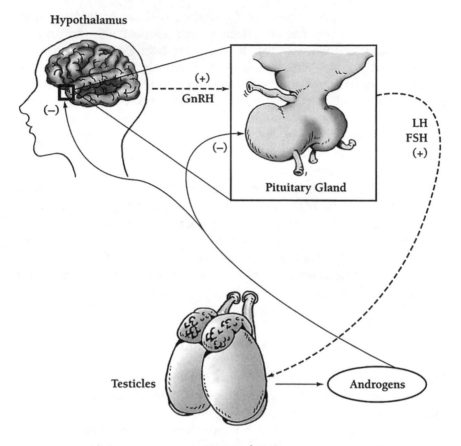

Figure 4.2
ANDROGEN ENDOCRINOLOGY: HORMONE FEEDBACK LOOPS
Higher centers in the brain send signals to the hypothalamus, which produces
pulses of gonadotropin-releasing hormone (GnRH). GnRH pulses stimulate the
pituitary gland to make follicle-stimulating hormone (FSH) and luteinizing hormone (LH), collectively known as gonadotropins. Gonadotropins stimulate the
testicles (or ovary) to produce androgens. Androgens "feed back" to the hypothalamus and pituitary gland, slowing gonadotropin production. Positive "feedback" is denoted by +, and negative "feedback" is denoted by –.

GnRH must be released by the hypothalamus in pulses. If a constant level of this hormone is produced, the pituitary will shut down. In fact, doctors use excessive doses of GnRH when they want to deliberately inhibit androgen production, in cases such as prostate cancer therapy. The signal from the pituitary gland to the testicle is removed, and the testicle will not make testosterone—and fortunately so, since testosterone helps prostate cancer grow.

Androgens are also made in the adrenal gland. There's another pituitary hormone, *adrenocorticotrophic hormone* (ACTH), which is better known for controlling cortisol production from the adrenal gland (see Chapter 8). ACTH also controls androgen production from the adrenal gland. This is more important in women than in men, where up to 50 percent of androgen production can come from the adrenal gland.

The brain can also prompt *more* testosterone production, of course. If it senses that the body needs more androgen—such as before an aggressive event such as a football game or boxing match, or if the testicles are failing—the brain will send the FSH/LH signal to the glands to produce more androgen. The opposite is also true: If the brain, via the pituitary, senses an abundance of testosterone, it can tell the glands to shut down.

Which brings us back to male bodybuilders, athletes, and other people who may use illegal steroids. Invariably, they all have small testicles. With all that extra testosterone floating around, the brain tells the testes that there is no need to produce more testosterone. The family jewels turn soft and shrivel.

It's generally easy for doctors to determine if someone is taking illegal steroids, even without checking his testicles. One basic test checks the levels of a person's brain hormones—the aforementioned FSH and LH. If they're very low, and the person is a bodybuilder, he's on steroids. On the other hand, if the same FSH and LH levels are low and the patient is flabby, tired, depressed, impotent, and/or weak, he's almost certainly *not* taking steroids—but may need to. Steroids aren't intrinsically bad, but they should be prescribed only for people who genuinely need them. In this case, where there may be a problem with his pituitary gland or hypothalamus that is causing the FSH and LH to be low—so his testicles aren't producing testosterone—steroid therapy may be recommended.

ANDROGEN DISORDERS IN MEN

These fall into six main categories.

- *Mild testicular failure.* This is what we refer to as "andropause," "viropause," "male climacteric," "male gonadopause," "male menopause," or "ADAM syndrome" (androgen deficiency of the aging male). Almost every man experiences a decline in testosterone as he gets older. Year by year, androgen levels slowly decline. By age 80, 60–80 percent of men have low testosterone levels.

   Many experts consider this a normal part of aging, but just how normal is it? Low testosterone levels are associated with decreased muscle size and strength, increased body fat, sexual dysfunction, cholesterol problems, and increased risk for heart disease. Studies have shown that very healthy men have fewer age-related declines in androgen levels. If you keep yourself healthy, eat properly, exercise, keep the stress down, and stay away from cigarettes and heavy alcohol, you can do a lot to lessen the inevitable decline in androgens as you get older.

   Declining androgen levels can occur slowly or abruptly, and the rate varies from person to person. If the symptoms come on abruptly, you may have a more serious form (see below). But at whatever rate it occurs, overtly low androgen levels are a concern.
- *Trauma or injury to the testicles.* Any injury to a gland can result in its dysfunction.
- *Infection.* Mumps is infamous for causing sterility in adult males; 25 percent of all cases are due to mumps. The AIDS virus also can cause male hypogonadism (low testosterone levels).
- *Autoimmune syndromes.* Along the same lines as type 1 diabetes and autoimmune thyroid disease, these are conditions whereby the body makes antibodies that attack itself. Any gland can be a target for attack, and the testicles are no exception.
- *Toxins, radiation, or chemotherapy.* Believe it or not, one of the most pernicious toxins to the testicle is alcohol. Drinking too much can permanently damage the testicle and inhibit testosterone production. Marijuana, cocaine, heroin, and other drugs have the same effect. Fat cells also produce toxins that damage the testicle, which leads to the increased risk of hypogonadism in overweight men.
- *Problems with the brain or pituitary gland.* The brain, pituitary gland, and testicles are intimately connected. Problems in one area affect the other.

Frank's Story

Frank seemed the very model of a successful, virile male. An executive with a chemical-manufacturing firm, he was 46, married with two children, and entering the stage of his life when he could afford to get out and play a little more. And play he did: Frank liked nothing better than escaping from the office on a Friday afternoon and getting in a round of golf with his colleagues.

But another form of play—that of sexual intimacy with his wife—wasn't going so well. Frank was having trouble getting and maintaining erections, and his sex life suffered. At the same time, he had put on a few pounds around the middle, his weekly round of exercise notwithstanding, and found himself feeling depressed. "I don't seem to have the same zest for life I used to," he said to me later. When first going through the symptoms, he had visited his family doctor for a checkup and a prescription for Viagra.

Not long after, Frank was on the golf course and tripped while leaving a bunker. The impact broke his wrist. When he went back to his doctor for a more thorough workup, the doctor discovered that Frank was suffering from osteoporosis—thinning and brittle bones.

Eventually, Frank came to see me. After a series of tests, I determined he was suffering from testicular failure—his testicles were simply not producing testosterone anymore. This being an easily treatable condition, I prescribed a testosterone gel. That only solved part of the problem, however. Frank later developed thyroid failure as well. It turned out that the same disease process, in which antibodies had disabled his testicles, had also affected his thyroid.

Cases of hypogonadism can go to extremes. In his book *Sexual Health for Men*, Dr. Richard F. Spark describes a twenty-something obese patient who came to him for help. The patient had not only developed breasts—not unheard-of in men—but those breasts were apparently producing milk.

The patient had started developing the breasts in high school, but managed to obtain doctor's excuses to avoid phys ed and other situations where he would have to disrobe. Later in life, when he finally (a process known as *gluconeogenesis*). Metformin does more than just treat diabetes, however. It lowers LDL cholesterol and triglyceride levels. Metformin has weight loss as a "side effect," but without improved nutrition and physical activity, this effect is minimal. Metformin reduces the risk of cardiovascular disease and the risk of type 2 diabetes. The original, short-acting version of metformin is better for weight loss and treating insulin resistance. The long-acting formulation is still good for treating insulin resistance, can be taken once a day, and has fewer side effects. If the pills are too big to swallow, a liquid form, called Riomet, is available.

The most common side effects of metformin are nausea, diarrhea, and upset stomach, which occur in about one of four people who take it. These side effects are almost always temporary and subside in three or four days, but can last for several weeks. To minimize side effects, start with the 500 mg tablet once a day with breakfast, and gradually increase the daily amount over several months. A fiber supplement can also be helpful for the side effect of diarrhea. The best dose for alleviating insulin resistance is 850 mg three times a day. It's important to take metformin with a substantial meal to minimize side effects. The manufacturer recommends that you do not drink alcohol while taking metformin, but many of my patients have an occasional alcoholic beverage without any problems. Metformin can cause problems in people who drink heavily or have a severe infection, or kidney or liver disease because of a rare but deadly side effect known as lactic acidosis. For the most part, however, metformin is a very safe drug.

Thiazolidinediones: Rosiglitazone (Avandia) and Pioglitazone (Actos)
A type of diabetes medication known as thiazolidinediones, "glitizones," or simply TZDs make cells more sensitive to insulin by regulating genes in the cells. They are excellent at improving insulin resistance and reversing many of its manifestations above and beyond their ability to treat diabetes. Their effects include lowering blood pressure and reducing inflammation and blood clotting. TZDs are ideal for treating the lipid abnormalities of insulin resistance because they decrease triglycerides, raise HDL levels, and can shift LDL from the dangerous "small dense" type to the less dangerous "large fluffy" type. These medications increase overall LDL cholesterol levels, however. TZDs are used as a treatment for fatty liver disease. A particularly interesting effect of TZDs is their ability to redistribute body fat, moving it from

dangerous areas, such as the belly and vital organs, to safer areas, such as the hips, buttocks, and under the skin. TZDs can prevent the high-risk people from getting diabetes and are used to treat a variant of insulin resistance seen in HIV patients known as *HIV lipodystrophy*.

The most publicized side effect of TZDs is weight gain, but the truth is that most people gain only a few pounds or none at all. If you follow the Hormonal Health Diet, it is more likely that you will lose weight while taking a TZD. Fluid retention is a more serious side effect, which can result in swelling of the legs and can be responsible for some of the weight gain. Heart failure is a contraindication to the use of TZDs because there can be a worsening of symptoms due to the fluid retention. (Some people with mild heart failure can take low doses of TZDs under close supervision.) The lowest doses (Avandia 2 mg or Actos 15 mg) are better for treating insulin resistance because there is less weight gain and less fluid retention. In May 2007, the safety of rosiglitazone came under question by the FDA when it was found to increase the risk of heart attack by as much as 30 to 40 percent. For this reason, endocrinologists use this class of drugs with extreme caution, and only if the benefits clearly outweigh the risks.

Metformin-TZD Combination Tablets (Avandamet—Rosiglitazone and Metformin; Actoplus Met—Pioglitazone and Metformin)

These medications are ideal for treating insulin resistance because of their synergistic actions. Metformin negates the weight gain seen when TZDs are used alone. For convenience, the manufacturers have combined them in one pill. Taking the medications as separate pills gives the exact same effect as the combination tablets.

Miglitol (Glyset) and Acarbose (Precose)

These diabetes medications work by blocking an enzyme in the intestine that breaks down carbohydrates, known as *alpha-galactosidase*. They slow, but do not prevent, the digestion of food, and foster a mild decrease in the absorption of carbohydrates. Their effect on weight loss is minimal.

Exenatide (Byetta)

This is a new hormonal medication that was listed as an experimental drug in the first edition of *Hormonal Balance*. Exenatide is now available and approved by the FDA for the treatment of diabetes.

Exenatide imitates the actions of the digestive hormone glucagon-like peptide-1 (GLP-1). (For more information on GLP-1, see Chapter 10.) The medication not only treats diabetes but also improves cholesterol and triglycerides, and has weight loss as a "side effect." Nausea is also a side effect because the drug slows down the digestive system, but as with metformin, the nausea is usually temporary. In rare cases, exenatide has been blamed for causing pancreatitis. The medication is given as an injection twice a day.

Pramlintide (Symlin)
Also listed as experimental in the first edition of *Hormonal Balance*, pramlintide is a newly approved hormonal diabetes medication. This drug works by mimicking amylin, a pancreatic hormone that regulates blood glucose. It is not widely used to treat insulin resistance, but can help people who have diabetes. The medication is given as an injection. Nausea, vomiting, low blood sugar, and headache are all possible side effects.

Lipid Medications

Lipid problems are a hallmark of insulin resistance, so it's not surprising that many people with insulin resistance end up taking medications. Combination drugs like Vytorin (a combination of ezetimibe and simvastatin) and Advicor (a combination of long-acting niacin and lovastatin) are convenient and may save on insurance co-pays, but offer no additional advantages to taking the medications as separate pills.

Statins: Atorvastatin (Lipitor), Pravastatin (Pravachol), Simvistatin (Zocor), Fluvastatin (Lescol, Lescol XL), Lovastatin (Mevacor, Altoprev), and Rosuvastatin (Crestor)
You can't watch the evening news nowadays without seeing a commercial for a class of drugs known as *statins* or *HMG CoA reductase inhibitors*. Statins work by inhibiting the enzyme HMG CoA reductase, which is needed to produce bad cholesterol. These blockbuster drugs are the most commonly used medications to treat high LDL cholesterol. But the amount of LDL cholesterol is not always the problem in insulin resistance. Insulin resistance causes the quality of LDL to shift to the dangerous "small dense" type. Statins have a small effect in lowering

triglycerides and raising HDL levels. Statins help in reducing insulin resistance because they improve the quality of LDL from the "small dense" type to the less dangerous "large fluffy" type. Statins have "antioxidant" properties, decreasing inflammation and blood clotting. Statins dramatically reduce the risk of cardiovascular disease, and can even reverse it. This is why statins are being prescribed more and more commonly and in higher doses than ever before.

The most common side effect is muscle problems, which can range from mild aches and pains to severe muscle damage. Any muscle pain or weakness should be reported to your physician. A test called CPK or CK can be done to determine if the drug is causing muscle damage. Because statins have such tremendous health benefits, most physicians now recommend that you continue taking the statin if it is causing only mild muscle pain. Inflammation of the liver is an infrequent side effect. Your doctor will need to monitor liver function periodically.

Fibrates: Fenofibrate (Tricor, Lofibra, Antara, Triglide) and Gemfibrozil (Lopid and Generics)

Also known as "fibric acid derivatives" or "fibrates," fenofibrate and the older, less effective gemfibrozil are cousins of the TZDs. Fibrates are a perfect choice for treating insulin resistance because they lower triglycerides and LDL cholesterol while raising HDL cholesterol. Side effects are uncommon, but muscle or liver problems can occur.

Niacin (Niaspan)

Also known as nicotinic acid or vitamin B_3, niacin, in high doses, simultaneously treats multiple lipid abnormalities by lowering triglycerides and LDL cholesterol while raising HDL cholesterol. Regular niacin is available as an over-the-counter supplement but is very hard to take because the doses needed (usually 1000–2000 mg per day) almost always cause side effects of flushing or tingling or redness of the skin. To reduce side effects, start with a low dose and gradually increase the dose over several months. The flushing can also be reduced by taking an aspirin and drinking a full glass of water one hour before taking the niacin. The slow-release prescription formulation of niacin known as Niaspan is easier to take because there are fewer side effects; however, there can still be significant flushing with this product.

A concern with niacin is that it can worsen insulin resistance and can raise blood sugar levels. For many people, the benefits outweigh the risks, and niacin can be beneficial in an overall plan of health and wellness. Even though niacin is available without a prescription, it should be taken only under medical supervision.

Omega-3 Fatty Acids (Omacor)
Omacor is a prescription formulation of the omega-3 fatty acids approved for the treatment of high triglyceride levels. This substance, found naturally in cold-water fish, also improves insulin resistance. The prescription formulation is better than over-the-counter preparations because it is purer and more potent.

Bile Acid Sequestrants: Cholestyramine (Questran, Questran Light), Colestipol (Colestid), and Colesevelam (WelChol)
These drugs, known as *bile acid sequestrants* or *bile acid resins*, lower LDL cholesterol by pulling it out of digestive juices, allowing it to pass in the stool. Cholestyramine and colestipol come in granular form and in packets or canisters, and are mixed with water for consumption. It is usually taken several times a day. Questran Light is a sugar-free version and is recommended for people with blood sugar problems. WelChol is a tablet taken once or twice a day. Some studies have shown that colesevelam (WelChol) can actually help lower blood sugar levels. It's thought to have an effect on the liver that improves glucose metabolism. Bile acid resins can raise triglyceride levels. The most common side effect is constipation. Fiber supplementation and proper hydration help control this problem.

Ezetimibe (Zetia)
This medication lowers LDL cholesterol by blocking absorption of cholesterol from the intestines. Ezetimibe doesn't do much for triglycerides or HDL cholesterol. Side effects are rare, but there can be abdominal pain or diarrhea.

Blood Pressure Medications

High blood pressure is a major feature of insulin resistance that frequently requires treatment with medications. Some of these drugs can improve insulin resistance and can reduce the risk for diabetes and cardiovascular disease. Other blood pressure medications can slow metabolism and worsen insulin resistance.

ACE Inhibitors: Ramapril (Altace), Perindopril (Aceon), Trandolapril
(Mavik), Lisinopril (Zestril), Benazepril (Lotensin), Quinapril
(Accupril), Enalapril (Vasotec), and Captopril (Capoten)
Angiotensin-converting enzyme, or "ACE," inhibitors slow the production of a hormone that raises blood pressure. ACE inhibitors are good at lowering blood pressure, but the benefits of this class of drugs go far beyond this. ACE inhibitors can improve insulin resistance. They have been shown to reduce the risk for diabetes, kidney disease, and cardiovascular disease. This is why ACE inhibitors are one of the best medications for people with insulin resistance. To obtain the protective effects from an ACE inhibitor, the maximum dose is needed.

One side effect is high potassium levels, so potassium should be monitored a few weeks after starting an ACE inhibitor. Other side effects include dry cough, fatigue, and headache. In rare cases, a serious allergic reaction can cause lip and tongue swelling, with sudden difficulty swallowing or breathing.

Angiotensin Receptor Blockers (ARBs): Losartan (Cozaar), Valsartan
(Diovan), Ibesartan (Avapro), and Candesartan (Atacand),
Olnesartan (Benicar), Telnisartan (Micardis), Eprosartan (Teveten)
ARBs, or angiotensin receptor blockers, operate on the same hormone system as ACE inhibitors but work by blocking the receptor for the same blood pressure–raising hormone. These drugs tend to be better at lowering blood pressure than ACE inhibitors. The beneficial effects of ARBs are similar to those of ACE inhibitors, but these medications don't have the long-term studies to support their use over ACE inhibitors. ARBs are traditionally recommended for patients who can't take ACE inhibitors, but are increasingly being used as first-line therapy. Side effects are unusual, but high potassium levels are sometimes seen.

Aliskiren (Tekturna)
Aliskiren is a new type of blood pressure medication known as a direct renin inhibitor. It works by blocking the enzyme, renin. Renin is part of the same hormone-enzyme system affected by ACE inhibitors and ARBs (see above). Although too soon to tell, it is hoped that this new

class of drugs will have similar beneficial effects as its cousins ACEs and ARBs.

Carvedilol (Coreg)
This medication is a second-generation beta-blocker. Carvedilol is a unique version called an *alpha-beta blocker* that tends to improve insulin resistance, whereas other beta-blocker medications make insulin resistance worse. Side effects include fatigue, slow heartbeat, and difficulty breathing. A once-a-day formulation of carvedilol, Coreg CR is also available.

Potassium-Sparing Diuretics: Spironolactone (Aldactone), Amilioride (Midamor), Triamterine (Dyrenium), and Eplerenone (Inspra)
Low potassium causes insulin resistance, so these mild diuretics help by lowering blood pressure and raising potassium levels. Side effects can include liver problems or elevation of potassium levels. Potassium levels and liver function should be monitored at regular intervals. Eplerenone blocks the adrenal gland hormone aldosterone, which is responsible for raising blood pressure and lowering potassium levels.

Weight Loss Medications

Weight loss medications can be helpful for treating insulin resistance when combined with proper nutrition and physical activity. Studies on weight loss medications show that most patients who lose weight gain it back when the medication is discontinued. There is no perfect medication, and the effects of available medications are mild at best.

Orlistat (Xenical, Alli)
Orlistat works by slowing or blocking the digestion of fat. This results in about one-third of the fat from the diet being passed in the stool. The typical weight loss with orlistat is about 25 pounds in 6 months. The most common side effect is oily diarrhea. This can be minimized by eating a low-fat diet and by taking a fiber supplement. Orlistat has a risk of blocking the absorption of fat-soluble vitamins, A, D, E, and K. I have seen a few patients who developed severe vitamin D deficiency (known as *osteomalacia*) from taking orlistat.

Sibutramine (Meridia)

Sibutramine is an appetite suppressant that works by altering the brain chemicals serotonin, norepinephrine, and dopamine. (See Chapter 10 for more information.) This drug is similar to venlafaxine and duloxetine in the way it achieves its effect. The main way it works is by increasing the feeling of satiety during a meal; it helps you feel full quicker. The average weight loss with sibutramine is 25 pounds in 6 months. High blood pressure, rapid heartbeat, insomnia, and agitation can be side effects. Blood pressure must be monitored regularly while you are taking sibutramine. Cardiovascular disease and uncontrolled blood pressure are contraindications to the use of sibutramine.

Phentermine (Adipex)

Phentermine is a weight loss medication that was one part of the "phen-fen" combination. Phentermine is approved only for short-term use, and people who take it routinely gain back all the weight they lost (or even more) after it is discontinued. Phentermine can cause agitation, insomnia, and elevated heart rate and blood pressure. For all of these reasons, I do not recommend its use.

Rimonabant (Acomplia)

Rimonabant has been called "anti-marijuana," because it acts by blocking the action of brain chemicals that have actions similar to marijuana (cannabis), known as *endocannabinoids*. The drug was developed with the knowledge that marijuana gives people the "munchies"; rimonabant blocks the reception of these hunger signals. Rimonabant causes people to lose these cravings to help prevent overeating. Rimonabant also helps reduce cravings for cigarettes and thus can help you quit smoking. Both smokers and overweight people have over-stimulated endocannabinoid systems. The endocannabinoid system is a system of natural brain chemicals that plays a role in maintaining metabolism through the regulation of food intake and energy expenditure. Rimonabant selectively blocks receptors in the endocannabinoid system, which puts the system in proper balance. Nausea, vomiting, and depression are possible side effects of rimonabant. Although available overseas, rimonabant is not available in the United States due to concerns about depression and possible suicide caused by the drug.

Antidepressants

Most antidepressants affect your weight in one way or another. This is because the brain chemicals related to depression—*serotonin, norepinephrine,* and *dopamine*—are the same brain chemicals that help regulate appetite. (See Chapter 10 for more information.) While some antidepressants typically cause weight gain, others can cause weight loss. The effect of antidepressants on weight is variable and may even be the opposite of what is typical for a particular drug. It is thought that antidepressants that improve insulin resistance do so because they make you lose weight. But depression itself raises cortisol levels, which can also cause insulin resistance, so treating the depression improves insulin resistance.

Venlafaxine (Effexor, Effexor XR) and Duloxetine (Cymbalta)
These medications alter the same brain chemicals (serotonin, norepinephrine, and dopamine) as the weight loss medication sibutramine (Meridia). The medications can decrease appetite and help with weight loss but may take several weeks to start working. The most common side effects are high blood pressure, rapid heartbeat, and insomnia. It is recommended that you have your blood pressure monitored regularly while taking these medications. These drugs can create a "withdrawal" syndrome if discontinued abruptly. If you need to stop taking venlafaxine or duloxetine, you should taper the drug slowly, under the supervision of your physician.

Bupropion (Wellbutrin, Wellbutrin SR, Wellbutrin XL)
Bupropion is a unique type of antidepressant that affects several brain chemicals, including dopamine and norepinephrine. Bupropion helps with weight loss by decreasing appetite. The weight loss seen with bupropion is similar to that characteristic of weight loss medications. Side effects of bupropion are related to its "stimulant" action and include agitation, insomnia, and in rare cases seizures.

Antiseizure/Antimigraine Medications

Zonisamide (Zonegran) and Topiramate (Topamax)
These medications are frequently used to treat seizures, chronic pain, and migraine headaches. They are now being prescribed for weight

loss because they can decrease appetite and prevent overeating. The exact way these medications work is unknown. This class of medications is especially helpful in reducing episodes of binge eating and nighttime eating. Higher doses of the medications are more effective for weight loss, but it is recommended that you start with a low dose and slowly increase the dose over several weeks. My experience is that many patients who tried these medications never took a high enough dose to result in any significant weight loss. Unfortunately, although higher doses are more effective for weight loss, they also increase the likelihood of side effects such as tingling of the hands, kidney stones, sedation, and memory problems.

Aspirin

Insulin resistance increases the risk of blood clotting and cardiovascular disease. This is why the current recommendation is that anyone with insulin resistance should take a baby aspirin (81 mg) every day.

Testosterone Replacement Therapy

This therapy is for men only. Testosterone deficiency, known as hypogonadism, is extremely common in men with insulin resistance. As discussed in Chapter 4, testosterone deficiency results in less muscle and more fat in the belly. Testosterone replacement therapy (TRT) improves insulin resistance by increasing muscle and decreasing fat. See Chapter 4 for more information.

Growth Hormone Replacement Therapy

Growth hormone deficiency results in loss of lean body mass, which causes insulin resistance. Growth hormone is considered a *counter-insulin hormone* because it can raise blood sugar, but the long-term effect is to lower insulin resistance. This is because growth hormone replacement therapy increases lean body mass and decreases fat mass. For more information, see Chapter 9.

MEDICATIONS THAT WORSEN INSULIN RESISTANCE

In order to achieve hormonal balance, it's important, whenever possible, to avoid medications that can intensify insulin resistance. Medications can make insulin resistance worse for a variety of reasons.

Corticosteroids (Glucocorticoids)

Common medications including prednisone, hydrocortisone, dexamethasone, and methylprednisolone work by mimicking the action of the hormone cortisol. Excessive cortisol causes severe insulin resistance and massive weight gain and promotes fat accumulation and muscle loss. Corticosteroids can cause diabetes and can increase the risk of cardiovascular disease and other ailments. For more information, see Chapter 8.

Sulfonylureas: Glyburide (DiaBeta), Glipizide (Glucotrol), and Glimepiride (Amaryl)

This class of drugs treats type 2 diabetes by stimulating the pancreas to produce insulin. They are great for blood sugar but make insulin resistance worse. Weight gain is a common side effect of sulfonylureas.

Diuretics: Furosemide (Lasix), Torsemide (Demadex), Bumetanide (Bumex), Indapamide (Lozol), Hydrochlorothiazide (HCTZ, Microzide, Hydrodiuril), and Chlorothiazide (Diuril)

Diuretics cause loss of potassium in the urine. When potassium is deficient from the body, insulin resistance gets worse. If you take diuretics, potassium supplementation is helpful.

Synthetic Progestins: Medroxyprogesterone (Provera), Norethindrone Acetate (Aygestin), Megestrol (Megace), Micronor, Nor-QD, Ovrette, Depo-Provera, and Norplant (as Well as Birth Control Pills That Contain Levonorgestrel, Norgestrel, or Norethindrone)

Progestins have high androgenic activity and produce side effects such as acne, bloating, weight gain, and elevated blood sugars. See Chapter 6 for more information.

Beta-Blockers: Propanolol (Inderal), Metoprolol (Toprol), and Atenolol (Tenormin)

Although sometimes necessary to treat conditions like high blood pressure, congestive heart failure, and abnormal heart rhythms, these medications can slow metabolism and worsen insulin resistance.

Calcium Channel Blockers: Amlodipine (Norvasc), Nifedipine (Procardia), Verapamil (Calan), and Diltiazem (Cardiazem)

Calcium channel blockers can sometimes worsen insulin resistance and can increase the risk of diabetes.

HIV/AIDS Medications: Amprenavir (Agenerase), Tipranavir (Aptivus), Nelfinavir (Viracept), Ritonavir (Norvir), Saquinavir (Invirase, Fortovase), Tipranavir (Aptivus), Indinavir (Crixivan), Fosamprenavir (Lexiva), Atazanavir (Reyataz), Darunavir (Prezista)

These life-saving drugs, known as *protease inhibitors*, cause severe insulin resistance and diabetes. They also cause a variant of insulin resistance known as *HIV lipodystrophy*, where people develop many of the physical features seen in Cushing's syndrome (see Chapter 8).

Antidepressants

Some antidepressants increase appetite and have weight gain as a side effect. The same brain chemicals involved in depression also regulate appetite (see Chapter 10 for more information). Older antidepressants, such as amitriptyline and nortriptyline, frequently cause massive weight gain. Mirtazapine (Remeron) is also notorious for increasing appetite and causing weight gain. Antidepressants such as fluoxetine (Prozac), sertraline (Zoloft), paroxetine (Paxil, Paxil CR), citolopram (Celexa), and escitalopram (Lexipro) have variable effects on weight.

Antiseizure Medications: Carbamazepine (Tegretol) and Gabapentin (Neurontin)

These medications can increase insulin resistance and cause weight gain and sedation.

Antipsychotic Medications: Olanzapine (Zyprexa), Risperidone (Risperdal), and Quetiapine (Seroquel)

These drugs can cause massive weight gain, insulin resistance, and diabetes and have been devastating for people with mental illness.

Antihistamines

Older antihistamines, such as diphenhydramine, and other antihistamines that make you sleepy can also worsen insulin resistance and cause weight gain. These antihistamines are a common ingredient in many over-the-counter allergy medications and sleep aids.

Unlike other androgens, DHEA is naturally made by the adrenal gland, not the testicle or ovary. There's also more than one kind of DHEA: Sometimes you'll hear of "DHEAS" or "DHEA-S." But that kind isn't much different from standard DHEA; all the "S" means is that a sulfate is attached to the DHEA, something that occurs naturally in the body.

DHEA has been called the "youth hormone" because levels peak when people are in their 20s, then decline dramatically with advancing age. The decline has been given a name, *adrenopause*. DHEA is available over the counter as a dietary supplement, and many people take it though we know very little about it. Among the claims: it's anti-aging, increasing lean body mass; it improves insulin resistance; it boosts energy levels and libido; it improves mood. One doctor, Dr. William Regelson, has made a cottage industry out of promoting DHEA as the "super-hormone." Yet almost all of these claims remain unproven, and the effect DHEA has on the body is mild at best.

But there are some troubling side effects. The most notable, though it also remains unproven, is a theoretical risk of prostate cancer in men and breast cancer in women. Those doctors who do recommend DHEA disagree on dosage levels, ranging from 10 mg on up to as high as 1,600 mg per day.

My belief? I think we need more research. DHEA may, indeed, be beneficial in some ways. But the jury is still out, both on its pros and cons. Fortunately, the National Institutes of Health is currently conducting a study, so we should have some results in the next few years.

MUSCLE BOOSTING TIPS

Although androgen replacement therapy isn't for everyone, there are still some things you can do to build up your muscle mass. Even if you do take androgens, these tips may help your hormones to work more effectively.

Weight training

In order to significantly improve your body composition, you must lift weights. There are many different weight-lifting techniques. If you have never lifted weights before, I recommend that you start with very low weights and slowly work your way up to higher weights. You may also want to consider two or three sessions with a personal trainer to perfect your technique. Many lifters debate which is better, free weights or machines. My answer: Both are great. Just remember, if you use free weights, you need to use a spotter. Many weight-lifting injuries can be prevented by the use of a spotter.

You should plan on hitting the gym at least twice a week. Consistency is key. A 30-minute weight-training session twice a week will have a significant effect on your body composition in as little as 4 weeks.

A new weight-training technique, known as **static contraction training** (SCT), may be an ideal form of weight training for many who have never lifted before. SCT uses very heavy weights (you must have a qualified trainer supervise you). The weights are held, motionless, until your muscles become completely fatigued. The weights are usually held for 5 to 15 seconds, only one set per exercise. This super-intense workout can be more effective than weight-training sessions that take hours—a true example of "less is more." Whether you use SCT or a more traditional approach, weight training is the best way to increase muscle mass. Remember, the more muscle you have, the better your metabolism.

Stress relief

Stress lowers androgen levels by reducing hormonal signals from the brain. Stress has a negative effect on many hormones, creating a hormonal imbalance that slows metabolism. Stress, either psychological or physical, will reduce muscle mass and increase fat mass. I have more suggestions for stress relief in Chapter 8.

Growth hormone

Growth hormone is another hormone that has a major effect on muscles. Growth hormone proper is only available by injection; however, a multitude of growth hormone "releasers" are available without a prescription. Growth hormone is not for everyone. Chapter 9 discusses growth hormone in more detail.

Get plenty of sleep

Your hormones are entwined in circadian rhythms. Androgens and growth hormone are both secreted while you sleep. When you don't get enough sleep, these hormones are not made in sufficient quantities.

Balanced diet

Stay away from fad, muscle-building diets. It is important to get the right number of calories and to have a healthy balance of carbohydrate, protein, and fat (see Chapter 11).

Protein supplements

Protein provides the building blocks for healthy muscles. Make sure you get your minimum protein requirements. Many body builders use protein supplements. Although these are not necessary, they can be a convenient way to make sure you get enough protein in your diet. Egg whites, low-fat dairy products, tofu, fish, and lean cuts of meat are excellent sources of protein.

ANDROGEN DISORDERS IN WOMEN

ANDROGENS ARE JUST AS IMPORTANT FOR WOMEN AS THEY ARE FOR MEN. Androgens follow the same rule as other hormones: Balance is critical. Too much or too little androgen can cause problems for women. Androgen deficiency, or *female low-androgen syndrome*, and androgen excess are both associated with metabolic problems and weight gain.

How do women get "male" hormones? Both the ovary and the adrenal glands make androgens. Problems with either one of these glands can result in an androgen disorder.

Both high and low androgen levels can cause weight gain. Despite this, there is very little awareness regarding androgens among women.

FEMALE LOW-ANDROGEN SYNDROME

Androgens help maintain muscle mass and determine body-fat distribution. Androgens are responsible for the appearance of body hair; they make the skin oilier; and, as in men, they contribute to sex drive. A deficiency of androgens can cause problems in women, just as in men. **Up to one-third of all women experience problems with androgen deficiency at some time in their lives.**

And just as in men, women's androgen levels decline with age. Androgen decline at menopause is considered part of the natural aging process. (It actually starts declining when a woman reaches her 30s.)

Symptoms of Androgen Decline

- Weight gain (or, sometimes, weight loss)
- Increased fat in the belly
- Loss of muscle, reduction in lean body mass
- Tiredness
- Lack of energy, leading to decreased activity and weight gain
- Loss of sexual desire
- Decreased sense of well-being
- Depression
- Decreased sexual responsiveness in the nipples
- Loss of shine in the hair, dryness of the skin
- Lack of mental clarity
- Irregular menstrual cycle
- Anemia
- Urinary incontinence, from loss of muscle tone in the pelvis and the bladder
- Osteoporosis or osteopenia

Overabundance of androgens can also cause problems, as I'll note later. The upshot is that hormonal *balance* is key.

Most problems with low androgens in women come from a failing ovary, but failing adrenal glands or even a failing pituitary gland can also cause problems. Testing for androgen deficiency in women is tricky. Blood tests usually don't help too much. If a woman has an excess androgen level, a blood test can be revealing, but low levels can be masked effectively by other conditions.

MENOPAUSE, ANDROGENS, AND HRT

During menopause, the ovary stops making its three hormones—estrogen, progesterone, and testosterone. (I'll discuss estrogen and progesterone in Chapter 6.) Estrogen replacement therapy (ERT), used in menopausal women, actually suppresses testosterone production by the ovary, so women on ERT have even *lower* androgen levels. ERT suppresses the brain signals FSH and LH, which are needed for ovarian hormone synthesis. Also, ERT increases SHBG, the blood protein that soaks up testosterone. (Only the "free" testosterone is active.) With more SHBG, there is less bioactive hormone. Adrenal gland production of androgens is not affected by ERT, however.

What's the point? Women on ERT are at high risk of having low androgens. Doctors are good about giving estrogen to women, but they forget about the testosterone component.

ANDROGEN THERAPY FOR WOMEN

Doctors are frequently afraid to prescribe androgens to women, although the treatment can be as beneficial as estrogen and progesterone therapy. They fear the side effects of testosterone, mainly the detrimental effects on cholesterol and possibly heart disease related to the cholesterol problems.

Originally, it was thought that androgens were helpful only for menopausal women who have symptoms of menopause not completely relieved by ERT. More and more studies are beginning to show that treating androgen deficiency in women has a wide range of benefits. Androgen therapy helps reduce fat and build muscle and bone, and it improves libido, energy level, strength, sexual function and overall quality of life.

Despite these benefits, androgen replacement therapy is still controversial. Some doctors fear that testosterone therapy could cause problems seen in androgen excess syndromes, such as weight gain, facial hair, and acne, and this can be true if testosterone is taken in excessive amounts. Typically, the testosterone therapies described in Chapter 4 are not used for women.

There are a number of drugs and therapies that are prescribed for women. Among them are the following:

- **Estratest**. Instead of giving just estrogen for menopause, Estratest combines the standard dose of conjugated estrogens with a small dose of testosterone (actually a form of testosterone known as methyltestosterone). Although testosterone pills are a concern in men because of the liver problems they can cause, the low doses in Estratest are unlikely to damage the liver. If you're going through menopause and your symptoms are not improved by estrogen alone, or you have a diminished sex drive, you may want to ask your doctor to switch you to Estratest. I recommend you start with **Estratest HS** (a "half-strength" version).

A study at Johns Hopkins School of Medicine recently showed that Estratest reduces fat by 2 to 4 percent and increases muscle mass by 4 to 6 percent after only 3 months. Further studies are needed to determine the long-term safety of Estratest in women.

- **Methyltestosterone (Android).** These capsules of pure methyltestosterone are 10 milligrams—four times the dose of methyltestosterone in Estratest. This makes dosing very difficult in women. Some compounding pharmacies can make smaller and more appropriate doses (1–5 mg) of methyltestosterone.

- **Birth control pills**. Most birth control pills contain estrogen and progesterone. Like estrogen, not all progesterone is created equal. Some pills have quite a bit of androgen activity, in fact. The ones that have the most are **norgestel** and **norethindrone**. Usually, this is responsible for some of the androgenic side effects of birth control pills, such as acne and hair growth. In women with low androgens, however, this can be an advantage. However, as I will discuss, these are exactly the types of progesterone that should be avoided in women with too much androgen.

- **Testosterone gel (AndroGel)**. Although not FDA approved for women, doctors have been giving women very small doses of this testosterone-containing gel. The doses of AndroGel currently available are too strong for women. New strengths may become available in the future. More research is needed on the use of AndroGel in women.

- **Testosterone creams.** Testosterone cream can be made by some compounding pharmacies, and as with other products of this nature, quality control can be variable.

- **Testosterone patches**. Currently available testosterone patches produce testosterone levels that are too high for women. Research is being done, however, on patches with testosterone doses more appropriate to women. Preliminary research has shown a positive benefit of the lower-dose testosterone patch.

- **Testosterone shots**. These are exactly the same as the ones given men and, as such, have some strong side effects. Women with severe androgen deficiency may benefit from injections of 50 mg testosterone propionate or testosterone cypionate every month or every other month.

- **Testosterone implants**. Although there have been doctors who implant testosterone pellets under the skin, I don't recommend it. They're hard to remove, and if there are side effects, you are stuck. Moreover, the effect is extremely variable.
- **Dehydroepiandrosterone (DHEA)**. DHEA is an androgen produced by the adrenal gland. As I noted in Chapter 4. DHEA is among the most abundant hormones in the body. In women, levels peak about age 30 and then decline progressively thereafter. By age 50, levels are about 50 percent of their peak.

  DHEA is one-twentieth as potent as testosterone. DHEA supplementation tends to boost all androgen levels because the body easily converts it to other hormones. Of course, this doesn't mean just testosterone; it can also be converted to estrogen.

  I have seen may women become "over androgenized" from taking too much DHEA. Side effects of too much DHEA include weight gain, increased facial hair, acne, cholesterol problems, and mood swings. DHEA can also have negative effects on cholesterol—raising bad cholesterol and lowering good cholesterol. A study on DHEA replacement in German women did not show any improvement in carbohydrate metabolism, body composition, or exercise capacity. The bottom line is, again, that DHEA remains controversial and is under little regulation by the FDA. DHEA clearly raises blood levels of androgens, but more research is needed to determine if it has any real benefit or, for that matter, long-term consequences—good or bad.
- **Androstenedione.** Androstenedione is another nutraceutical hormone that is available in most health-food stores. Androstenedione is a weak androgen that is easily converted by the body to other hormones. I do not recommend its use. For more information on androstenedione, see Chapter 4.
- **Tibolone.** This is a hormone in development that combines the effects of estrogen, progesterone, and testosterone. Early reports indicate that it seems to protect against osteoporosis, helps with vaginal dryness, stops hot flashes, and is generally beneficial. Currently labeled with the brand name Livial, it has yet to be released in the United States.

SIDE EFFECTS OF ANDROGEN THERAPY IN WOMEN

Androgen therapy can have many side effects. Among the most concerning are the negative effects on the cholesterol profile and a possible risk of heart disease. Anyone who takes androgen replacement therapy should do so under the supervision of a qualified physician. Other side effects include

- Acne
- Hair growth in male areas, such as face, chest, nipples, and back
- Voice deepening
- Overactive sex drive
- Menstrual irregularities
- Balding on the head
- Enlargement of the clitoris
- For women on thyroid medication, thyroid medication dosage may need to be increased

ANDROGEN EXCESS IN WOMEN

Androgen excess (known as *hyperandrogenism*) is the most common hormonal disorder in young women. Although common, it is a serious problem that should not be ignored. Elevated androgens can be a signal of other problems in women including high blood pressure, high cholesterol, insulin resistance, diabetes, and heart disease. As with most health problems, the first step is admitting there is a problem. After that, you can be treated.

The side effects of androgen therapy described above can also be symptoms of androgen excess. In general, these symptoms manifest themselves slowly over the years; hair growth in "male areas"—those listed above, as well as the lower stomach, upper arms, chin, and upper pubic triangle—is a prime indicator.

- *Weight gain or difficulty losing weight.* Elevated androgen levels lead to insulin resistance and weight gain. Many women with androgen excess are unable to lose weight despite valiant dieting attempts. Correction of the androgen problem can make weight loss easier.

- *Hair growth in male areas (hirsutism).* The hair follicle is sensitive to androgens. Hyperandrogenism can cause hair growth on the upper lip, chin, sideburns, neck, chest, arms, nipples, back, buttocks, stomach, shoulders, arms, legs, and inner thighs. It is important to note that not all hairiness is a sign of an androgen problem. This can be normal, especially for women of Mediterranean or Middle Eastern heritage. Hair on the lower back, chest, stomach, shoulders, buttocks, and inner thighs is *always* considered abnormal, however.
- *Hair loss.* Although excess hair grows on the face and body, androgen excess can cause hair loss from the scalp.
- *Acne.* Up to 50 percent of teenagers have acne; so just having acne doesn't necessarily mean that someone has hyperandrogenism. Persistence of acne into the late teens or 20s, however, is of concern and may be a sign of hyperandrogenism. This type of acne is usually very hard to treat and often requires the expertise of a dermatologist.
- *Acanthosis nigricans.* A darkening of the skin, usually neck and armpits, associated with insulin resistance (see Chapter 3).
- *Menstrual irregularities.* The most common scenario is skipping periods. However, androgen excess can lead to a variety of problems including light or heavy flow and periods that are missed, late, or even too frequent.
- *Infertility.* Women with hyperandrogenism can have difficulty getting pregnant.
- *Psychological problems.* Androgen excess has been associated with both anxiety and depression. Many women with androgen excess also have problems with poor body image that can lead to social isolation.
- *Premenstrual syndrome.* PMS is common in women with androgen excess.
- *High blood pressure*
- *High cholesterol*
- *Insulin resistance or type 2 diabetes*

If these symptoms arise suddenly, don't even think of hesitating; get right to a doctor. *A sudden onset of an androgen disorder is a warning sign for cancer, either the adrenal gland or the ovary.* Severe androgen excess, like that caused by cancer, can also cause a condition in women known as *virilization*. Features of virilization include:

- *Balding,* such as in male pattern baldness, with a receding hairline
- *Deepening of the voice*
- *Masculinization of the body*—extensive muscle growth, shrinkage of the breasts and hips
- *Severe hirsutism*
- *Cessation of the menstrual cycle*
- *Excessive body odor*
- *Clitoromegaly*—an enlarged clitoris, bigger than 1 cm in length. It may even begin to take on the appearance of a small penis.

Anita's Story

Anita was a woman in her early 40s. She came to me full of attitude, very angry and aggressive. Every question I asked had a retort; every comment was met with a glare. (Aggressiveness, as noted earlier, can be a sign of too much testosterone.) She told me that all she needed was her choles- terol checked; why was I wasting time with all these questions?

But, once I managed to get past her embarrassment, I noticed Anita had hair on her chin. Intrigued, I asked her about it. She hadn't had the growth long, she told me. She also admitted that she had stopped having periods a few months earlier, but birth control pills had taken care of this. As I asked her about other symptoms of sudden-onset andro- gen disorder, she nodded her head. She had almost every one.

I performed a physical exam and detected a mass in her belly. Anita had a very large adrenal gland cancer. To com- bat it, we tried every therapy known to science. Still, two years later, she died. It was a long time to live with this kind of cancer, but that's little solace. It's never long enough.

Early detection saves lives. If your symptoms have come on sud- denly, or the symptoms are severe—virilization, as mentioned above— seek attention immediately.

Polycystic Ovary Syndrome (PCOS)

PCOS, also known as Stein-Leventhal syndrome, is the most common cause of androgen excess in women. It happens in as many as 10 percent of reproductive-age women. It's also a very common cause of weight gain. Most women are diagnosed with PCOS in their late teens or early 20s (or even later). Research has shown, however, that the problem begins in the early teens (or earlier). Every attempt should be made to diagnose and treat PCOS as early as possible.

Dr. Sibodh Verma has called PCOS a "multifaceted metabolic disease": It's got a very broad spectrum of problems and an equally broad spectrum of symptoms. Moreover, women with PCOS may have one or all of the symptoms. Menstrual irregularity is the most widespread, but even women with normal cycles can still have PCOS. PCOS is associated with a vast array of hormonal problems. Although androgens receive most of the attention, insulin resistance may actually be at the heart of PCOS. High insulin levels stimulate the production of androgens by the ovaries. High androgen levels cause insulin resistance. It's the chicken and the egg.

The "O" in PCOS stands for "ovary"; however, excess androgen actually comes from both the adrenal glands and the ovaries. This double source of androgens prompts the brain to send mixed signals back to the ovaries. Ovary walls become thickened—eggs cannot be released at their normal time of the month. This condition, known as *anovulation*, is the reason why women with PCOS have trouble getting pregnant. In some, the menstrual cycle becomes abnormal. Women with PCOS start developing symptoms not long after puberty, but they usually aren't diagnosed for 5 or more years.

Meanwhile, with the hormones out of whack, metabolism is also thrown out of balance—and usually slowed down. As we've seen, this is a recipe for weight gain. The medical community now universally recognizes that PCOS is associated with serious metabolic problems including insulin resistance, type 2 diabetes, obesity, high blood pressure and elevated cholesterol. Together, these metabolic consequences lead to an increased risk for developing coronary heart disease. In recent years, treatment for PCOS has changed from treating the complications to treating the cause of PCOS.

Jennifer's Story
A secretary-receptionist in (of all places) a doctor's office,
Jennifer was 43 years old when she had a heart attack. She
weighed close to 200 pounds, had a diet high in sugars,
starches, and fats, and an exercise regimen limited to walking
from her car to wherever she was going. She was also afflicted
with PCOS, which didn't help matters any; in addition to
being overweight, she was insulin resistant and at strong risk
for diabetes. She took metformin, but ignored her doctors'
advice on diet and exercise.

Jennifer was lucky in one way: Her heart attack happened
at work and she was treated immediately. And, of course, she
lived. But, unless she changed her lifestyle, she knew she may
not be so lucky next time. With encouragement and guidance
from her employers, as well as no small amount of willpower
on her own, she adopted a regular exercise regimen, cut back
on the junk food, added more vegetables and fruit to her diet,
and started paying attention to all aspects of her life. She lost
60 pounds and has emerged a healthier, happier person.

Jennifer's story is an extreme example of what PCOS can do to you, but not always typical. So, who is the typical PCOS woman? Probably somebody like Beth, another patient of mine. Beth is in her early 30s, overweight, and with an extra down of hair on her chest, face, and pelvic region. Her chief complaint was the inability to lose weight. She told me, "I diet and exercise and I just can't seem to lose any weight. I think my metabolism is too slow." Beth also had irregular menstrual cycles, a condition that concerned her because she'd always been "as regular as a clock," as she put it.

After conducting some tests, I noticed a few things. Beth had elevated blood sugar levels, for one—something she wasn't even aware of. She was also suffering from mild high blood pressure and problematic cholesterol levels. Had she not come to me with the weight problem, I would have first thought that her problems were almost exclusively insulin related. But hormones, as I've noted, often react with one another—and the brain—and therefore conditions often cannot simply be boiled down to one specific hormonal imbalance. However, the wonderful thing is that treatment for one condition—such as obesity—often has positive effects throughout the body.

Further testing confirmed that Beth had PCOS. Beth started medications and began following the meal plan suggested in Chapter 11. Six months later, Beth had lost 20 pounds and had normal blood sugar levels, cholesterol levels, and blood pressure.

Testing for PCOS

It is important to let your doctor know if you have any symptoms of androgen excess. Your doctor should perform a careful physical exam, looking for signs of hirsutism or virilization (see above). Hirsutism can be graded using a scale known as the Ferriman-Gallwey scale. Do not be shocked if your physician requires a pelvic exam or asks to inspect your vulva and clitoris. Tell your doctor if you have a family history of obesity, diabetes, high cholesterol, or high blood pressure.

When specific hormones are measured, it should be done within the first 7 days of the menstrual cycle.

- **Testosterone**. Most of the patients I see with PCOS have *total testosterone* levels at the "upper range of normal." Some, however, have overtly high total testosterone levels. Remember that excess androgen levels lead to low levels of the blood protein SHBG and that SHBG soaks up free testosterone. The point is, obese women with PCOS may have a normal total testosterone because of the lower SHBG levels, but *free testosterone* levels can still be very high. Even *that's* no guarantee—a significant percentage of women with PCOS have a normal free-testosterone level. Many laboratories have inaccurate "normal values" for testosterone levels in women. In fact, the authors of a 1999 study at the University of Texas Health Science Center have urged that new reference ranges be established by some of the commercial laboratories to better measure total and free testosterone. One sad fact: Very high testosterone levels (above 300 ng/dL) are suggestive of ovarian cancer.
- **Androstenedione**. In women, this is a lesser-known and weaker ovarian androgen. Levels are usually high or at the high end of normal.
- **DHEA and DHEA-S.** These can be normal or occasionally slightly elevated. This hormone, you'll recall, is made in the adrenal gland and not the ovary. Very high levels are a tip-off to an adrenal gland problem such as congenital adrenal hyperplasia or adrenal gland cancer.

- **Sex hormone binding globulin (SHBG).** SHBG is a blood protein that binds both testosterone and estrogen. PCOS can cause low SHBG levels.
- **LH/FSH ratio.** The classic finding is that the LH level is at least double that of the FSH level—*even if both are in the normal range*. This test, if positive, is highly suggestive of PCOS. However, one-third of PCOS patients do not have an elevated LH/FSH ratio. NCAH (see below) can also cause an elevated LH/FSH ratio.
- **Progesterone.** Progesterone levels should be measured on day 21 of the cycle. A progesterone level of less than 2 ng/mL suggests that you are not ovulating.
- **17-hydroxyprogesterone (17-OH-P).** This blood test should be done to eliminate the possibility of NCAH, an imitator of PCOS that has markedly different treatment (see below).
- **Glucose and cholesterol profile.** All women suspected of PCOS should be checked for diabetes and elevated cholesterol. Tests such as the fasting plasma glucose (FPG) test or the oral glucose tolerance test (OGTT) should be conducted. Because higher cholesterol and triglyceride levels are also associated with PCOS, a fasting lipid profile is mandatory. Diabetes and high cholesterol are two of the most serious metabolic consequences of PCOS and demand immediate treatment.
- **Pelvic ultrasound.** Some doctors encourage their patients to have a test known as pelvic ultrasound. This test helps detect abnormalities in the ovary. Conditions other than PCOS cause problems in the ovary, and not all women with PCOS have detectable ovarian cysts. Most experts agree that the pelvic ultrasound should *not* be used as a criterion for the diagnosis of PCOS. A pelvic ultrasound is important, however, to make sure there is not a tumor or other serious problem.

Treatment of PCOS

There are several available treatments for PCOS—many of which are better known for treating other conditions.

Diet and exercise
The diet I recommend for PCOS can be found in Chapter 11. Many women with PCOS have had tremendous relief with diet and exercise

alone. The key is lowering insulin resistance. For a variety of reasons, when insulin resistance is lowered, the androgen levels follow.

Diet and exercise are especially important because of all the health problems that go along with insulin resistance. Diet and exercise help with all these problems. Many women with PCOS have full-blown diabetes; given this fact, diet and exercise are even more critical. A 1997 study published in the *Annals of Internal Medicine*, in fact, has linked PCOS to coronary artery disease.

Stress relief
This goes hand-in-hand with a good diet and regular exercise. Remember, stress creates a hormonal imbalance that lowers metabolism and causes weight gain.

Self-confidence
Many women with PCOS have issues with "poor body image." The fear of social rejection can make some women become socially isolated. Poor self-esteem and self-image can even lead to depression. Work on developing social skills and self-confidence. It is often helpful if you can understand PCOS as a medical/hormone problem. It is not a woman's fault that she has PCOS. Many mental health professionals now specialize in treating body image problems related to PCOS.

Metformin (Glucophage)
In 1996, Dr. John Nestler published a landmark study in the *New England Journal of Medicine* which showed that treating PCOS with metformin significantly "ameliorates hyperandrogenism." Since then, many major studies have shown a dramatic improvement in PCOS when treated with metformin. The combination of clomiphene citrate and metformin appears to be a particularly potent treatment in inducing fertility in women with PCOS. Many women with PCOS have experienced tremendous benefit from metformin. I recommend this as an excellent treatment option. See Chapter 3 for more information on metformin.

Birth control pills
The Pill—along with suppressing production of reproductive hormones—also decreases both ovarian androgen production and adrenal androgen production. However, avoid birth control pills that contain androgenic progestins such as **levonorgestrel, norgestrel,** or

norethindrone. These progestins have high androgenic activity. And that's what's responsible for many of the side effects of birth control pills, such as acne and bloating. These progesterones can also cause insulin resistance. The least androgenic synthetic progestins are **deso-gestrol** and **norgestimate**. Birth control pills with desogestrol or norgestimate include **Apri, Desogen, Otho-Cept, Ortho-Cyclen,** and **Ortho Tri-Cyclen. Yasmin** is a birth control pill with a new progestin, **drospirenone**, which actually has anti-androgen properties and can be extremely helpful in PCOS. See Chapter 6 for more information on birth control pills.

Medroxyprogesterone acetate (Provera)

Given at a dose of 20 to 30 milligrams a day, this drug can be used to help increase the breakdown of testosterone by the liver. Side effects include vaginal bleeding, liver problems, depression, and hot flashes. In general, I rarely use this as a treatment for PCOS.

GnRH (Gonadotropin releasing hormone) agonists or analogues

The hypothalamus, as I noted near the beginning of this chapter, normally produces GnRH in short pulses or bursts. When high doses of GnRH agonist medication are given—usually a long-acting shot given once a month—the pituitary gland shuts down its production of FSH and LH. This causes all ovarian hormones to be suppressed—estrogen, progesterone, and androgens—and can make a woman feel like she is going through menopause.

Antiandrogen medications

These include spironolactone (Aldactone), a mild diuretic that also competes for androgens at the androgen receptor; cyproterone acetate, a strong progesterone medication that also acts as an antiandrogen (not available in the United States); flutamide (Eulexin), which blocks the androgen receptor; and finasteride (Proscar), which I discussed earlier, and has not been approved by the FDA for use in women. These medications all have side effects, ranging from greenish urine to irregular periods to possible birth defects, and all should be thoroughly discussed with your doctor before beginning treatment. Incidentally, a common antacid medication—cimetadine (Tagamet)—also blocks the androgen receptor but is not as strong as other blockers. I recommend it *not* be used for treating PCOS.

Rosiglitazone (Avandia) and pioglitazone (Actos)

These medications, known as "PPAR agonists" or "glitazones," are approved by the FDA for the treatment of diabetes. These medications help PCOS by ameliorating insulin resistance. Unlike metformin, they cause weight gain. Glitazones work at the level of the fat-cell DNA, making insulin work better. So insulin resistance is improved, but at the expense of making a bigger, healthier, and more efficient fat cell. These "super fat cells," which have a renewed ability to respond to insulin, get bigger and bigger.

Clomiphene citrate (Clomid)

A medication usually used as a fertility drug, it's an effective treatment for PCOS in women who want to get pregnant.

D-Chiro-insoitol

This experimental medication, not yet available, improves PCOS by improving insulin resistance. More research is needed before it is made available in this country.

Chromium

This medication improves insulin resistance, as noted in Chapter 3. Any therapy that improves insulin resistance will help PCOS.

OTHER DISORDERS RELATED TO ANDROGEN EXCESS

Cancer

Remember, if the symptoms of an androgen disorder come on suddenly or are severe, it could be an indication of ovarian or adrenal cancer. See a doctor right away.

Cushing's syndrome

See Chapter 8, on cortisol, for more information.

Hyperandrogenic-insulin resistant acanthosis nigricans (HAIRAN) syndrome

This is a mouthful to say, but it refers to a "malignant" form of PCOS. It's everything bad about PCOS magnified, and it's very destructive to the body.

Congenital adrenal hyperplasia (CAH)

Endocrinologists refer to the adult variety of this genetic condition as "21-hydroxylase deficient non-classic adrenal hyperplasia," or NCAH. A more severe form of this disorder causes what is called ambiguous genitalia, in which little girls are born with a clitoris so enlarged that it looks like a penis. A milder form of CAH causes 1 to 2 percent of androgen disorders in women. CAH is particularly common in the Ashkenazi Jewish population. The source of the excess androgens is the adrenal gland. Doctors (even endocrinologists) commonly miss CAH because it isn't usually tested for. Results of standard blood tests for male and female hormone levels can appear identical in CAH and PCOS.

I recommend testing for CAH in any woman with an androgen excess problem. The treatment for CAH is markedly different from the treatment for PCOS.

Ask your doctor for the 17-hydroxyprogesterone (17-OH-P) blood test. However, even this test is not perfect; many CAH patients frequently fall into a gray zone. If this happens, more sophisticated testing is needed. There is a genetic test to diagnose this disorder, but as with most genetic tests, it is rarely covered by insurance.

If the disorder is mild, treatment is not mandatory. Sometimes women use shaving, creams, or electrolysis to control hair growth. In more severe cases, a cortisol-like medication called dexamethasone (Decadron) is used to treat the condition. This blocks the adrenal gland's production of androgen.

Arlene's Story

Arlene had NCAH. She had the symptoms: She was overweight and slightly hirsute. But she was never diagnosed with the disorder.

Arlene got pregnant. Her child, a girl, was born with full-blown CAH—a genetic condition. (Given the severity of her child's condition, the father must have been a carrier of the gene.) The little girl required extensive plastic surgery to make her vagina appear normal, and she was undoubtedly subjected to high testosterone levels during her fetal development.

None of this is the end of the world, of course. But if Arlene had been screened and diagnosed with NCAH, she could have been treated with dexamethasone during her pregnancy, and it's likely the baby's problems could have been avoided. If you've been told you have PCOS and plan to get pregnant, please get checked for NCAH.

Idiopathic hirsutism

If the answer "none of the above" fits, doctors use the term "idiopathic." This is a diagnosis of exclusion after the more serious conditions are ruled out. Ironically, in this case it's not idiopathic at all. It turns out that idiopathic hirsutism is a disorder of the 5-alpha reductase enzyme, but this is an enzyme that is in the skin. The rest of the body is normal. In the skin, testosterone is converted at an abnormally high rate to the more active dihydrotestosterone, causing male-pattern hair growth. It's sometimes referred to as "benign familial hirsutism" because it doesn't seem to be associated with any other problems, other than cosmetic issues, and it runs in families.

The condition is genetically transmitted, so if your mother and grandmother are hairy, or the women on your father's side are hairy, you also have a good chance of being hairy. It also is more common in women of Mediterranean ancestry.

Local hair removal treatments are all that is necessary to handle this condition (see below). Some doctors use spironolactone, but I rarely recommend it. Shaving, electrolysis, and other simple forms of hair removal are much more effective.

Getting Rid of Excess Hair

For many women, hirsutism is seen as cosmetically disfiguring as well as detrimental to one's emotional and social life. It is important to note that all of the above treatments may slow the progression of hirsutism, but may not make the hair go away entirely. The best and most effective ways of doing so are mechanical.

- Electrolysis is the best method known to permanently remove the hair.
- Shaving is fine. Incidentally, hair will *not* grow back thicker. This is a myth.
- Plucking and waxing can lead to inflammation and infection in the skin and are not as good as shaving.
- Bleaching and depilatory creams are helpful but can also cause inflammation of the skin.

- Laser hair removal has still not been perfected. It's expensive, and the hair tends to grow back with time. In the future, better laser techniques may make this the hair-removal therapy of choice.
- Eflornithine hydrochloride (Vaniqa) is a cream recently approved for the treatment of unwanted facial hair. The medication works by inhibiting the biosynthesis of hair proteins. Unfortunately, if the cream is stopped, the hair grows back.
- Finasteride is approved only for use in men and is only available in pill form. Despite this, Dr. Jean Lucus reported in the journal *Endocrine Practice*, that the pills can be ground and mixed into a cream. She was able to demonstrate that the cream decreased hair growth and had very few side effects.

CHAPTER SIX

WOMEN'S
HORMONES

ESTROGEN IS CONSIDERED A "FEMALE" HORMONE, BUT THAT'S REALLY A VAGUE
TERM. After all, both men and women have estrogen (and the other
major "female" hormone, progesterone) just as both men and women
produce testosterone, which is traditionally associated with men. And,
as we've seen, it's androgens like testosterone that are the source of
libido and sexual feelings in both men and women.

Yet estrogen is the hormone that, until recently, was more whis-
pered about and maligned. It doesn't help that men's attitudes aren't
usually the most helpful: It was probably a man who gave estrogen its
name, which is derived from the Greek for "mad with desire." Men
often find the topics of menstruation and menopause a sexual turn-off
or even repulsive. So women don't talk about their hormonal problems
with their male partners, and when those problems start manifesting
themselves in symptoms such as food cravings, mood swings, or
depression, a couple's relationship starts suffering from a great deal of
stress—much of it due to lack of communication.

Well, estrogens can cause problems. And sometimes those problems
aren't just in women. Take this case from the *New England Journal of
Medicine*: A 60-year-old man started gaining weight, stopped needing to
shave, became impotent, and grew "breasts." What was his problem? He
had a form of testicular cancer known as a "leydig-cell tumor of the
testis," a cancer that produced excessive amounts of estrogen. The
excess estrogen was "feminizing" the man. He even began taking on the
shape of a woman, gaining weight in his hips and buttocks.

That's rare, of course. But the point is that high levels of estrogen can cause you to gain weight and that estrogen exists in both men and women. And the better estrogen is understood, the more we understand some of the problems humans, particularly females can have with high or low levels of the hormone.

WHAT IS A "FEMALE" HORMONE?

Estrogen and testosterone are more closely related than people think. Both are steroid hormones, and estrogen is chemically almost identical to testosterone. It's only small changes in the structure of the molecule that make it act differently. And estrogen has its own "steroid hormone receptor," known as the estrogen receptor. Humans actually have two kinds of estrogen receptors, and different receptors have different levels of activity in various parts of the body.

A second "female" hormone is **progesterone**. Though I'll discuss it in more detail later, there are a few things I'd like to bring up now—the main point of which is to indicate that many concepts associated

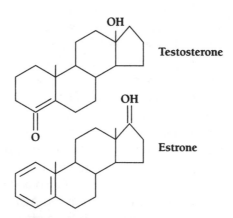

Figure 6.1
CHEMICAL STRUCTURES OF TESTOSTERONE AND ESTRONE
All steroid hormones are built around the same basic structure: a 4-ring framework known as the *steroid nucleus*. Note the minute differences between the testosterone and the estrone.

with estrogen, such as fluid retention, bloating, weight gain, and PMS, are all actually closely linked with progesterone. Think about the name: pro-gesterone—gestation, preparation for pregnancy. In fact, progesterone is thought of as the "pregnancy hormone," but it's much more than that. Unlike estrogen, which is at the end of the line in the steroid synthesis pathway, progesterone is made very early in that process. It can be converted to just about any steroid hormone (see Figure 4.1.).

Two lesser female hormones are **pregnenolone** and **prolactin**. Pregnenolone, in recent years, has been advertised as a cure-all: It's been thought to be a weight-loss medication and an anti-aging hormone, but all we really know is that it's made by the adrenal gland. Alternative-medicine proponents encourage pregnenolone consumption to heal various ills, but I don't encourage it, particularly since it's likely to be converted into other hormones. Prolactin, which is made by the pituitary gland, is responsible for breast milk production. Pituitary gland problems can raise prolactin levels, which can lead to problems with estrogen and progesterone leading to weight gain. High prolactin can also cause a woman (or a man) to produce breast milk, a condition known as *galactorrhea*.

But the focus always returns to estrogen, and we shall do the same. It is estrogen, after all, that helps mold a girl into a woman during puberty. The breasts form, the hips, thighs, and buttocks take their adult shape, and vaginal lubrication increases. (Ironically, other changes in puberty—the growth of pubic and underarm hair, skin oiliness, and certain body odors—are due to androgens, ones more closely associated with males.)

There are three major types of estrogen:

- **Estrone** (E1; -one = one) is produced by fat. Yes, fat makes hormones just like any other gland. (See Chapter 10 for more on fat as an endocrine organ.) Unlike other types of estrogen, estrone promotes storage of fat in the belly and around the organs. As discussed in Chapter 3, this type of "metabolically evil" fat causes insulin resistance. This is why many doctors refer to estrone as a "bad" estrogen. Young women have low levels of estrone because the ovaries can easily convert estrone into estradiol. After menopause, the ovaries lose this ability.
- **Estradiol** (E2; -di = 2) is produced by the ovary and is the predominant estrogen in young women. Estradiol promotes storage of

"healthy" fat around the hips and buttocks. This fat distribution improves insulin resistance and helps stabilize blood sugar levels. Estradiol is responsible for the majority of the positive benefits attributed to estrogen and is known as a "good" estrogen.

- **Estriol** (E3; -tri = 3) is produced by the placenta during pregnancy and is made from other types of estrogen. This is a weaker form of estrogen that has little effect on metabolism.

Each type of estrogen prompts slightly different actions, and each one can be converted into the other. As a rule, that's why they're generally thought of as, simply, estrogens. But, as you can see, all estrogens are not the same. This has led to some of the misunderstandings about estrogen. The estrogen level is not as important as the relative amounts of estrone, estradiol, and estriol. Menopause is associated with a decline in healthy estrogen (estradiol) and a rise in unhealthy estrogen (estrone). Many women have problems with estrogen replacement therapy because they take estrogens that disrupt the normal healthy balance of estradiol and estrone.

YOUR FAT CELLS AND ESTROGEN

Your body contains more than 30 billion fat cells. They're there for a reason: to store fat. When you eat more than your body needs, the fat cells go into storage mode (lipogenesis); when you eat less than you need, the fat cells release fat (lipolysis) to be used for energy.

In women, the fat cells in the hips and buttocks are particularly sensitive to estradiol. You may have heard the old joke about eating fatty foods: "You may as well apply it directly to my hips." That's not far off the mark, actually. Estradiol causes weight gain in a particular body distribution. It's the hips and buttocks that tend to get bigger. When estradiol is low, fat accumulates in the belly.

Ironically, however, the fat in the hips and buttocks is "safe fat." It may not be aesthetically pleasing to many women, particularly given the emphasis on thinness in our society, but that fat is there as protection. When women lose too much weight, the free fatty acids in the blood increase because of the breakdown of this fat. That can be as unhealthy as being overweight.

If you had to choose between lipogenesis and lipolysis, your gut reaction would be to choose the latter—fat breakdown. The truth is, however, that balance is critical. Too much lipolysis can be harmful. Free fatty acids released into the blood as a result of excessive lipolysis can cause insulin resistance. As we've discussed in Chapter 3, that's a recipe for weight gain.

The fat cell contains the aromatase enzyme, which converts androgens to estrogens—primarily estrone. Estrone is the estrogen that gains dominance after menopause, when the ovaries shut down; before that, estradiol is the primary form of estrogen in the body. Given that fat cells convert androgens to estrogen, and that estrogen is primarily estrone, people who are overweight also have—guess what?—a lot more estrone than average. And remember, estrone is the "bad" estrogen that causes insulin resistance.

There's an irony here. The fat cell makes estrogen, but it's also influenced by estrogen. You've probably seen this theme before in the book: that circle of hormones being made by a certain organ, and that certain organ being influenced by the hormone it produces. The body is truly one big feedback machine.

(Incidentally, the metabolically evil fat in your belly also results in too much cortisol—see Chapter 8.)

In terms of weight gain, men and women are not alike. Young women tend to gain weight where they already have fat—the buttocks and hips. Older women and men tend to gain weight in the belly. The former, the classic pear shape, is thought of as *gynoid*; the latter, the apple shape, is called *android*. So, when estradiol production declines and estrone levels rise during and after menopause, fat in women tends to follow the same pattern as fat in men—going to the belly. This shape is associated with a greater risk of heart disease, hypertension, diabetes, and insulin resistance.

(Once again, fat is usually thought of as a bad thing, but when it comes to men and women there are distinct differences in percentage of body fat—and those differences are key. Women need more fat than men. A man with 18 percent body fat is above normal in this department, but a woman with less than 18 percent is on the low side. In fact, women tend to have a number of biological problems when their body fat percentage is less than 18 percent.)

Men and women have about the same number of fat cells, but the enzyme systems between the two sexes have subtle differences. The female fat cell is bigger and has more fat-storage enzymes. Estrogen stimulates fat-storage enzymes and directs where fat will be stored, and it also directs where fat will be lost when a woman diets—making it difficult to lose weight where you want it. (Every woman knows that hips and thighs can be particularly resistant to weight loss.) And men have more muscle than women: Androgens create muscle, and muscle burns fat.

Women's fat cells are also more efficient than men's at storing fat. But consider: fat is protective, a reserve of energy for times of need. Back in the Stone Age, when finding food was a daily gamble, having this reserve meant the difference between life and death—between having the support system for fertility and pregnancy and wasting away.

Estrogen, however, does not make you fat. It's more complicated than that. The point I'm trying to make is that there are differences between men and women with respect to the fat cell and how it responds to estrogen. Besides, estrogen levels have different effects on fat during the course of a woman's life. In some cases, in fact, estrogen can help women lose fat. In the course of this chapter, I'll develop these ideas further.

ESTROGEN AND CANCER

Without question, hormone-related cancers have risen since World War II. Incidences of breast cancer, uterine cancer, colon cancer, prostate cancer, and testicular cancer have all increased—despite advances in medicine and food production. Ironically, some of these advances may have contributed to the increase: Studies indicate that the earlier onset of puberty in boys and girls—and thus an earlier increase in hormonal levels—has been coincident in the rise of hormone-related cancers. The invention of synthetic hormones is also thought to play a role. While these hormones may have short-term pluses, they're not exactly what the body would produce on its own, and the body reacts with increased toxicity.

Obesity tends to indicate the body's hormones are out of whack already and, of course, brings on a host of other ailments—heart disease, stroke, diabetes, you name it. Studies have also shown a connection between obesity and cancer. For women, the number-one threat is breast cancer.

BREAST CANCER AND ESTROGEN

There are more than 180,000 new cases of breast cancer every year; it's second only to lung cancer for cancer-related deaths in women. Moreover, the rates are skyrocketing. Breast cancer is closely linked with the hormones estrogen and progesterone and is being seen with increasing frequency. Cancer cells may contain estrogen receptors and/or progesterone receptors, making its growth dependent on these hormones. It is a disease of Western civilization, just like colon cancer and heart disease. Our environment is full of chemicals that mimic estrogens, and our diet is a high-fat diet, one that leads to fat-cell production of estrogen in the form of estrone. *Obesity dramatically increases a woman's risk of getting breast cancer.*

As has been noted, more fat means more estrogen, and high estrogen levels are associated with breast cancer. However, it's not just the estrogen: Obesity itself increases the risk of breast cancer. Being overweight can also hamper the accuracy of mammograms, making it hard to pick up tumors in their earlier stages.

Alcohol has a mixed role. It has plenty of positive health benefits, including prevention of heart disease and stroke, but it also increases the risk of breast cancer. Like estrogen, alcohol is broken down in the liver. The two compete for metabolism and, essentially, alcohol makes estrogen levels rise. Then we're back on the same road.

Interestingly, the fat in your diet may make your estrogen more dangerous in regard to breast cancer. High-fat diets increase metabolism of estrogen to an "active" form and may be responsible for increasing breast and uterine cancer rates.

If there's a silver lining in a breast cancer discussion, it's that treatments are getting better. Today, more than 90 percent of women with breast cancer survive longer than 5 years after detection.

UTERINE CANCER, COLON CANCER, AND ESTROGEN

As they can with breast cancer, high estrogen levels can also cause uterine cancer; obesity can as well. Elevated estrogen levels cause growth of the lining of the uterus, the part known as the *endometrium*, which increases cancer risk.

However, estrogen may help *prevent* colon cancer, according to a study by the American Cancer Society. The reason, it is suggested, may be that estrogen reduces the concentration of bile acids in the colon. Another study, by the University of Southern California School of Medicine, indicated that menopausal women on estrogen replacement therapy had a one-third lower risk of colon cancer than menopausal women not on estrogen replacement therapy.

ENVIRONMENTAL ESTROGENS

One reason for the increases in breast and uterine cancer rates may be an increase in "environmental estrogens," also known as *xenoestrogens*. These are chemical compounds that have a structure similar to that of natural estrogen. Like estrogen, they can turn on the estrogen receptor. Many modern chemicals—particularly pesticides—are similar in chemical structure to estrogen and have impacts we're only beginning to see. For example, in 1980 a toxic DDT spill in Lake Apopka, Florida, killed off the majority of alligators in the area. The surviving alligators suffered a biological defect due to the estrogen-like properties of the DDT. They had penises 75 percent shorter than the average. Although DDT was banned in the United States in 1972, the pesticide, and its breakdown product DDE, still persists in the environment. Plastic and detergents also contain chemicals similar in structure to estrogen. These substances are stored in your fat and are non-biodegradable.

And it's not just chemicals in the great wide open; it's chemicals where we live. Some tooth fillings have xenoestrogens; so do the linings of cans, meat and milk products, even marijuana. Some of these estrogens come about because of the environmental circle: We spray a field with a pesticide, the cow eats the grass from that field, we drink the milk from the cow, we end up consuming a form of that pesticide. But other estrogens are formed naturally; bacteria inside cow intestines, for example, ferment clover to form natural estrogens. And some estrogens, such as those in many plants, are considered healthy. I'll talk more about healthy estrogens later in this chapter.

ESTROGEN AND YOUR BRAIN

Your brain controls estrogen production and estrogen controls your brain—the feedback loop found with so many hormones and hormone-producing glands. Hormones such as GnRH, FSH, and LH act on the ovary just as they act on the testicle (see Chapter 4). GnRH is produced by the hypothalamus in a pulsatile manner, and the small bursts of this potent hormone stimulate the pituitary gland to make its two hormones—FSH and LH. These hormones work collectively to control the production of hormones from the ovary (see Figure 6.2).

The three main hormones made by the ovary are estrogen, testosterone, and progesterone. Each of these hormones feeds back to the brain in a check-and-balance-type system.

Several other hormones, some of which have been mentioned in this book, also communicate with various parts of the brain. They include **DHEA**, **androstenedione**, **pregnenolone**, **activins**, and **inhibins**. The latter two do exactly what their names state. Activins tell the brain to step up production of FSH and LH; inhibins do the opposite. When everything is working properly, the ovary makes more inhibins, keeping brain stimulation to a low level. When the ovary is in trouble—or when the body needs extra hormones during times like pregnancy—it cranks up production of activins. During menopause, inhibins drop and activins rise, so the pituitary gland pumps out more LH and FSH. High LH and FSH levels, in fact, are the primary indicator of menopause.

Estrogen deficit is also thought to play a role in dementia and Alzheimer's disease. Estrogen replacement at menopause may prevent Alzheimer's, and it's been shown that estrogen improves memory in a typical postmenopausal woman. However, estrogen therapy does *not* improve patients who already have Alzheimer's.

And, just as testosterone makes men (and women) more aggressive, improving libido but also creating shorter fuses, estrogen can help prevent mood swings, anxiety, even depression. For women taking antidepressants, this is important information: The prescribed levels of each substance must be balanced to prevent one or the other throwing moods out of whack.

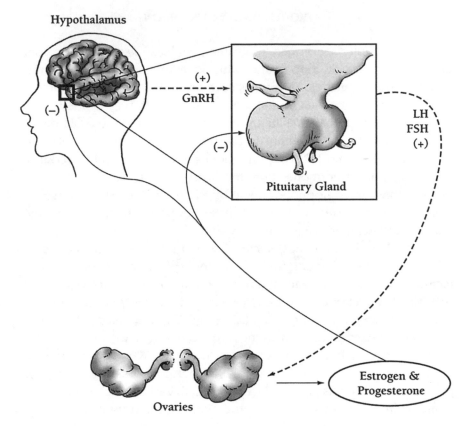

Figure 6.2
ESTROGEN AND PROGESTERONE ENDOCRINOLOGY:
HORMONE FEEDBACK LOOPS

Higher centers in the brain send signals to the hypothalamus, which produces pulses of gonadotropin-releasing hormone (GnRH). GnRH pulses stimulate the pituitary gland to make follicle-stimulating hormone (FSH) and luteinizing hormone (LH), collectively known as gonadotropins. Gonadotropins stimulate the ovaries to produce estrogen and progesterone. Estrogen and progesterone "feed back" to the hypothalamus and pituitary gland, slowing gonadotropin production. Positive "feedback" is denoted by +, and negative "feedback" is denoted by –.

HORMONES CONTROL THE MENSTRUAL CYCLE

It's no secret that the menstrual cycle, with its ebb and flow of estrogen and progesterone production, has a great effect on the rest of the body—particularly mood and appetite. The standard cycle, in terms of hormone production, works like this:

- Day 1 of the cycle is considered the first day of menstrual flow. During and after menstruation, brain FSH levels rise, stimulating the ovary to produce estrogen, thus stimulating the lining of the uterus to proliferate, preparing it for possible pregnancy. This phase, known as the follicular phase, is marked by rising estrogen levels and low progesterone levels.
- About 13 days into the cycle, brain levels of LH and FSH abruptly rise, signaling a critical event in a woman's monthly cycle—ovulation. Women who want to know exactly when they will ovulate can use test strips to test their urine for LH. When urine LH levels spike, ovulation is hours away.
- After ovulation, estrogen levels drop slightly and progesterone levels rise markedly. Progesterone is produced by the ovary in preparation for possible pregnancy. If the egg is fertilized, the lining of the uterus will be healthy and thick, and ready for implantation. If fertilization does not occur, progesterone and estrogen levels drop and the uterus sheds its lining—menstruation. The high progesterone levels just prior to menstruation are responsible for food cravings, mood swings, and many other problems associated with premenstrual syndrome (PMS).

Why bring all this up? Well, the normal hormonal fluctuations of menstruation are perhaps the most elegant hormonal systems in the entire human body (see Figure 6.3). The timing of the GnRH pulses from the hypothalamus controls it all like a conductor of a symphony. Also, if you're a woman, it may help you understand your hormone fluctuations and, in particular for this book, why you have the two most well known side effects of menstruation: cravings and bloating, or fluid retention. Both are related to the very high progesterone levels during the second half of the cycle.

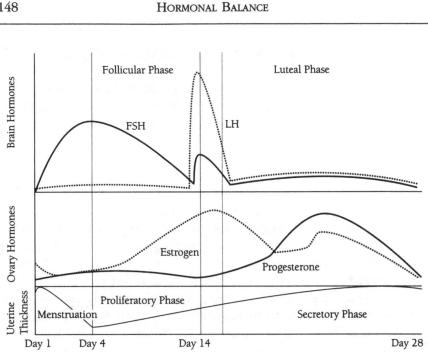

Figure 6.3
HORMONAL CHANGES DURING THE MENSTRUAL CYCLE
The hormonal rhythms of the menstrual cycle. Graph depicts a 28-day cycle.

FOOD CRAVINGS

Many women know about the intense craving for food—particularly chocolate and sweets—that hits during the second half of the menstrual cycle, the time before menstruation. There are a number of theories about this, but essentially it comes down to one simple fact: *Progesterone makes you hungry.*

Why chocolate and sweets? Chocolate—the sweetened, Hershey bar or M&M form we're used to—contains the three most valuable food groups if you're craving food: fat, sugar, and mood-affecting chemicals. Fat, as we know, provides comfort. Sugar offers energy. And the chemicals, which include phenethylmine and theobromine, have the same effect on the brain as more expensive antidepressants, offering a rush of serotonin and a calming influence.

Chocolate gets a lot of guff, but it won't get it from me. Not only does it taste great, it's not the major bugaboo that some health authorities would have you believe. Chocolate was considered an aphrodisiac a few hundred years ago (and there are more than a few people who will tell you it's a worthwhile forerunner to sex today). It doesn't necessarily lead to weight gain, either: The French and Swiss, who eat far more chocolate than Americans do, have less obesity than Americans. Chocolate is rich in substances called *phenolics*, the same chemical in red wine, and may decrease the risk of heart disease as wine does. And chocolate cravings may not necessarily be a sign of weakness, but merely a result of acylethanolamines, chemicals that may have a similar effect on the brain as marijuana. Marijuana has been known to create a condition known as "the munchies," a sudden craving for food. Chocolate can do the same thing.

On a larger level, women may have carbohydrate cravings just before or just after the menstrual period begins. This is because the second half of the menstrual cycle is associated with altered glucose metabolism. As we've seen in previous chapters, a slowdown in metabolism is often answered by a desire for more food, not less—at least until the body exhausts itself. The body wants energy, and the quickest energy is in sugars and starches. The diet I have provided at the end of this book will help eliminate food cravings.

PROGESTERONE MAKES YOU HUNGRY

I mentioned that progesterone is the primary culprit for the cravings that come during the second half of the menstrual cycle when progesterone levels are high. So many diets and explanations focus on estrogen, but it takes both progesterone and estrogen, working together, to coordinate many of the processes important for women. And it's progresterone that is the hormone that provokes appetite. Progesterone also makes you sleepy and less likely to want to exercise. Progesterone causes insulin resistance and makes blood sugar levels rise. This can enhance weight gain, especially during the second half of the menstrual cycle.

The synthetic form of progesterone, incidentally, is called *progestin*, and it's a progestin medications that are used to stimulate appetite in cancer and AIDS patients. Progestins are sometimes used as birth control, the most common forms being Depo-Provera and Norplant. These two forms of birth control cause insulin resistance and weight gain. Progestins are also used to prevent uterine cancer in women who take hormone replacement therapy. There are also other types of progesterone medications, which I'll get into later.

Synthetic progestins have properties similar to those of androgens. In many women, these synthetic hormones cause symptoms of androgen excess such as acne, facial hair, and weight gain. Progesterone—especially in its synthetic forms—can cause insulin resistance and elevated blood sugars.

As I noted earlier, progesterone is a steroid hormone, just like estrogens, androgens, and cortisol. However, though it's similar in chemical structure, it's very different in chemical activity. Progesterone is made very early in the steroid synthesis pathway. In fact, most other steroid hormones can be made from progesterone.

A cousin of progesterone, pregnenolone, is sometimes referred to as "the mother of all hormones." Pregnenolone is very similar to progesterone in structure and can be found in health-food stores in pill form, usually touted as having magical qualities. My guess is that it's nothing special; like progesterone, it's probably just converted into all of the other end-of-the-line hormones, like cortisol, estrogen, testosterone, and progesterone itself.

BLOATING AND FLUID RETENTION

The root of the word *menses*, as in menstrual cycle, comes from "month"—which, in turn, comes from "moon." The moon has a 29-day cycle, more or less; the menstrual cycle is 28 days. In ancient times, the body was considered a miniature universe, and from what we know now, the ancients weren't far wrong. After all, life began with water and the chemical reactions of a developing planet, including the cycles of the moon and the tides. Today, we carry around that history in our DNA.

Unfortunately for many women, water and the menstrual cycle are still closely related. Many women suffer from fluid retention and bloating, conditions that occur just before menses. Not coincidentally, this is a time of high progesterone levels.

Progesterone causes muscle relaxation, particularly in the smooth muscle—the type of muscle found in the uterus and bowels. The uterus relaxes from progesterone as does the smooth muscle of the bowels. During the second half of the menstrual cycle, when progesterone levels are high, the smooth muscle relaxation causes the bowels to expand, stretching the belly and causing the sensation of bloating. The belly sticks out because the muscle tone of the bowels is not as good and cannot keep everything in tight. Bloating is rarely associated with serious disease, though—it is an uncomfortable symptom, but is usually not a symptom of a serious hormonal disorder. Nevertheless, it is a common concern of women. Men can have fluid retention too, but it's usually related to heart, kidney, or liver disease.

Progesterone is also responsible for preparing a woman's body for pregnancy. The same factors are responsible for stimulating appetite and salt cravings. After all, pregnant women need to gain weight.

What can be done about fluid retention and bloating? Here are a few tips:

- *Avoid salt and prepared foods.* Salt makes you retain water. Do not reduce your water intake, though: This will not help, and it can make you dehydrated.
- *Eat fresh fruits and vegetables, and stick to a low-carbohydrate diet.* A high-carbohydrate diet means more insulin and more fluid retention. The eating suggestions I have recommended will lower insulin levels and help with fluid retention.
- *Don't adhere to a no-carbohydrate diet.* A diet with no carbohydrates can cause extreme loss of fluids and salts, and the low-carb diet can cause a milder form of this. With a no-carbohydrate diet, a major problem is dehydration and depletion of body salts—the opposite of what we're talking about here.
- *Avoid foods high in fat, especially high in animal fat.* Fat slows the movement of the intestinal tract and makes bloating worse.
- *Avoid too much fiber.* Although I advocate plenty of fiber, if you have bloating, fiber should be minimized. Fiber swells in the intestines and worsens the sensation of bloating. Beans in particular are high in fiber but also cause gas, which could worsen bloating.
- *Eat small, frequent meals.* Nibbling or "grazing" is good. See my nibbling suggestions in Chapter 2.

- *Don't skip breakfast.*
- *Eliminate—or at least moderate—caffeine and alcohol.* Both have diuretic effects, and both function as stimulants, which artificially raise the body's levels of various hormones, only to send them crashing when the effect wears off.
- *Exercise.* Progesterone tends to make you sleepy—reducing your activity level. Muscle activity is important for reducing fluid retention. As muscles are worked, they force blood into the heart. Swimming can be very good, because the pressure of the water in the pool forces tissue fluid back into the general circulation where it can be eliminated by the kidneys.
- *Use a heating pad.* Yes, heating pads may actually reduce PMS bloating, and they're inexpensive.
- *Lose weight.* All of the above should help you do so, but don't just do these things during "that time of the month." Obesity contributes to fluid retention by increasing pressure inside the abdomen, making it harder for blood to return to the heart.
- *Diuretics.* Diuretics should only be used under the careful supervision of a physician.

Incidentally, fluid retention may not be from progesterone. Idiopathic cyclic edema is an extreme form of menstrual fluid retention. (*Idiopathic* is medical jargon for "we don't know what's causing this.") Severe edema can be a sign of more serious diseases such as heart failure, kidney disease, and liver disease.

PREMENSTRUAL SYNDROME (PMS)

It's the subject of jokes—by both men and women—and remains a misunderstood part of women's biology. It's a time when tempers can get short, appetite can increase, depression can set in . . . and it can all fade away after a few days. It's PMS, premenstrual syndrome (aka premenstrual dysphoric disorder), and it effects as many as 60 percent of all women.

Darlene's Story
Darlene is 38, a mother twice over, a middle manager in a paper company. Every month before her period, she becomes irritable and depressed. She lashes out at her children, her

*husband, her pets, and the slightest incident—a dropped glass,
a car cutting in front of her on the expressway—becomes
cause for a huge blowup. She's collapsed in tears and practically slugged a co-worker. Sometimes this period can last for
more than half the month.*

*Darlene laughs off the symptoms—after they've safely gone
away—and calls it PMS. "Oh, you'd better not get near me
when I'm PMSing," she'll tell others, but she wonders: Is this
really PMS? Or is she being affected by something more serious?*

*It doesn't help that there are physical problems, too. She
feels achy. Her breasts swell. She gets occasional panic attacks.
And the problem has only gotten worse as she has gotten older.*

*Is there hope for Darlene? Does she indeed have PMS, or is
it something else?*

From a medical standpoint, the problem with PMS is that it's such
a broad designation. There are several common symptoms—food cravings, food binges, bloating and fluid retention, weight gain, increased
hunger, depression, crying spells, fatigue, and headaches. But we're
still not sure what causes PMS. Many physicians blame progesterone,
but hormonal theories remain controversial. PMS may also be a sign of
an androgen disorder (see Chapter 5). What is known is that PMS is a
problem in the brain and that it's caused by the brain's response to hormones.

The good news is that PMS can be tamed, if not cured:

- Stick to the eating suggestions recommended in this book.
- Exercise and try to reduce your stress.
- Stop smoking.
- Minimize caffeine intake.
- Get plenty of sleep.
- And you're allowed a little chocolate. Just don't overdo it.

A number of medications and vitamins help improve PMS symptoms. These include

- *Calcium supplements.* Calcium is recommend to help prevent
  osteoporosis, but it also helps decrease the symptoms of PMS. I recommend taking 1,500 mg each day. I discuss calcium in more detail
  later in this chapter.

- *B-complex vitamins,* especially vitamin B6, increase brain serotonin levels. This helps reduce symptoms of moodiness, irritability, and carbohydrate cravings.
- *Vitamins C and E* (fruits and vegetables are an excellent source of both).
- *Spironolactone* (a prescription diuretic—use with caution).
- *Natural progesterone.*
- *Estrogen.*
- *Selective serotonin reuptake inhibitor,* or SSRI, antidepressants, such as Celexa, Prozac (also marketed as Sarafem specifically for PMS), Paxil, Zoloft, and Luvox. These medications are gaining increasing popularity among physicians for treatment of PMS.
- *Evening primrose oil* (which contains vitamin E) tends to help with the symptoms of PMS. The dose is 3–4 grams per day.
- *Birth control pills,* with many caveats: particularly that women should use the one with the least possible progestin and must not smoke. If the pills are too high in synthetic progestin or are the wrong type for a particular woman, they can make symptoms worse.

BIRTH CONTROL PILLS AND HOW THEY WORK

The birth control pill has become a regular part of care for millions of women all over the world. Ten million U.S. women take the Pill, and despite 40 years of hand-wringing and doomy warnings from anti-birth-control forces, it has become an accepted part of the American scene.

But the Pill is not without its side effects. It's been blamed, somewhat justifiably, for weight gain—a condition due to the synthetic progesterone rather than the estrogen. It also raises the risk of stroke or heart attack in women over 35 who smoke. (Women in this demographic group should not take the pill.) It's also not a cure-all: For example, it does nothing to stop the transmission of AIDS.

On the positive side, however, those same hormones clear up acne and help prevent ovarian and uterine cancer. The newer versions of birth control pills also don't prompt the same weight-gain problems earlier pills did.

How do birth control pills work? They work by following part of the feedback loop that creates so many of the conditions of the human body. The relatively high doses of estrogen in the pill suppress FSH and LH surges. In turn, this suppression prevents ovulation and pregnancy. Women on the Pill must take it regularly, of course: These hormones return to normal levels very quickly, and once a woman goes off the pill her regular menstrual cycles will resume.

Incidentally, there are literally dozens of brands of birth control pills on the market, in price ranges from less than $10 a month to almost $50. Each of these brands contains different types and/or amounts of estrogen and progestin.

Oral contraceptive pills or (OCPs) come with estrogen in varying amounts: low, medium and high (see Table 6.1). When your weight is concerned, the **medium-dose estrogen is the best** (30–40 mcg ethinyl estradiol). High-dose estrogen (50 mcg) can cause nausea, headaches, and weight gain. The low-estrogen pills may also cause weight gain.

The dose and type of progesterone in these pills varies considerably. All the progesterones are synthetic. As I have discussed, these synthetic progesterones can cause weight gain, bloating, edema, and depression. Some of the progestins have more androgenic properties than others (see Chapter 5). Many birth control pills contain androgenic progestins such as **levonorgestrel, norgestrel,** or **norethindrone**. These are the progesterones that have the most androgenic activity. And that's what's responsible for some of the side effects of birth control pills, such as acne and bloating. These progesterones can also cause insulin resistance. The best synthetic progestins are **desogestrol** and **norgestimate**. They are associated with less weight gain and lower risk of blood clots. Ortho-Cyclen and Ortho-Tri-Cyclen contain norgestimate. Apri, Desogen, Ortho-Cept, and Mircette contain desogestrel.

Yasmin contains a unique progestin, drospirenone, which may actually block androgens. Drospirenone is similar to a medication, called spironolactone, which blocks testosterone action (known as an antiandrogen), blocking both the production and action of androgens. Drospirenone also blocks the hormone aldosterone, which influences the regulation of water and electrolyte balance in the body. This means less fluid retention and bloating when compared to other progestins. It also means that if you take Yasmin, your doctor should periodically check blood electrolyte levels.

Table 6.1
TYPES OF BIRTH CONTROL PILLS

Low-Estrogen OCPs (20 mcg ethinyl estradiol)

Alesse	Loestrin 1/20
Levlite	Mircette

Medium-Estrogen OCPs (30–35 mcg ethinyl estradiol)

Apri	Nordette
Brevicon	Norinyl
Demulen 1/35	Norethin 1/35
Desogen	Ortho Tri-Cyclen
Estrostep	Ortho-Cept
Genora 1/35	Ortho-Cyclen
Jenest	Ortho-Novum 1/35
Levlen	Ortho-Novum 10/11
Levora	Ortho-Novum 7/7/7
Lo/Ovral	Ovcon 35
Loestrin 1/30	Tri-Levlen
Low-Ogestrel	Tri-Norinyl
Modicon	Triphasil
Necon .5/35	Trivora
Nelova 1/35	Yasmin
Neocon 1/35	Zovia 1/35
Neocon 10/11	

High-Estrogen OCPs (50 mcg ethinyl estradiol or mestranol)

Demulin 1/50	Ogestrel
Genora 1/50	Ortho-Novum 1/50
Nelova 1/50	Ovcon
Neocon 1/50	Ovral
Norinyl 1/50	Zovia 1/50

Birth control pills come in two main classes, *monophasic combination pills* and *multiphasic combination pills*. This refers to the dose of estrogen and progesterone. Monophasic pills keep the dose of estrogen and progesterone the same throughout the entire month. Multiphasic pills vary the dose of estrogen and/or progestin throughout the month. The rationale for multiphasic pills is that they more closely simulate the hormonal fluctuations of a normal menstrual cycle. There is no evidence, however, that there is an advantage to taking a multiphasic over a monophasic pill.

For most women, I recommend Desogen, Otho-Cept, Ortho-Cyclen, Ortho Tri-Cyclen, or Yasmin because these birth control pills contain both an ideal level of estrogen and the less-androgenic progestins.

SIDE EFFECTS OF BIRTH CONTROL PILLS

The major side effects are as follows:

- *Weight gain.* This is usually seen with the very high and very low dose birth control pills. To avoid this side effect, stick with a dose of ethinyl estradiol in the 30–40 mcg range.
- *Acne.* Most pills will improve acne, but sometimes the acne gets worse before it gets better. This is because the pill raises blood protein levels, especially sex-hormone binding globulin (SHBG). Increased SHBG means lower "free testosterone" levels and less acne. Pills that contain the third-generation progesterone, **norgestimate**, such as Ortho-Cyclen and Ortho Tri-Cyclen, have been shown in two clinical trials to improve acne. Sometimes, however, acne may get worse with the pill.
- *Insulin resistance.* To a small extent, all of the progestins in birth control pills cause *some* low-level insulin resistance. Birth control pills with levonorgestrel, norgestrel, or norethindrone may cause more insulin resistance than others.
- *Blood clots.* Life-threatening blood clots are a real risk with birth control pills. The risk is highest if you smoke cigarettes. If you smoke, I recommend that you do not use birth control pills.
- *Other side effects.* Birth control pills may make PMS worse and may cause nausea, breast swelling and tenderness, headache, and depression. If you get nauseated, try taking the pill in the evening instead of the morning.

PROGESTERONE-ONLY BIRTH CONTROL

Other forms of hormonal contraception—usually pure progesterone in one form or another—work by making the uterus unfavorable for pregnancy. With progesterone-only birth control, *ovulation can still occur and so can fertilization.* The woman can actually be "pregnant" for 2 to 3 days, but since the embryo cannot grow in the unfavorable conditions of the uterus, it dies.

There is, technically, a third class of birth control pills, the progesterone-only "minipill." It's rarely used because of the weight gain and other side effects of progesterone. The progesterone most regularly used is called norethindrone, which has more androgen activity than other progesterones. It may temper some of the weight-gain problems but comes with other side effects, including irregular bleeding. Progestin-only OCPs include Micronor, Nor-QD, and Ovrette. My advice is: If you're thinking of going on the minipill, think about condoms instead. You'll be better off.

A handful of birth control medications are designed to be taken periodically instead of daily. These include Depo-Provera and Norplant. Depo-Provera is a shot given once every 3 months, though a monthly version is also in trials. It tends to cause weight gain and depression more than most birth control medications. Some physicians push it because it's cheap, easy, and effective, but the side effects aren't worth it. Avoid Depo-Provera at all costs. Norplant gained a lot of notoriety several years ago when it was first produced. It's a series of tiny capsules that are implanted under the skin—usually in the forearm—and slowly release progesterone for up to 5 years. In the short run, it's a very cheap and effective birth control method. But in the long run, it causes a lot of weight gain and bloating. It's also been seen as a classist type of birth control, since it's routinely given to poor or underprivileged women.

Progesterone-containing intrauterine devices (IUD) (Progestasert and Mirena) release small amounts of progesterone into the lining of the uterus. Little progesterone is transferred to the rest of the body. They are useful for birth control and cause less side effects than other types of progesterone-only birth control. A 2001 study found that these devices may be an excellent alternative to hysterectomy for women who have excessive menstrual flow.

DOES MENOPAUSE CAUSE WEIGHT GAIN?

The average woman goes through menopause at age 50 and dies at age 80. That's 30 years of postmenopausal life. On average, women gain about 10 pounds in the first few years after menopause. Moreover, the body shape may change, with more weight going to the belly.

Why this weight gain? Is it the fault of menopause?

Doctors refer to menopause as a state of "estrogen deficiency." Most physicians agree that if you are postmenopausal, taking estrogen replacement therapy (ERT, or HRT for hormone replacement therapy) has many health benefits. But the therapy is not without risks. For some it is a smart move, while other women are better off not taking hormones. The biggest concerns about hormone replacement therapy in the eyes of women include weight gain, cancer, blood clots, heart attacks, and strokes, all of which are possible, and all of which have scared women off HRT at one time or another.

In fact, most postmenopausal women still do not take hormone replacement therapy (HRT). It is estimated that only 20 percent of women who could take hormones are given the opportunity to do so by their physician. And among those who are prescribed HRT, half stop taking the hormones within the first year.

Estrogen has both positive and negative effects on other parts of the body. To the heart, estrogen is generally positive. For years, doctors have thought that estrogen is good for the cardiac muscle. It has a beneficial effect on cholesterol and insulin resistance, and with its decline during menopause, the risks of heart disease and diabetes immediately increase.

So, it seems that HRT would be a good thing—that putting some estrogen back in the body would be just as beneficial as when it was there in the first place. But it's a controversial subject. Estrogen may have links to uterine cancer, breast cancer, and other ailments, so some doctors see HRT as a trade-off.

Although it's wise to keep these concerns in mind, remember this: Estrogen replacement therapy, when taken in the proper dosage and form, improves insulin resistance and body fat distribution. (The key is "taken in the proper dosage and form"—if estrogen medication is taken in higher dosages or the wrong form, it can *worsen* insulin resistance; and if it is taken via "the patch" as opposed to pills, some positive effects are diminished as well.)

HORMONE FLUXES AND WEIGHT GAIN
DURING THE TRANSITION TO MENOPAUSE

Perimenopause is the time of transition just before a woman enters menopause. It's not always a gentle time. For a time—years in some

women—a woman may have alternating periods of low estrogen, leading to the symptoms listed below, mixed with surges of very high estrogen levels. These symptoms wax and wane, causing even more problems. It's commonly misdiagnosed as depression.

Perimenopause is also a time when many women gain weight,
especially in the belly. Women who have always carried their weight
on their hips and buttocks may now experience a shift in the distribution of body fat to the middle section.

When estrogen levels become low, women frequently experience
vasomotor symptoms. The most common of these is called the "hot
flash" or "hot flush," the latter term preferred by endocrinologists. Sleep
disturbance is one of the most common symptoms of perimenopause.
Sleep problems then cause disruption in growth hormone production
(see Chapter 9).

Meanwhile, menstrual cycles may become irregular. Estrogen will
surge at times, causing episodes of very heavy bleeding. The estrogen
surges can also contribute to the growth of benign uterine tumors known
as fibroid tumors, simply called "fibroids" or "fireballs." They almost
never cause cancer, but they are one of the most common reasons for
needing a hysterectomy. Some can become quite large, up to 30 or 40
pounds. One patient of mine gained 40 pounds when she was in her
early 40s. All the weight was up front, leading her (and many of her
friends) to believe she had become pregnant. The truth turned out to be
far less joyous—she had a 40-pound fibroid uterine tumor. She underwent a successful operation and her weight is now back to normal.

Meanwhile, along with the estrogen surges—which cause weight
gain and bleeding—come periods of low estrogen levels. It's at this
time women begin to lose the protective effect of estrogen. The risk of
heart disease increases, bad cholesterol goes up while good cholesterol
tumbles, osteoporosis sets in, and fat distribution begins to change.

Usually, estrogen (especially estradiol) causes fat to go to the hips,
buttocks, and under the skin. But, as estradiol levels drop in the early
stages of menopause, and estrone takes on increasing importance, fat
moves to the belly. This "visceral fat" or "abdominal adiposity" is the
metabolically evil fat I have discussed in earlier chapters. Many women
note their breasts and hips get smaller, but they gain weight in their bellies during this time. When menopause is complete, this effect on
weight distribution is even more pronounced.

Menopause is a stressful situation. Stress causes hormonal changes that slow metabolism and promote weight gain including insulin resistance, low thyroid hormone activity, high cortisol, and low growth hormone.

Other symptoms kick in. Progesterone production declines, followed by erratic estrogen fluctuations. In many women, loss of androgens that begins during perimenopause is associated with symptoms of female low-androgen syndrome (see Chapter 5). Menstrual cycles become irregular; hot flashes, sleep disturbances, vaginal dryness, weight gain in the belly, and shrinkage of breasts may occur. The fluctuations in hormones cause emotional fluctuations.

It's at this time women should carefully consider starting hormone replacement therapy or even low-dose birth control pills. This is because changes due to *estrogen deficiency* begin in the body during the perimenopause. In particular, bone begins to thin, brain cells begin to die, and arteries begin to accumulate blockages.

So there are many reasons why you start to gain weight as you near menopause. All are intimately related to your hormones. But you are not doomed. Estrogen therapy can help reverse these effects.

MENOPAUSE MAKES WOMEN LOOK AND FEEL OLDER

The average age of menopause is 51. This hasn't changed since records were first kept about this life change, about 600 A.D. In the perimenopausal years, estrogen production has been declining; now the aging ovary shuts down and stops making estrogen entirely. Progesterone deficiency occurs as well, though its significance is less well understood.

With estrogen deficiency now a fact of life, the symptoms of menopause start in earnest. They include

- *Weight gain*, especially around the belly
- *Hot flashes*, also known as "hot flushes" because the woman may become red and flushed
- *Vaginal dryness* and *pain with intercourse* (dyspareunia)
- *Urinary tract infections*
- *Dry skin*
- *Depression*

- *Loss of memory*
- *Migraines*
- *Sleeping problems* and *insomnia*
- *Fatigue*
- *Irritability*
- *Osteoporosis or osteopenia*
- *Heart disease*

MENOPAUSE AND YOUR BONES

Ironically, women who are overweight before menopause do have an advantage: They have stronger bones. All the extra estrogen from the excess fat they carry has helped the bones stay strong; moreover, carrying around all that weight has made bones stronger as well.

Think of a person in space. Routinely, astronauts who go up in space for long lengths of time come back to earth having lost bone mass; without gravity, the bones aren't used as much as they are on earth, and they start to thin out. It's the "loading" of bone that makes them healthy and strong. Overweight men and women, in general, have stronger bones than thin people.

Despite this, overweight women can still have *osteoporosis* (thinning of the bones). Many doctors urge menopausal women to enter into HRT, partly because the estrogen helps stop the progression of osteoporosis.

Osteoporosis is a painless, silent disease. Unless tested for it, most people have no idea they even have it unless they break a bone. And once a bone is broken, the chances of acquiring another illness—such as pneumonia or a blood clot—are greatly increased if the person isn't able to get up and move around. Fractures of the spine known as compression fractures make women shorter as they age, and give them that all-too-familiar humped back, known as *kyphosis*. Indeed, many women with osteoporosis die within a year of their first broken bone.

But osteoporosis is preventable. Among the treatments are the following:

- **Estrogen and SERMs.** Estrogen stops the progression of osteoporosis and helps firm bone matter. Despite a number of new therapies for osteoporosis, in fact, estrogen is still the best. SERMs are a new type of "designer estrogen," discussed later in this chapter.

- **Calcitonin**. A synthetic form of a thyroid hormone, this is taken by nasal spray, and when taken in addition to calcium, can increase bone density. It does have side effects.
- **Bisphosphate medications**. These are medications, including alendronate (Fosamax) and risedronate (Actonel), which work directly on bone.
- **Vitamin D**. Vitamin D is actually a steroid hormone, and one that allows your gut to absorb calcium. Without it, most of the calcium you eat passes right out into your stool. Most people get their dose of vitamin D from sunlight and dairy products, yet many women remain deficient in this vitamin. Like most vitamins and minerals, it's available in supplement form: 800 IU—two multivitamin pills—is the dose I recommend.
- **Exercise**. Weight-bearing exercises, such as walking and lifting weights, are best for rebuilding bone. They also help add lean body mass, losing fat and improving insulin resistance.
- **Calcium**. This key mineral becomes even more important to women as they age. If a person suffers from a lack of calcium, the body will take the difference directly out of the skeleton. Physicians recommend at least three 8-ounce glasses of milk each day (skim milk and whole milk have the same amount of calcium, incidentally) or their equivalent.

How much calcium?

- Before menopause, a minimum of 1,000 mg in food and/or supplements per day
- During and after menopause, at least 1,000 mg per day—if you're taking estrogen
- Without estrogen replacement therapy, at least 1,500 mg per day

---

Keep in mind that the average American consumes less than 800 mg per day.

Calcium should be consumed over the course of the day, not all at once, and always with plenty of water. (All humans should drink plenty of water *anyway*—not only does it help with absorption, as in the case of calcium, but it flushes the system.) Unfortunately, high-fiber diets prevent the absorption of calcium, so you should take this into consideration when taking calcium supplements. Better to get your calcium as *part* of such a diet, not *in addition* to it. Calcium itself interferes with the absorption of iron, so iron supplements and calcium supplements should not be taken at the same time.

All calcium preparations contain "elemental calcium" for a simple reason: calcium is an element, number 20 on the periodic table. But it cannot exist alone, and must be bound to another atom or molecule to be stable. For this reason, not all calcium supplements are created equal. Calcium carbonate, for example, is about 40 percent calcium, so the typical 1,250-mg tablet has about 600 mg of elemental calcium. But calcium citrate, however, contains only *21 percent* calcium—so an equivalent tablet has almost 300 mg less elemental calcium. It's an old saw, but true: Always read those labels!

Calcium carbonate is the most common calcium preparation available. It's got the highest percentage of calcium and is readily available in sources ranging from oyster shells to antacid tablets. Calcium itself is a mineral in milk, cheese, yogurt, collard greens, kale, broccoli, and sardines.

EARLY MENOPAUSE

For some women, menopause doesn't begin at age 50 or so, but more than 5 years earlier, before the age of 45. What causes this condition?

There are several reasons. Since the essential result of menopause is that the ovaries stop functioning, most of these reasons have a direct effect on those organs. (Early menopause is also called POF, for *premature ovarian failure*.) It may be that the ovaries are simply depleted of eggs. It may be that the woman has taken medication that has damaged the ovaries. A woman may have an autoimmune condition that has damaged the ovaries with various antibodies. Or, finally, a woman may have what is known as "Savage syndrome," in which the ovarian follicles are in an immature state and do not respond to the brain hormones, LH and FSH.

One thing to keep in mind: Not all of these reasons happen because of severe illness or a congenital condition. Smoking is a source of damage to the ovary as well. Women who smoke go through menopause 1 to 2 years earlier than women who do not smoke.

Other disorders that cause early menopause include

- *Pituitary disorders.* Tumors and other causes of high prolactin levels are associated with cessation of periods and sometimes galactorrhea (breast milk production).
- *Hypothalamic amenorrhea.* This is caused by brain tumors, starvation, or excessive exercise. When a woman's body fat drops below a certain percentage, you'll recall, the brain shuts the ovary down as a form of self-protection. It's the reason why many women with *anorexia nervosa*, as well as female athletes, stop having periods.

TESTING FOR MENOPAUSE

From previous chapters, you'll recall that many hormone tests aren't the be-all and end-all for diagnoses. So many variables come into play, so many mistakes can be made, that you should always make sure that (1) your doctor is very familiar with your diet and lifestyle and that (2) your doctor is aware of how to properly interpret test results, before you allow the diagnosis to stand.

In women, there are additional variables. Levels of female hormones undergo tremendous fluctuations over the course of a month, something that is simply part of the female cycle. **Symptoms of menopause—such as vaginal dryness, hot flashes, and a loss of sex drive—in combination with cessation of menstrual periods, are about as good an indicator as any blood test.** Most women do not need, and have never needed, a blood test to tell them they are menopausal.

Nevertheless, here is information on the basic tests used to determine menopause:

- *FSH level.* The most common blood test used. As the ovary makes less and less estrogen, the brain responds by increasing FSH levels. Although both LH and FSH come from the pituitary gland to control the ovary, FSH is the first hormone to rise in menopause. Doctors call this a "monotropic FSH rise."

The elevation of FSH with a normal LH is a common situation in early menopause. If you are still menstruating, the best time to measure an FSH level is on the second day of the menses. If the FSH level is more than 10 mIU/mL, it means the ovaries are beginning to fail. An FSH level over 40 mIU/mL suggests menopause, but should be confirmed by a second test. FSH levels fluctuate wildly, so repeat testing often gives very different results.

- *LH level.* LH is another brain hormone. Eventually LH will rise, but FSH is the first indicator. Moreover, by the time LH rises, menopause is obvious, so there's really no reason to do blood tests for it.

- *Estradiol level.* This is an indicator of "healthy" estrogen levels. Estradiol levels drop in menopause, but estrone (the estrogen made from fat) may actually go up. Estradiol should be checked on day 2 or 3 of the menstrual cycle (follicular phase; see Figure 6.3). An estradiol level less than 80 pg/mL is suggestive of estrogen deficiency, and levels below 50 pg/mL are highly suggestive of estrogen deficiency. Levels up to 200 pg/ml are considered normal. Remember, levels can fluctuate wildly during perimenopause. High estradiol levels do not mean that you do not have an estrogen problem.

Estradiol levels can also be used to monitor the adequacy of hormone replacement therapy (HRT). If you are on HRT and are tired, gaining weight, or have other symptoms of menopause, your dose may be too low. Many women have symptoms of menopause (including weight gain in the middle) when estradiol levels are below 80 pg/mL.

TREATMENT OF MENOPAUSE: ESTROGEN REPLACEMENT THERAPY

Menopause is frequently associated with weight gain—on average, several pounds. But not all women gain weight, and some women gain quite a lot. Obviously, other factors come into play: heredity, weight distribution, diet, physical activity.

Estrogen replacement therapy does not necessarily help women lose weight. It may only redistribute weight (fat) to the chest and hips, places where it was in more youthful days, instead of the stomach, where it tends to go during and after menopause. And a quarter of women who take estrogen actually gain weight, even if only a couple pounds of fluid retention. This is one of the reasons that only 30 percent of all menopausal women take HRT.

But what estrogen *can* do is improve vitality and insulin resistance, two key factors in battling the bulge. Estrogen can help a woman feel younger, helping her to maintain a more active lifestyle—as well as muscle. Although estrogen does not have a major effect on weight, it does on body composition. Studies confirm that women who take estrogen have more muscle and less fat than those who do not. Keep that in mind: If you're overweight and start estrogen, you will lose fat and gain muscle but your weight may not change.

Estrogen Medications for Menopause

Estradiol pills *(Estrace and generics)*
This is pure **estradiol** in the form of 17-beta estradiol. Micronization is a special manufacturing process that produces a pill that dissolves into very small pieces. This allows the estradiol to be easily absorbed into the system. Estradiol is called a "natural" estrogen because it is the most abundant in the body during the reproductive years and is responsible for many of the positive benefits attributed to estrogen. Estrace is available in 0.5 mg, 1 mg, and 2 mg tablets and is available as combination estradiol/progesterone products Activella, FemHRT, and Ortho-Prefest. Estradiol is also available as cream, patches, and a vaginal ring (see below).

Estradiol patches *(Estraderm, Alora, Climara, and Vivelle)*
This is also known as *transdermal estrogen therapy*. As we discussed earlier, the patch has both advantages and disadvantages. The patch has less benefit when it comes to insulin resistance and improving cholesterol. On the other hand, the patch is associated with fewer blood clots. The blood clot issue makes the patch a better alternative for smokers.

The patch provides the steadiest levels of estrogen. Estrogen levels spike then fall after taking the pill, but remain constant on the patch. But there are problems to be aware of: The patch can fall off or irritate the skin. Dosing is inflexible—if you need something in between the available patch doses, you are out of luck. You can't take half a patch like you can take half a pill. Climara patch and Vivelle patches have partially addressed this issue by making four different dose strengths available.

Conjugated equine estrogens (CEE) *(Premarin and generics)*
Many consider this a synthetic estrogen, but Premarin is a natural form of estrogen (just not natural to humans). CEE is a collection of estrogens extracted from the urine of pregnant mares, thus "pre-mar-in." Because it comes from horses, it is "natural." The exact components of Premarin have never been completely characterized, but the substance contains at least 10 different estrogens. The most abundant of these is estrone. Estrone is the type of estrogen that is associated with insulin resistance and weight gain. Premarin is by far the most commonly prescribed estrogen for menopause, and it's the form of estrogen doctors are most experienced with. Another concern with CEE is that besides estrone, CEE contains other forms of estrogen not natural for humans; these are estrogens for horses known as *equilenin* and *equilin*.

To date, horse estrogens have not been shown to have any harmful effects, but still, many women claim they feel better taking other types of estrogen.

Conjugated synthetic estrogens *(Cenestin)*
Cenestin is a *synthetic* form of CEE and also contains high levels of estrone. Because Cenestin is so new, no one has any long-term experience with this hormone.

Esterified estrogens *(Estratab and Menest)*
These contain several types of estrogens derived from plants. Estrone is the primary ingredient.

Estropipate *(Ogen, Ortho-Est, and generics)*
This type of estrogen is very similar in chemical structure to estrone. As discussed, estrone is a "bad" estrogen and can contribute to insulin resistance and weight gain, but there is no proof, in the proper doses, that estropipate does this. It's another natural estrogen and worth a try if other estrogens have not worked.

Low-dose birth control pills

These are probably not good for menopausal women, but peri-menopausal women may consider taking a low-dose birth control pill as their form of hormone replacement therapy. Pills containing the 20 mcg dose of ethinyl estradiol are OK, but the progesterone in these pills may cause weight gain.

Estrogen injections

These are available from some doctors. I rarely recommend injections except under very unusual situations.

Estrogen implants

These are small pellets of estradiol, which are implanted under the skin and last about 3 months. Some physicians have made a whole career into implanting these pellets into women. I do not recommend hormone implants. There is too much variability in the blood levels of estrogen and levels can skyrocket.

Vaginal estrogen creams

Among the forms are micronized estradiol cream (Estrace cream), estropipate cream (Ogen cream), conjugated estrogen cream (Premarin cream), and dienestrol cream (OrthoDienestrol cream). However, the only thing the cream is good for is vaginal and urinary symptoms (known as *atrophic vaginitis*). Only small amounts of estrogen enter the general circulation via the vagina, which means patients lose most of the benefits (though, of course, most of the problems as well). The creams are *not* an equivalent of a pill or a patch.

Vaginal ring

Estring is a flexible, time-release source of estrogen that is inserted into the vagina like a diaphragm. It can be left in place for up to 3 months. Like the cream, the estrogen from the ring is not absorbed into the bloodstream and is therefore good only for vaginal symptoms (dryness) and urinary problems.

Natural menopause supplements

Many of the natural menopause products available in grocery stores, drug stores, and health food stores contain soy isoflavones. *Isoflavones* are chemicals extracted from plants (like soybeans) that are similar to (but not exactly the same) as estrogen. A recent study in monkeys showed that "soy protein isolates" were better than CEE in preventing hardening of the arteries. More studies are needed. For the most part, at this time, I am hesitant to recommend these products. Concentrations of isoflavones can vary tremendously from brand to brand and from pill to pill. In addition, because isoflavones are not identical to estrogen, their effects are not identical to those of estrogen. I do recommend consuming foods high in plant estrogens to help with menopausal symptoms (see below).

Here are some things to think about if you're considering estrogen replacement therapy:

- *What about estrogen's side effects?* Nausea and breast tenderness are the most common side effects of estrogen. It usually helps to start at a very low dose and increase gradually. Also, weight gain, vaginal discharge, acne, and headaches may accompany HRT.
- *Estrogen and your weight.* Estrogen medications do not cause significant weight gain; however, you may notice a change in body composition. You will have an increase in lean tissue (muscle and bone) and a decrease in fat. This may lead to a small increase in weight (but a smaller body).
- *"Natural" vs. "synthetic."* Most estrogens come from natural sources but natural does not always mean better. As mentioned earlier, Premarin, which is considered a "natural" hormone, is extracted from the urine of pregnant horses and contains estrogens that are foreign to humans.
- *Dosing and brands.* There is no "cookbook" dose of estrogen. In my experience, women usually have to try two or three (sometimes more) different doses or brands of estrogen until they find the one that suits them. If you've had problems with estrogen in the past, don't give up—it's likely you'll find a regime that works for you. I usually start a patient with a low dose of estradiol and increase the dose over the next 6 to 12 months. If this doesn't do the trick, I will switch her to a different form of estrogen.
- *Pills vs. patch.* Each has its advantages and disadvantages. Estrogen pills are absorbed through the intestines to the bloodstream and then transported to the liver, where they are metabolized. This is known as the *first-pass effect.* (Remember: The liver is an important

organ in the insulin resistance game; it's through the liver that estrogen improves insulin sensitivity. (See Chapter 3.) For the most part, estrogen pills improve insulin resistance. The estrogen patch avoids the liver and has less effect on insulin. Estrogen in patches is absorbed through the skin and then transported directly into general circulation, so the effects on the liver are greatly diminished, though not eliminated. Estrogen pills decrease LDL (bad) cholesterol and increase HDL (good) cholesterol, but the patch's impact is, again, diminished. Estrogen pills, ironically, can increase triglycerides, but the patch can lower them. The patch causes fewer blood clots, and possibly fewer migraine headaches and gallbladder problems, than the pill.

- *Menstruation or not?* With **cyclic dosing**, a larger dose of progesterone is added to the daily estrogen for 5 to 14 days a month. You will continue to have monthly cycles. The natural hormonal cycles are mimicked in this regime, but it is far from being exactly like the natural hormonal ebb and flow. Expect to have a short and light menstrual period 6 hours or so after the last dose of the month. The periods will be very regular. This form of HRT can also result in PMS, something most women would like to avoid. Twenty percent of women taking cyclic dosing will stop having periods after a while. This is OK: The lining of the uterus has simply become inactive.

  With **continuous dosing**, a smaller dose of progesterone, in combination with estrogen, is taken every day. You may have irregular and unpredictable spotting for up to 6 months, but then there should have no further bleeding. Most women prefer this to the cyclic dosing. Continuous dosing protects from uterine cancer better than cyclic dosing.

  Combination medications containing both continuous and cyclic progesterone regimes are available, including **Activella, FemHRT, Prempro,** and **Premphase**. A combination patch, **CombiPatch,** is also available.

  A new regime for HRT is known as **pulsed progestin HRT**. Here the progesterone is given for 3 days on, 3 days off. The difference is perhaps fewer side effects and better protection against uterine cancer than traditional continuous dosing, without the withdrawal bleeding you will have with cyclic dosing. **Ortho-Prefest** is a combination estrogen/progestin product that alternates 3 days of estradiol alone with 3 days of estradiol plus the progestin, norgestimate.

HRT IS NOT FOR EVERYONE

Women should **not** take estrogen when these circumstances occur:

*   *Estrogen-responsive cancers, especially breast and uterine (endometrial) cancer.* The line is becoming blurred here, though, especially with breast cancer. Some doctors will prescribe estrogen for a woman who is considered "cured" of breast cancer (usually 5 to 7 years out without evidence of recurrence). Often, the tumor tissue is tested for the presence of an *estrogen receptor.* If the tumor did not have an estrogen receptor ("estrogen receptor negative") and it looks like the cancer is gone, some doctors will prescribe estrogen under very close supervision. Though family history of breast cancer is not an absolute contraindication of estrogen use, many women choose not to take estrogen for this reason. If you do have a family history of breast cancer and you take estrogen, careful monitoring by your physician is imperative.
*   *Blood clots (aka "thromboembolic events").* As mentioned earlier, estrogen can make the blood clot more easily, leading to blood clots in the legs, lungs and brain. Smoking further enhances this risk. If you take estrogen, you should not smoke. Moreover, women who take estrogen and get sick and can't get out of bed may want to consider not taking their estrogen until they are on their feet again. Being bed-bound increases the risk of blood clots, and estrogen can magnify it.
*   *Liver disease.* Remember, estrogen is metabolized in the liver. Women with severe liver disease should avoid estrogen pills. Patches, however, may be considered.
*   *High triglycerides.* Estrogen pills can raise levels of this blood fat.
*   *Severe high blood pressure.* Estrogen can raise blood pressure, so if your blood pressure is high, and not controlled with medications, beware.
*   *Pregnancy.* If you are pregnant, you should never take estrogens.
*   *Long-term use.* The Woman's Health Initiative, a large, long-term, government sponsored study, was halted prematurely in 2002 because combination estrogen/progesterone HRT was found to increase a woman's risk of breast cancer, stroke, and heart disease. Because of this finding, most doctors will only prescribe HRT for three to five years.

PROGESTERONE AS A COMPONENT OF HRT

Progesterone (or progestins) is added to hormone replacement therapy for only one reason: to prevent uterine cancer (endometrial cancer). Most women who take progesterone for long periods of time experience weight gain around the middle, develop insulin resistance, and may be at increased risk for developing diabetes. If you have had a hysterectomy, there is no need to add progesterone to your HRT.

In the section on birth control pills, I noted that some progestins such as **levonorgestrel, norgestrel,** and **norethindrone** can act like the male hormone, testosterone. And that's what's responsible for some of the androgenic side effects of birth control pills, such as acne and bloating. These progestins can also cause insulin resistance. Medroxyprogesterone acetate, Provera, also causes extreme hunger, insulin resistance, and weight gain. The synthetic progestins **desogestrol** and **norgestimate** are less androgenic and cause less insulin resistance; however, these are generally not available for use in HRT. I recommend natural progesterone such as Prometrium or Crinone as the best choice for the progesterone component of HRT.

Among the commonly prescribed progesterones are the following:

Micronized progesterone (Prometrium)
The process of micronization allows the tablet to break down into smaller pieces, so the progesterone dissolves easier and is more easily absorbed into the body. This natural product comes from yams and is dissolved in peanut oil. It causes less weight gain, but also makes you sleepy. Take it before you go to bed.

Progesterone gel
Crinone is a vaginal gel made of natural micronized progesterone (also derived from yams). A premeasured applicator ensures that you get the right amount into the vagina. The progesterone is absorbed through the lining of the uterus and works quite well at protecting the lining of the uterus. Only about 4 percent of the medication is absorbed into general circulation, so there is much less hunger, fluid retention, and weight gain compared to progesterone taken by mouth. Crinone is not approved for use in HRT, but it's sometimes used for this purpose. To induce a menstrual cycle, use one applicator of Crinone gel every day for 6 days each month.

Medroxyprogesterone acetate (MPA) *(Provera, Cycrin, and generics)*
Provera is the most widely used progesterone. It's a synthetic progesterone and has many side effects including increased appetite, weight
gain, bloating, fluid retention, mood swings, and insulin resistance.

Norethindrone acetate (Aygestin)
This synthetic progesterone comes in a 5 mg tablet, which is five times
the dose used in birth control pills. It has a high androgenic activity and
can cause all of the side effects associated with progestins. Weight gain
may be less with norethindrone than with medroxyprogesterone acetate.

Megestrol (Megace)
Not commonly used for HRT, but it is used for treatment of endometrial cancer and as an appetite-stimulant medication for AIDS and cancer patients.

Cyproterone acetate (CPA) (Androcur)
Not routinely available in the United States, this form of progesterone
is also an anti androgen.

Progesterone creams
Extracted from Mexican yams, this natural alternative is reported to be
effective in helping relieve the hot flashes of menopause. These creams
are made up by a variety of local pharmacies, so there is tremendous
variability among different preparations. Some creams can be exceptionally potent, 10 to 20 times more potent than pills. I have seen many
women gain weight with progesterone creams and do not recommend
their use.

    Combination estrogen/progesterone products include:

- *Ortho-Prefest,* a combination of estradiol and norgestimate (progestin). This is a good choice for a combination product because it
  contains healthy estrogen in the form of estradiol and norgestimate,
  one of the better progestins. Ortho-Prefest is a combination estro-
  gen/progestin product that alternates 3 days of estradiol alone with
  3 days of estradiol plus progestin. This is a new method of HRT
  called pulsed progestin HRT.
- *Activella,* a combination of estradiol and a low dose of norethindrone that works well for some women.

- *FemHRT*, a combination of ethinyl estradiol (synthetic estradiol) and norethindrone (progestin). One of the downsides of this combination is the low dose of estrogen and the higher dose of the norethindrone (which has high androgen activity) component used as the progesterone.
- *Prempro* and *Premphase*, a combination of Premarin (CEE) and Provera. Prempro provides daily progesterone (continuous progesterone therapy), and Premphase provides Premarin only for 14 days followed by Premarin and progesterone for the next 14 days (cyclical progesterone therapy).
- *CombiPatch*, a combination of pure estradiol and progestin (norethindrone) in a patch form providing constant levels of both hormones.
- *Tibolone*, a product that has the effect of estrogen, progesterone, and testosterone. It is available only in Europe at this time.

These products come with all the same progesterone problems: increased hunger, weight gain, fluid retention, mood swings, and insulin resistance. As with estrogen, if you have problems with one form of progesterone, it's worthwhile to try a different form.

BENEFITS OF HRT

- *Cancer prevention*. Most women fear breast cancer, and that is a real risk. But estrogen protects against ovarian cancer and may also protect you from colon cancer.
- *Proper fat distribution*. Estrogen lets overweight women have more "safe" fat. Without estrogen, metabolically evil belly fat and blood levels of free fatty acids grow. Taking the hormone prevents the toxic effect of fat, which produces insulin resistance.
- *Cholesterol*. HRT raises HDL (good) cholesterol and lowers LDL (bad) cholesterol. Despite improvements in cholesterol, HRT may increase your risk for heart attack or stroke.
- *Osteoporosis prevention*. Three-quarters of the bone loss that occurs in women during the first 20 years after menopause can be attributed to hormone loss, according to Dr. Leon Sperloff, who did a study of the benefits of estrogen in the mid-1980s. The earlier hormone loss is treated—through taking estrogen, among other supplements—the less bone loss will occur.

- *Lower blood pressure.* Studies show that women who take HRT have lower blood pressure than those who do not.
- *Better memory.* This remains a controversial area, however most studies seem to show less dementia in women who take HRT.
- *Improvement in menopausal symptoms.* The many symptoms that accompany menopause—hot flushes, poor sleep, depression, lack of energy—can be alleviated by estrogen. This is the most widely agreed upon and least controversial benefit of HRT.
- *Prevention of tooth loss.* Estrogen helps bones, we know that—and that probably helps women hold on to their teeth. At the least, a study of women on HRT showed that they kept their teeth more than women not on HRT.
- *Keeps skin young.* Estrogen helps skin retain collagen and prevents early wrinkling.
- *Quality of life.* Most women who take HRT feel younger and more vibrant. HRT is considered one of the critical elements in a new form of hormone therapy known as anti-aging medicine.

RISKS OF HRT

Should you take HRT? The American Association of Clinical Endocrinologists "believes that menopause is a state of hormone deficiency that should be treated." There are risks to HRT and you should carefully consider your individual risks and benefits with your physician. If you choose to take HRT, you should probably do so for a maximum of three to five years.

- *Breast cancer.* Fear of breast cancer is the number-one reason why women fear HRT. The risk, however, is not as bad as you think: It increases by only 1 or 2 percent per year. It's the same as if you drink one or two alcoholic beverages a day. (Yes, alcohol increases your risk of breast cancer, too.) What are your chances of getting breast cancer, on or off HRT? The lifetime risk is 1 in 8, though it does increase as you get older. At age 30, for example, the risk is 1 in 2,525; by age 50 it's increased to 1 in 50. Estrogen replacement therapy, by liberal estimates, may increase the risk up to 30 percent—but, again, this isn't as high as it seems. Say the risk is 1 in 10 (10 percent) at age 80; HRT will increase this to 13 percent, or about 1 in 8. Interestingly, although the risk of getting breast cancer increases, the risk of dying from the cancer does *not* increase.

Note the following facts regarding breast cancer in women who take HRT: Breast cancer tends to be picked up earlier, when there is less chance that it has spread. The tumors are less aggressive—they grow slower and don't like to spread as easily as the breast cancer that develops in women not taking HRT who get breast cancer. The bottom line is that, although the risk for breast cancer goes up, the risk of *dying* from breast cancer may actually go down if you take HRT. This may be due to early detection, or it may be the effect of HRT itself. Some experts believe that taking estrogen actually does not increase the risk of breast cancer; simply, women on HRT are tested for breast cancer more often, so more cases are picked up earlier.

And remember, being overweight is a major risk for breast cancer. Many cases of breast cancer are preventable by simple weight loss.

A 2000 study published in the *Journal of the American Medical Association (JAMA)* has found that progesterone medications markedly enhance the risk of breast cancer when added to estrogen for hormone replacement therapy. The increased breast cancer risk seems to be with the sequential progesterone dosing, where a woman has a monthly period. The other methods of dosing, continuous combined HRT and the pulsed regime of progesterone, may not further increase risk of breast cancer.

- *Uterine cancer.* The evidence here is a little more clear-cut. Estrogen replacement does increase the risk of uterine cancer, actually called *endometrial cancer* after the lining of the uterus. As a woman's body goes through the menstrual cycle, estrogen makes the uterine lining grow thick. When estrogen is given on a daily basis—known as "unopposed estrogen therapy"—the lining gets thicker and thicker and can become cancerous.

But there is a counter to this process, and that's progesterone. It can completely prevent endometrial cancer caused by estrogen. However, progesterone does have a lot of weight-related side effects, so it's a trade-off—but a worthy one to make to avoid the risk of cancer.

Treatments for PCOS That Help Insulin Resistance

All of the treatments for insulin resistance discussed in Chapter 3 can improve the symptoms of androgen excess.

Metformin (Glucophage, Glucophage XR, Fortamet, Riomet, and Generics)
Although metformin is approved by the FDA for the treatment of type 2 diabetes, it is the most prescribed medication for treating PCOS. Metformin attacks the primary cause of PCOS—insulin resistance. Metformin can improve many symptoms of PCOS, including menstrual cycle problems and skin problems, and can help women lose weight. Metformin increases fertility and has been responsible for many "PCOS babies." For more on metformin, see Chapter 3.

Rosiglitazone (Avandia) and Pioglitazone (Actos)
These medications help alleviate androgen excess by ameliorating insulin resistance. They are approved by the FDA for the treatment of diabetes but have become widely used to treat PCOS. Rosiglitazone and pioglitazone can improve all of the symptoms of androgen excess and can increase fertility and lower the risk for diabetes. In May 2007, the safety of rosiglitazone came under question by the FDA when it was found to increase the risk of heart attack by as much as 30 to 40 percent. Better long-term safety studies are needed for this class of drugs before routine use is recommended for treating androgen excess in women. For more information, see Chapter 3.

Birth Control Pills
Birth control pills, or oral contraceptive pills (OCPs), are a tried and true way of treating androgen excess. OCPs decrease androgen levels because they shut down androgen production in the ovary as well as increase the production of blood proteins, such as sex hormone–binding globulin (SHBG). SHBG binds to androgens, making them inactive. Birth control pills contain synthetic versions of the hormones estrogen and progesterone. The amount of estrogen and the type of progesterone are what make each pill different.

Synthetic progesterone, called *progestin*, is not exactly like real progesterone. Progestins stimulate both the progesterone receptor and the androgen receptor and are said to have *androgenic activity*. When it comes to PCOS, I recommend birth control pills that have progestins, like *drospirenone, desogestrel,* or *norgestimate*. These progestins have the least amount of androgenic activity. The best progestin, drospirenone, actually blocks the androgen receptor. It was developed specifically for women with androgen excess. Drospirenone is found in the product Yasmin, which is the most frequently prescribed pill for PCOS. It has a chemical structure similar to the androgen-blocking medication spirono-lactone. It also has mild diuretic properties, so there's less fluid reten-tion and bloating than with other OCPs. Yasmin can also raise potassium

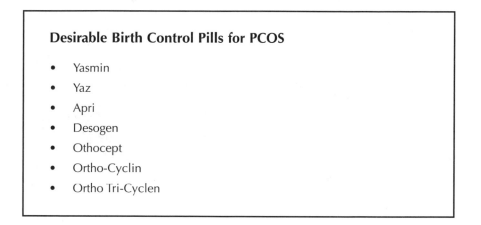

Desirable Birth Control Pills for PCOS

- Yasmin
- Yaz
- Apri
- Desogen
- Othocept
- Ortho-Cyclin
- Ortho Tri-Cyclen

levels, which can improve insulin resistance (see Chapter 3). A side effect can be potassium levels that are too high, so regular blood tests are necessary. Because Yasmin and spironolactone have similar actions, it is inadvisable to take both of these medications at the same time.

The progestins *levonorgestrel, norgestrel,* and *norethindrone* have high androgenic activity. OCPs with these progestins have side effects including acne, bloating, weight gain, and insulin resistance.

Side effects of all birth control pills include acne, headaches, breast tenderness, nausea, PMS, and depression. OCPs with the androgenic progestins levonorgestrel, norgestrel, and norethindrone can increase insulin resistance, raise blood sugar, and cause weight gain. OCPs with high doses of estrogen may also cause weight gain, but the medium-

and low-dose pills do not cause weight gain. Life-threatening blood clots, heart attacks, and strokes are a real risk with birth control pills. The risk is highest if you smoke cigarettes. If you smoke, you should not use birth control pills.

Progesterone and Progestins

Progesterone and progestins (synthetic progesterone) are used in the treatment of PCOS primarily to induce a menstrual cycle. Not having a cycle for 3 months or more is a risk factor for cancer of the uterus. Progesterone is usually given for 10 days every 3 months to induce a menstrual cycle. Other than stimulating a menstrual cycle and lowering the risk of uterine cancer, progesterone does not do much to help PCOS. In fact, progestins with high androgenic activity make PCOS worse. Most physicians prescribe *medroxyprogesterone acetate (Provera),* which is a highly androgenic progestin that causes side effects like weight gain, bloating, depression, and hot flashes. Androgenic progestins can make insulin resistance worse. If progesterone therapy is necessary, I recommend one of the following products.

Micronized progesterone (Prometrium) is natural progesterone that is a good choice for women with androgen excess. The process of micronization allows the tablet to break down into smaller pieces, so that the progesterone dissolves easier and is easily absorbed into the body. This product comes from yams and is dissolved in peanut oil. It causes less weight gain but also makes you sleepy. Take it before you go to bed.

Progesterone gel (Crinone, Prochieve) is a vaginal gel made of natural micronized progesterone (also derived from yams). A pre-measured applicator ensures that you get the right amount into the vagina. The progesterone is absorbed through the lining of the uterus and works quite well at protecting the lining. Only about 4 percent of the medication is absorbed into general circulation, so there is much less hunger, fluid retention, and weight gain compared with progesterone taken by mouth.

Progesterone-containing intrauterine devices (Progestasert and Mirena) release small amounts of progesterone into the lining of the uterus. Little progesterone is transferred to the rest of the body.

Spironolactone (Aldactone)

Spironolactone has two different effects that work together to improve androgen excess. It is a *potassium-sparing diuretic* medication that also blocks the androgen receptor. The anti-androgenic effect is mild and works best in combination with a birth control pill. As a potassium-sparing diuretic, spironolactone helps the body retain potassium. Potassium is required for proper insulin action, and low potassium can lead to insulin resistance. Spironolactone can be taken one to four times a day. Blood tests are required to monitor potassium levels and to check for liver problems, which are a rare side effect. Spironolactone can cause birth defects and should not be taken unless a woman is using some form of birth control.

Flutamide (Eulexin)
Flutamide is a potent androgen-blocking medication that is best for treating excessive facial hair. This drug is not used very often because it can cause liver problems. Like all other androgen blockers, it can cause birth defects.

Finasteride (Proscar, Propecia) and Dutasteride (Avodart)
Although approved for use in men, these medications are sometimes used to treat androgen excess in women. Finasteride and dutasteride work by blocking the enzyme *5-alpha reductase,* which converts testosterone into the more active form, *dihydrotestosterone* (DHT). Although effective, these medications can cause birth defects and should be used only with careful supervision.

Clomiphene Citrate (Clomid)
A medication usually used as a fertility drug, clomiphene citrate is an effective treatment for PCOS in women who want to get pregnant.

GETTING RID OF EXCESS HAIR

For many women, hirsutism is seen as both cosmetically disfiguring and detrimental to one's emotional and social life. It is important to note that all of the preceding treatments may slow the progression of hirsutism, but may not make the hair go away entirely. The best and most effective ways of doing so are mechanical.

- **Electrolysis** is claimed to permanently remove the hair, but multiple treatments are usually necessary.

- **Shaving** is one of the best ways to remove excess facial hair. (Incidentally, the hair will not grow back thicker; this is a myth.)
- **Plucking** and **waxing** can lead to inflammation and infection in the skin and are not as good as shaving.
- **Bleaching** and **depilating creams** are helpful but can also cause inflammation of the skin.
- **Laser hair removal** has still not been perfected. It's expensive, and the hair tends to grow back with time. In the future, better laser techniques may make this the hair removal therapy of choice.
- **Eflornithine hydrochloride (Vaniqa)** is a cream approved for the treatment of unwanted facial hair. The medication works by inhibiting the biosynthesis of hair proteins. The cream must be applied twice a day for at least 2 months before you will see an effect. Unfortunately, if the cream is stopped, the hair grows back.

FEMALE LOW-ANDROGEN SYNDROME

Although androgen excess receives more attention, low androgen levels can also be problematic for some women. Up to one-third of all women experience problems with androgen deficiency at some time in their lives. Androgens help maintain muscle mass and determine body fat distribution. Androgens are responsible for the appearance of body hair; they make the skin oilier; and, as in men, they contribute to the sex drive.

Also just as in men, women's androgen levels decline with age. Androgen decline at menopause is considered part of the natural aging process. (The decline actually begins when a woman reaches her 30s.) Estrogen medications suppress testosterone production by the ovary, so women on estrogen replacement therapy or birth control pills usually have low androgen levels. Symptoms of androgen decline include loss of sexual desire (libido), weight gain (or sometimes weight loss), increased fat in the belly, loss of muscle, tiredness, lack of energy, decreased sense of well-being, depression, loss of shine in the hair, dry skin, lack of mental clarity, anemia, urinary incontinence (from loss of muscle tone in the pelvis and the bladder), and osteoporosis.

Androgen therapy for women is considered controversial by most endocrinologists. The only androgen products approved for use in women are *Estratest* and *Estratest HS* (a "half-strength" version), which combine conjugated estrogens and testosterone (*methyltestosterone*). These products are used as *hormone replacement therapy* for women who have symptoms of menopause that are not completely relieved by estrogen alone.

Testosterone gels (*Androgel, Testim*) are approved for use in men but are being prescribed more and more for female low-androgen syndrome. The dose is one-tenth that for a man. Dosing is difficult because of the way testosterone gels come packaged. A 2.5-gram Androgel packet should last 5 to 10 days, but once opened, the gel dries out in a few days. The Androgel pump dispenses a pre-measured amount, so it's hard to get the right amount for a woman. Testim comes in 5-gram tubes with a screw top, which makes it more practical for women to use. One tube (which is one day's dose for a man) should be used by a woman over 10 days. Testosterone creams can be made by some compounding pharmacies, and as with other products of this nature, quality control can be variable. A testosterone patch for women holds promise but has had problems getting approval by the FDA.

Androgen therapy can have many side effects. Among the most serious are the risk of birth defects, negative effects on the cholesterol profile, and a possible risk of heart disease. Anyone who takes androgen replacement therapy should do so under the supervision of a qualified physician. Other side effects include acne, hair growth in male areas (face, chest, nipples, and back), voice deepening, overactive sex drive, irregular bleeding, hair loss, and enlargement of the clitoris. For women who take other hormone medications, such as thyroid medication, the dosage may need to be adjusted after initiation of androgen therapy.

CHAPTER SEVEN

THYROID HORMONE

ALL ABOUT YOUR THYROID

It is a small, butterfly-shaped, brownish-red organ located at the base of the throat. It weighs only about an ounce, and secretes and contains relatively small amounts of two hormones. But this small structure, the thyroid gland, and the substances it produces have a wide-ranging impact on your weight—an impact that is often misunderstood or ignored.

Millions of Americans suffer because their thyroid hormone levels are too low. It's easy to overlook the effects of a healthy thyroid gland, as easy as overlooking simple good health. The thyroid helps regulate body temperature. The thyroid controls metabolism. The thyroid helps maintain psychological well-being, appetite, energy level, sex drive, and sleep ability.

But if you develop thyroid dysfunction, body systems can go haywire. An underactive thyroid (*hypothyroidism*) can lower your energy level. Suddenly, your metabolism slows down. You're tired, so you don't feel like exercising. Coupled with the lowered metabolism, this lack of activity promotes depression and anxiety and begins a vicious circle, which—pardon the term—feeds on itself. You become irritable, unhappy, and overweight.

Many people have heard about underactive thyroid as a cause of being fat. They know an underactive thyroid makes them tired and depressed, makes their hair fall out, and gives them dry skin. But when they go to the doctor, they get a standard "TSH" test and are told everything is OK—if that. For doctors often overlook the role of the thyroid in this vicious cycle. Nowadays, it's easy enough to suggest psychotherapy and prescribe a pill, such as Prozac or Zoloft, for depression. Certainly, many things can bring on depression, and a capable psychiatrist can help patients come to terms with their issues and thought processes. But this "it's all in your head" diagnosis ignores the importance of the thyroid in affecting mood, appetite, and metabolism.

However, every day, more and more physicians are becoming aware of underactive thyroid and the role it can play. Endocrinologists, such as myself, are treating milder and milder cases all the time, and scientific data is finally coming out confirming what clinicians have known all along—that you can have normal thyroid tests and still have thyroid dysfunction. There are many reasons this can occur, ranging from brain tumors to environmental toxins to nutritional problems and even stress.

Given the thyroid's importance to metabolism, any insult to the system—whether it be stress, other hormonal problems, improper diet, nutritional or vitamin deficiencies, or toxins—can block the critical conversion of one type of thyroid hormone to another, a conversion key to metabolism regulation. Without a diagnosis and treatment that includes the thyroid, many patients—who could be well on their way to better health and losing weight—may remain in that vicious cycle for years. And that's something no diet can cure.

This chapter will outline modern thought on hypothyroidism and other forms of thyroid dysfunction. I will stress symptoms you may have that may be a clue to thyroid dysfunction. This chapter will be helpful if you suspect you have thyroid disease, or if you've been diagnosed with hypothyroidism, are taking medications, but still don't feel well.

THE FACTS ABOUT THYROID DISEASE

Thyroid disease is much more common than most people realize. It is estimated that more than 10 million Americans have some form of thyroid disease. (Some estimates say the figure is as many as 1 in 10, or almost 30 million Americans.) Women are 10 times more likely to get thyroid disease than men. And thyroid disease is more likely to affect you as you get older. Given the current demographic trend of the United States—with more and more of the 75 million baby boomers (persons born between 1946 and 1964) passing age 50 each year— there's a strong possibility that thyroid disease may be on the rise.

But thyroid disease is difficult to pin down. Thyroid problems tend to present themselves in a wide variety of medical complaints. Each person is affected differently: There may be one, two, or many symptoms. Any or all of the body's organ systems may be influenced by the changes in the thyroid.

When weight problems begin, many people suspect that the thyroid gland may be at fault. They may have noticed other symptoms, such as a diminished sex drive or simple fatigue. But their doctors tell them that everything is OK; the problem lies elsewhere. This isn't necessarily the physician's fault. Traditional thyroid tests often do not detect subtle or even not-so-subtle forms of thyroid disease.

How Thyroid Hormones Are Made

Let me take a minute to discuss how thyroid hormones are made. The backbone of thyroid hormone is an amino acid called tyrosine. Tyrosine is found naturally in protein (amino acids such as tyrosine are the building blocks of protein) and is also available in capsule or pill form from many health-food stores. It's made by the body by converting another amino acid, phenylalanine. Iron is necessary for this process to occur. Two of these tyrosine molecules are linked together to form a double ring structure.

There are two types of thyroid hormone, *triiodothyronine* (T3) and *thyroxine* (T4), (see Figure 7.1). The "3" and the "4" refer to the number of iodine molecules attached to the double ring structure. A healthy thyroid gland makes about 80 percent T4 and 20 percent T3.

T4 is considered an "inactive" hormone. In order for the T4 hormone to become activated, one of the iodine molecules on the outer ring must be removed by special enzymes. This process is known as T4 to T3 conversion, or *deiodination*. The three-iodine version, triiodothreonine, or T3, is the active and most potent form of thyroid hormone. An inactive form of thyroid hormone, known as *reverse T3*, is created when the iodine molecule is removed from the inner ring

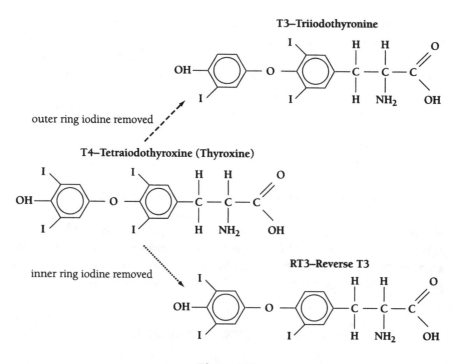

Figure 7.1
THYROID HORMONE STRUCTURES
Note the similarities among thyroid hormones. T4, thyroxine, is a mostly inactive hormone that is converted by enzymes to its active form, T3 (triiodothyronine), by removing an iodine molecule from the outer ring. If an iodine molecule is removed from the inner ring, T4 is converted to "reverse T3," an inactive hormone.

instead of the outer ring. **Many people have thyroid problems related to this conversion process.**

The enzymes responsible for removing this outer-ring iodine from T4 are known as *selenodeiodinases*. Selenodeiodinases, incidentally, are known by that name because they contain the element selenium, a trace mineral necessary for the enzyme to function properly. Another trace mineral, zinc, is also important for proper enzyme function. **Diets low in selenium or zinc cause problems converting T4 to T3.** Too much copper in the diet can also block the conversion process.

Low T3 levels slow metabolism and cause weight gain.

A common blood pressure medication known as propanolol (Inderal) can inhibit this process. Propanolol comes from a class of drugs known as *beta-blockers*. Another medication, amiodarone, also causes conversion problems. Amiodarone (Cordarone) is a heart medication currently growing in popularity. Interestingly, amiodarone has been found to cause a variety of thyroid difficulties, including over- and underactivity.

THE BRAIN REGULATES THYROID HORMONE PRODUCTION

Your body is a collection of systems constantly changing based on the short-term and long-term messages it receives from the brain. As your senses come into contact with new information—as you hear a baby's coo, for example, or see a car up ahead stop short, or even if you simply feel hungry—your brain puts the various systems to work. Because of the hormones it secretes and those hormones' importance in dealing with stress, the thyroid is a key link in making those systems work.

It starts with signals from the brain. Your body is undergoing a stressful event; the brain immediately starts sending messages to parts of the body in the form of hormones. The hormones originate in the section of the brain known as the *hypothalamus*, the part of the brain which regulates the internal activities of the body. Along with hormone production, these activities include sexual behavior, emotions, and the autonomic nervous system. The hypothalamus, which is located roughly behind the eyes, is hard-wired to almost the entire nervous system and directs the "fight or flight" impulse that puts such stress on the body.

To get to the thyroid, the hypothalamus sends a message to the pituitary gland in the form of a hormone—TRH, or *thyrotropin-releasing hormone*. The pituitary gland reacts to the influx of TRH by releasing a second hormone—TSH, or *thyroid-stimulating hormone* (aka *thyrotropin*). TSH travels through the bloodstream to the thyroid gland. TSH directs the thyroid gland to produce thyroid hormones. The pituitary is responsible for making sure the level of thyroid hormones in the blood remains constant, so if thyroid hormone levels fall, the pituitary gland increases its production of TSH. Figure 7.2 illustrates this process.

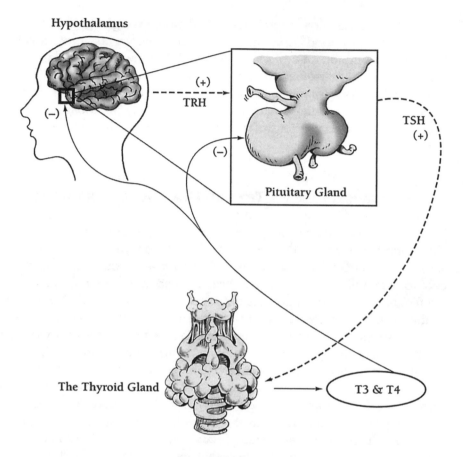

Figure 7.2
THYROID HORMONE ENDROCRINOLOGY: FEEDBACK LOOPS
Higher centers in the brain send signals to the hypothalamus, which produces
thyrotropin-releasing hormone (TRH). TRH stimulates the pituitary gland to
make thyroid-stimulating hormone (TSH). TSH stimulates the thyroid gland to
produce thyroid hormones. Thyroid hormones "feed back" to the hypothalamus and pituitary gland, slowing TSH production. Positive "feedback" is denoted by + and negative "feedback" is denoted by –.

Because of its impact on the thyroid, the pituitary's production of TSH has a profound effect on the body, particularly in regard to diet. If the body is starving, the pituitary produces less TSH, prompting the thyroid to produce less T4, slowing metabolism. However, the body doesn't make distinctions about why it's starving: The same decline in T4 production will happen whether a person is on a crash diet, suffers from an eating disorder, or is simply malnourished.

STRESS AND YOUR THYROID

Just as thyroid dysfunction can have an effect on the mind, so the mind can have an effect on the thyroid gland. Stress, in particular, is a major catalyst in disrupting the normal performance of the thyroid.

When under stress, the body sends messages triggering responses from many hormones. Many of these responses are short-lived and beneficial: The production of adrenaline (epinephrine), for example, provides people with the extra shot of energy and excitement often needed to get through a stressful situation. (Think of how you feel when making a public speech: The palms sweat, the heart beats faster, you feel very afraid and very alive—all part of the "fight-or-flight" instinct developed over millions of years.)

But if the stress lasts for a long time, such as the kind felt after surviving a tragedy or losing a loved one, the endocrine system becomes overburdened. Naturally, this can lead to health problems. In particular, the immune system is weakened, because the brain—using the flood of stress-inspired chemicals as a guide—is focusing its responses elsewhere. With the weakening of the immune system, the body is helpless against viruses, antibodies, and other chemicals that attack the thyroid.

Moreover, stress isn't just psychological. The wrong type of dieting can cause physical stress because the body believes it is starving. The resulting impact, however, is similar: The immune system is weakened and the thyroid comes under attack.

But when the body is under stress, other problems can occur. In one scenario, the wrong iodine—the inner-ring iodine—can be removed from the T4 hormone. This creates a totally inactive form of the hormone called *reverse T3*. Given the inert state of reverse T3, metabolism is slowed to a crawl.

Sloan's Story

Sloan went on a crash diet. She quickly lost 10 pounds, but also became fatigued, depressed, and discouraged. Moreover, despite her continuing efforts, she couldn't lose any more weight, exacerbating the cycle. She stopped exercising and whatever positive results she had gained from the diet went by the boards.

Sloan visited a doctor for a consultation. The doctor tested her, but all her thyroid hormone levels appeared normal. Eventually, Sloan got another diagnosis. Because of the stress of her crash diet, her body was fooled into thinking that it was starving and it lowered its metabolism—via its thyroid hormones— accordingly to protect itself. This condition, known as sick euthyroid syndrome, has normal thyroid tests in the early stages. Modification of Sloan's diet (and a modest increase in calories) allowed her to resume exercising, lose weight, and feel better.

A Word about Iodine

Iodine, element 53 on the periodic table, is a dark-gray to purple-black solid that is used in activities ranging from photography (silver iodide) to medicine (tincture of iodine, commonly used as an antiseptic). In the body, this element is contained in thyroid gland hormones. If it's lacking in your diet, a goiter—the swelling of the thyroid—will result. Obviously, iodine is an important part of a functioning thyroid and a healthy body.

The average person requires 150 micrograms of iodine a day. However, in the United States, the usual consumption ranges between 300 and 700 micrograms a day—a testament to our love of salt and salty products, for most of the salt used in the United States is iodized. (Salt without iodine is called "free running.") Too much iodine can be as harmful as too little; high iodine intake may lead to thyroid cancer or thyroiditis.

Iodine also comes from seafood, sea vegetables, and certain medications—the best known being amiodarone, used to treat heart arrhythmia.

Iodine is found in a variety of "thyroid support" formulas in the form of kelp, bugleweed, and bladderwrack. These so-called support formulas often try to foist iodine supplements—kelp is particularly pop-ular—on people as a way of staying healthy. "Look at the Japanese," you might hear, referring to that nation's traditional reliance on seafood and relatively low incidence of obesity and certain illnesses. But thy-roid-support supplements can put thousands of milligrams of iodine into a healthy system—way too much for the thyroid to process. (Incidentally, the Japanese also have a relatively high rate of autoim-mune thyroid disease.) So, if it's one thing Americans generally *don't* need, it's iodine supplements—but you see that claim all the time. Sources of dietary iodine include kelp, salt (iodized), saltwater fish, shrimp, milk, cheese, eggs, and crops grown in iodine-rich soil.

Tina's Story

Tina thought she had thyroid problems. Her doctor did the routine, TSH test, and it was normal. Tina started taking kelp on the recommendation of her local health-food store. Shortly after starting the kelp, her symptoms became much worse. In one month, she gained 15 pounds. Although she had normal thyroid tests prior to starting the kelp, a repeat test showed a high TSH and extremely low thyroid hormone levels. Tina quit taking the kelp. She started feeling better, and her thyroid tests returned to normal after a few weeks.

If the thyroid gland is overwhelmed with iodine, it shuts down, inhibiting production of thyroid hormone. Sometimes a different con-sequence of thyroid overload, iodide-induced *hyper*thyroidism, has also been known to occur. If you have a smoldering, low-level thyroid dis-ease and then consume a large amount of iodine (like taking kelp), the consequences can be devastating. The effect is like spraying a fire with gasoline: Huge amounts of thyroid hormone are suddenly produced, resulting in severe hyperthyroidism. Either way, it is not a good idea to flood your system with iodine.

HYPOTHYROIDISM

How do you know if you have hypothyroidism? There are literally dozens of signs and symptoms. In general, these symptoms occur because metabolism is slowed.

Weight gain

As I noted in the previous section, lack of production of T4 plunges the body into a vicious cycle. Chief among this cycle's indicators is simple weight gain. The lack of T4 prompts the body to slow its metabolism, so the body processes food more slowly. Ironically, many people then start a crash diet, which only speeds up the cycle: The stress of the diet forces the body to underproduce T4 even more, so metabolism continues slowing, and other symptoms start cropping up.

Women who have trouble losing weight after giving birth may have a form of hypothyroidism. Transient hypothyroidism lasting about 1 year is common after pregnancy and is known as **postpartum hypothyroidism**. The condition may be misdiagnosed as **postpartum depression** and never properly treated. Most of the time, the hypothyroidism improves by itself and is forgotten. But the afflicted woman, by this time, has been miserable for about a year and has likely gained tremendous amounts of weight. This condition occurs in as many as 5 percent of American women after giving birth.

Fatigue

Reduced metabolism leads to low energy levels. People with low thyroid levels are tired all the time. They simply have no energy. Many report sleeping 12 to 14 hours each night.

Aging

Cosmetically, hypothyroidism may cause people to look older. One need not look any further than the case of Boris Yeltsin, the former president of Russia. In 1991, when he took over the country, Yeltsin was the very picture of vigor: Who can forget the then-youthful 60-year-old rallying people in the streets of Moscow after an aborted takeover by Soviet hard-liners?

But within 5 years, Yeltsin appeared old, tired, and out of touch. He slurred his speech; his face was puffy and bloated. In 1996, prior to a heart bypass operation, he was diagnosed with hypothyroidism. The diagnosis was almost certainly overdue, since the disease had probably started much earlier—perhaps brought on by the stress of his job and exacerbated by Yeltsin's alcoholism. Interestingly, once Yeltsin's thyroid was treated, his heart problems got worse. This is not uncommon. Thyroid hormone accelerates metabolism throughout the body, including the heart. The accelerated metabolism increased the amount of oxygen his heart demanded, and because of his coronary artery disease, not enough blood could get to heart muscle.

Menopausal symptoms

As many as 18 percent of menopausal women have an underactive thyroid gland. Symptoms of weight gain, mood swings, depression, hair loss, and dry skin attributed to menopause could actually be due to undiagnosed thyroid disease.

Goiter

A goiter is not necessarily an indicator of hypothyroidism; it means only that the thyroid is enlarged. However, a goiter with any one of the other symptoms on this list is highly suggestive of thyroid problems. Goiters can cause a feeling of fullness in the neck. Some people with goiters report a choking sensation, hoarseness, or difficulty swallowing.

Joint and muscle aches

Hypothyroidism causes joints and muscles to feel stiff, painful, and sore—symptoms that can be misdiagnosed as arthritis.

Feeling cold or being cold

The thyroid regulates body temperature, so any sign of that temperature being "off" can be a sign of a diseased or dysfunctional thyroid gland. However, so many other things can cause fluctuations in body temperature that doctors often overlook the thyroid. Doctors understand an increase in body temperature: That's a common sign of fever and sickness. But a decrease in body temperature can be associated with slowed metabolism, poor diet, or simply a bad chill—in other words, other symptoms of hypothyroidism, but not ones doctors usually pay attention to.

Body-temperature measurements have been touted as an early indicator of thyroid dysfunction. Many thyroid experts recommend taking your temperature first thing in the morning. Normal body temperature is between 97.8 and 98.4 degrees. Some experts believe that a temperature below 97.6 is suggestive of low thyroid activity.

Constipation

Hard, painful bowel movements or bloating are signs of hypothyroidism, but again, like many others on this list, these signs are often dismissed as something else.

Loss of memory and inability to concentrate
Given the relationship between hypothyroidism, slowed metabolism, and fatigue, the memory is often sacrificed in favor of other brain functions. The body becomes obsessed with its drives, most notably sleeping and eating. Concentrating and remembering take a back seat.

Depression
This is one of the most common misdiagnoses of hypothyroidism. Nowadays, it's easy to blame depression for so many things. We all have moments when we're feeling down, and for a sizable minority of Americans, full-blown depression is a real threat and illness. But though it's as important to look at the physiological roots of depression as it is to look at the psychological roots, many physicians don't look in that direction. And one of the indicators of depression can be hypothyroidism.

Dry, pale, yellowy skin
A person with hypothyroidism finds that the body isn't doing many things it should and, in fact, is attacking itself. Skin becomes dry and flaky and due to carotene buildup, takes on a yellow tinge.

Facial puffiness, thickened lips, bloating, or edema
Hypothyroidism causes fluid retention resulting in bloating and edema.

Gruff voice
Many people with hypothyroidism report that their voice becomes hoarse, husky, and gravelly or simply sounds deeper. This is caused by thickening of the vocal cords.

Menstrual problems and infertility
Hypothyroidism can cause havoc with the female reproductive system. Periods may be longer and heavier, and periods may become prolonged—more time between each one—or irregular. Increased blood flow, or menorrhagia, is common; the thyroid controls muscle contraction in the uterus. Without the proper contracting of the muscle, the uterus cannot clamp off the bleeding blood vessels. Hypothyroidism can also prompt "anovulation," a situation where the ovary does not release an egg at all.

Some women actually have reduced menstrual flow, or lose their periods altogether. Loss of menstrual cycle with symptoms of low thyroid could mean "central hypothyroidism," explained below, where the pituitary gland does not make enough TSH. Despite this situation, however, traditional thyroid testing may come up normal.

Slow reflexes

This symptom can be a key to diagnosing hypothyroidism, and endocrinologists examine reflexes very carefully when determining if a patient may have thyroid disease. In hypothyroidism, the "relaxation phase" of the reflex is slowed. For example, in the standard knee-jerk reflex, a doctor hits a knee with a reflex hammer and the knee kicks out. In a patient with hypothyroidism, the return of the knee to a resting position is delayed. The delay may not be apparent to the untrained eye, but an experienced endocrinologist knows that this is the most sensitive way of determining subtle thyroid deficiencies at the bedside. Through its effects on the nervous system, hypothyroidism can also cause problems like muscle cramps, numbness or tingling in the hands and feet, or even carpal tunnel syndrome.

Snoring or sleep apnea

Sleep apnea is a situation that occurs when excess tissue in the neck cuts off breathing during the night, leading to snoring, poor sleep, daytime sleepiness, high blood pressure, and—if left untreated—eventual heart and lung failure. Sleep apnea is not uncommon among overweight people, and the slowing of metabolism caused by hypothyroidism can contribute to this condition.

Hair, eyebrow, and fingernail problems

A lowered metabolic rate brought on by thyroid hormone underproduction can slow the growth of hair and cause it to become coarse and brittle. Hypothyroidism also causes hair to fall out, sometimes in clumps. People with hypothyroidism frequently lose the hair in the outer third of the eyebrows. Fingernails can also become brittle with hypothyroidism.

Decreased sweating

Sweating is another area where metabolism plays a role, because the body will shut down systems it deems unnecessary.

Allergies or hives
Many people with thyroid problems can have worsening of their allergies. Treating the thyroid makes the allergies better.

Breast milk production
This is a rare event, but it does happen. As the brain vigorously tries to produce more TSH, more of another hormone, prolactin, can also be produced. Prolactin stimulates breast milk production and can cause menstrual abnormalities. In some cases, this situation is misdiagnosed as a brain tumor and patients have been known to have an unnecessary removal of the pituitary gland, when all that was needed was thyroid hormone replacement.

HYPOTHYROIDISM CAUSES HEART DISEASE

Studies have linked hypothyroidism to heart disease. An underactive thyroid lets the body's cholesterol levels climb, particularly so-called bad cholesterol (LDL, or low-density lipoprotein cholesterol). In combination with high blood pressure (also caused by hypothyroidism), this puts a person at increased risk for heart attack.

Recent studies have also linked elevations of homocysteine levels with hypothyroidism. Homocysteine is an amino acid found in the blood and is linked to heart disease. Hypothyroidism makes the levels of homocysteine increase, just as it does cholesterol levels. Treatment of hypothyroidism tends to lower cholesterol and homocysteine levels, and thus is good for the heart.

In patients with normal thyroid levels, elevated homocysteine may be the result of dietary deficiency of folate (vitamin B1) or vitamin B6, so increasing fruit and vegetable intake also helps reduce homocysteine levels.

Thyroid hormone has direct effects on the heart. Underproduction of thyroid hormone prompts the heart to beat less strongly, and more slowly, and may cause fluid to build up around it. Thyroid hormone speeds up the heart and makes it pump stronger. For these reasons, doctors must be very careful when giving thyroid hormone replacement to people at risk for heart problems. A sudden increase in metabolism can strain the heart and cause a heart attack. (Think of Yeltsin.)

THYROID HORMONE MAKES YOU HUNGRY

*Hyper*thyroidism is the opposite of *hypo*thyroidism: Instead of the body producing too little thyroid hormone, it's producing too much. Its symptoms are usually the reverse of hypothyroid symptoms. Instead of metabolism slowing, it speeds up. So hyperthyroidism usually produces weight loss, not weight gain.

But there's a twist. One of hyperthyroidism's major effects is increasing appetite. If appetite increases faster than metabolism, guess what? Weight gain.

The primary symptom of hyperthyroidism is uncontrollable appetite. Patients complain of never eating enough, of always being hungry, of waking up ravenous and going to sleep the same way—even if they've eaten far more than recommended during the day.

You might recognize other symptoms as reverse images of hypothyroid symptoms. They include feeling hot, hyperactivity, increased sweating, irritability, nervousness, tremor, heart palpitations, insomnia, brittle nails, diarrhea or increased frequency of bowel movements. Interestingly, fatigue is a symptom of both hypo- and hyperthyroidism.

One extreme form of hyperthyroidism is called *thyroid storm.* Patients can have vomiting, fever, mental confusion, and—sometimes—seizures. This form requires hospitalization.

Like hypothyroidism, hyperthyroidism is frequently caused by an attack of an overactive immune system on the thyroid gland. The most common cause of hyperthyroidism is *Graves' disease.* Graves' disease is an attack on the thyroid gland by the immune system usually kicked-off by stress. The most famous case of recent years occurred in 1991, when President George Bush came down with the ailment in the aftermath of the Persian Gulf War—the war having likely put the president under extreme stress for several months. The disease caused heart fibrillations, forcing the president into the hospital. Eventually, after observation and tests, President Bush's Graves' disease was treated with medication. Even *subclinical hypothyroidism* (discussed below) has its companion in *subclinical hyperthyroidism.* The tip-off for this diagnosis is low TSH and normal thyroid hormone levels. Treatments for hyperthyroidism include radioactive iodine, antioxidants, a healthy diet, antithyroid drugs such as Tapazole or propylthiouracil (PTU), and—in some cases—surgical removal of the thyroid.

THE BODY'S ATTACK ON ITSELF

Like Graves', most hypothyroidism cases are caused by an autoimmune attack of the thyroid by the body's immune cells. This is known as *Hashimoto's thyroiditis*. In some cases, a short period of thyroid overactivity is seen during the initial attack of the thyroid when the thyroid hormone stores are released into the bloodstream. Imagine the thyroid as a gas tank that has been ruptured: First, all the gas is released, sometimes causing an explosion if there's a spark around; then, with all the gas either spilled or vaporized, there is no gas left. In some people, this kind of attack can come and go, causing waxing and waning of the symptoms.

Symptoms of hypothyroidism are related to the severity and duration of the disease, the rapidity with which it occurs, and the individual characteristics of the person who has it. One common feature of hypothyroidism, however, is weight gain.

It is estimated that 2 percent of the population has severe hypothyroidism. But 7 to 12 percent of the population—maybe more—suffers from low-grade hypothyroidism known as *subclinical hypothyroidism*. Stress or a diet low in iodine, selenium, or zinc can worsen subclinical hypothyroidism.

Linda's Story

Linda, a 32-year-old mother of two, came to see me after having been diagnosed with chronic fatigue syndrome. Her doctor had done extensive blood testing, including Linda's thyroid hormone level, and assured her that everything was normal. She wanted a second opinion.

A former college athlete, Linda had not been active in years. She admitted she had less energy since she had stopped exercising, but suddenly all the energy was gone. At first, Linda blamed her fatigue on her job, her kids, and her age. But deep down she knew something was wrong. Linda had gained a remarkable 45 pounds in one year. She stated, "No matter what I do, I can't lose weight. I have cut way back on what I am eating, but it is not doing any good. I am tired all the time. I never feel like exercising any more."

She went on to describe a frightening story. "I was out running errands last week and suddenly I just broke down crying. I did not know why I was crying; I just couldn't help myself. I sat in the car and cried all afternoon. Then, as I was pulling myself together, I realized that I had forgotten to pick up my oldest son from basketball practice. By the time I got to the school, the coach had already driven him home."

I reviewed Linda's blood tests. Although her thyroid hormone level was normal, her TSH test was slightly elevated, a sign of early thyroid dysfunction. I explained to her that TSH, or thyroid-stimulating hormone, is produced by the pituitary gland, which is located in the brain. When the brain senses thyroid dysfunction, it increases its production of TSH. The increased levels of TSH try to stimulate the thyroid gland to make more hormone. The diseased gland eventually gives up and hormone levels drop. In the early stages of thyroid disease, it is very common to have normal thyroid hormone levels despite significant symptoms. I performed a **thyroid antibody** test, which was incredibly high. This meant that Linda's immune system was attacking her thyroid gland. It was only a matter of time before her thyroid gland would fail completely.

Linda was treated with a thyroid hormone medication known as levothyroxine. Her mood and memory improved, and she regained her energy. After 4 months on the medication, Linda had shed 25 pounds. She had reached a plateau and wanted to lose the remaining 20 pounds. I recommended dietary changes and added a specific vitamin and mineral supplement to her weight-loss program. Linda now had enough energy to start exercising again.

At her last visit she admitted, "I haven't felt this good in years. I don't know what to do with all this energy. I actually played basketball with my son the other day. I've only got 5 pounds to go, and I know I can do it."

Linda had a classic example of **mild thyroid failure**, one of the most common hormonal problems in women. The underproduction of thyroid hormone slowed her metabolism to a virtual crawl. Since her thyroid hormone test was normal, the diagnosis was initially missed. Thyroid hormone pills returned Linda's metabolism to near normal. As is typical of many thyroid patients, the medication alone was not enough. Lifestyle, diet, and nutritional modifications were also required for Linda to achieve normal thyroid function and to optimize her metabolism.

TESTING FOR THYROID DISEASE

Testing for thyroid imbalance is a tricky business. Most doctors rely on a simple blood test, the TSH test, to determine if a patient is suffering from hypo- or hyperthyroidism; however, the range for such a determination can be so narrow some doctors may dismiss a patient as normal even if a thyroid imbalance exists. At the other extreme are physicians and healers who, without taking a blood test, note a patient has one or more of the indications of thyroid imbalance and treat these symptoms with prescriptions of thyroid hormone (a medication available in both natural and synthetic varieties). Patients with these symptoms, however, may not be suffering from hypo- or hyperthyroidism at all, or certainly not to the degree the ailment is being treated. Thus, neither group is well served by their medical care.

The TSH Test

Thyroid experts recognize the TSH test as the test of choice when thyroid disease is suspected. The primary reason is that TSH begins to rise *before* thyroid hormones drop below the normal range. As such, it's a better indicator of *early* thyroid dysfunction.

TSH is the hormone that comes from the pituitary gland and communicates with the thyroid gland, stimulating it to make and release thyroid hormones. Early in hypothyroidism, TSH goes up, trying to coax the thyroid to do its job. As noted previously, if hypothyroidism is present, the thyroid won't be able to do that job properly. Meanwhile, TSH levels keep going up, continually trying to prod the thyroid back to normal production of thyroid hormones; the thyroid continues declining. After a while, the thyroid hormones levels will drop below normal—but by that time, hypothyroidism has already taken effect and is likely getting worse. Figure 7.3 illustrates this progression of hormone decline.

The TSH test is a good (but not perfect) test for thyroid disease. TSH values *above* the normal range indicate *hypo*thyroidism, and the higher the number, the more severe the hypothyroidism. *Low* TSH values are usually caused by an overactive thyroid (*hyper*thyroidism).

Early hypothyroidism, when TSH is high, but thyroid hormone levels are normal, is known as *subclinical hypothyroidism* or *mild thyroid*

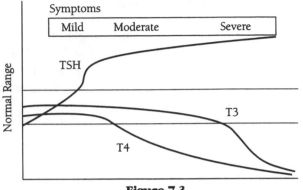

Figure 7.3
PROGRESSION OF HORMONE DECLINE IN HYPOTHYROIDISM
In the evolution of hypothyroidism, subtle deficiencies in thyroid hormone levels are sensed by the brain and pituitary gland. The TSH rise is generally detectable before thyroid hormone levels fall below the normal range. During this phase, symptoms are generally mild. As T4 and T3 levels fall, symptoms worsen.

failure. Many physicians are reluctant to treat this condition. Mild thyroid failure is increasingly being recognized as a real disease and is being treated. A 2000 article in the *Annals of Internal Medicine* found that mild thyroid failure more than doubles your risk of a heart attack.

Most of the time, if your TSH is mildly elevated, the usual diagnosis is mild thyroid failure. There are exceptions, however, to this rule. All of these exceptions are possible, but rare.

- *Tumor.* If the pituitary gland has a tumor, it may overproduce TSH on its own. Patients with this problem usually have symptoms of an overactive thyroid (hyperthyroidism), but those symptoms may overlap with those of an underactive thyroid.
- *Medication.* Anti-nausea medications (e.g., Phenergan and Reglan) and psychiatric medications (e.g., Haldol and Prolixin) can throw TSH tests out of whack.
- *Timing.* TSH should always be tested during the day. TSH levels often surge at night, and testing at this time can give an indication of TSH levels being high—when, actually, they're normal.
- *Immune problems.* TSH antibodies can give false readings in the lab test, making a normal test appear high.

TRH Stimulation Test

This test measures the ability of the pituitary gland to respond to an injection of TRH (thyrotropin-releasing hormone). TSH is measured, TRH is injected, and TSH is measured again, 30 minutes later. If the TSH does not increase, a pituitary gland problem is suspected. If the TSH rises to a level of greater than expected, it can indicate hypothyroidism. Because of the accuracy of the TSH test, the TRH stimulation test is rarely used today.

Total Thyroxine (TT4)

This test measures the level of all thyroxine (T4) in the blood. More than 99 percent of thyroid hormone is bound to the blood protein, TBG. This bound hormone is inactive. Problems with TBG can invalidate this test. Estrogen-containing medications such as those used in HRT or birth control pills increase TBG levels, making the TT4 test of limited usefulness in women who take these medications. Other tests can be done to correct for protein problems.

Free Thyroxine (FT4)

This test measures only the 1 percent of thyroid hormone that is unbound. This "free hormone" is the active hormone. Bound hormone has no biological activity. By testing for free thyroxine, the possibility of being mislead by a protein problem is eliminated. In general, *free* hormone levels are more accurate than *total* hormone levels.

Total Triiodothreonine (TT3)

As with total thyroxine, this test measures both bound and unbound T3 levels. TBG problems can lead to problems with this test.

Free Triiodothreonine (FT3)

This test measures only the unbound portion of T3 and is not subject to protein problems. This is an important test for people who have problems converting T4 to T3.

Reverse T3 (RT3)

This test measures levels of an inactive hormone produced when T4 is improperly processed. Physicians rarely order this test. It is very expensive and is usually not helpful in determining if you have problems converting T4 to T3.

Thyroid Binding Globulin (TBG)

This test measures actual levels of binding proteins in the blood. TBG problems cause false readings for total, but not free, hormone levels.

One cause of elevated TBG, incidentally, is a high estrogen level. This can be caused by pregnancy, birth control pills, estrogen replacement therapy, environmental estrogens (see the section on estrogen and menopause), and high consumption of soy products.

Antithyroid Antibodies (ATA)

Antithyroid antibodies indicate whether or not you have an autoimmune thyroid disorder (the most common cause of hypothyroidism). There are two tests available: antithyroglobulin and antimicrosomal (also known as antithyroid peroxidase—TPO antibodies). Thyroid antibodies indicate the level of attack the immune system is waging on the thyroid gland. High levels in any of these tests indicate a more intense attack and, if your TSH is already high, signify a greater chance of progressing to severe disease.

Many people with symptoms of hypothyroidism but a normal TSH test have a positive antibody test. Thyroid antibodies may be a clue to thyroid disease; however, they do not guarantee this.

Several other factors can cause problems with thyroid hormone measurements:

- *Antibodies.* Sometimes the T4 is falsely elevated because of antibodies that cause problems in the actual laboratory measurement of the hormone levels. In some cases, the T4 may be low, but missed because the test showed normal levels. In actuality, the hormone levels were low, but the test was falsely reading the antibodies as actual hormone. These antibodies are different from those that attack the thyroid gland itself.

- *Normal range.* Another problem of measuring hormone levels alone is that even normal thyroid hormone and TSH levels may not exclude a thyroid problem. As discussed, the pituitary hormone TSH (thyroid-stimulating hormone, or thyrotropin) begins to rise long before T3 and T4 falls into what is said to be the "low range." What's happening is that the body senses low levels of thyroid hormone and compensates by cranking up the signal from the brain. These higher-than-normal levels of TSH further stimulate the thyroid gland to keep up with the demand. But, at the same time, the thyroid gland is failing. Technically, thyroid hormone levels are in the normal range, but they are lower than they used to be. Even these mild drops in hormone levels can lower metabolism. Eventually, all the TSH in the world won't be able to stimulate the gland enough to make it work properly. This is when T3 and T4 levels finally drop below the "normal range."

Rebecca's Story

Rebecca, a sales rep for a software company, came to visit her doctor. In her mid-20s, this vivacious, attractive young woman was complaining of irritability, fatigue, and weight gain— symptoms that could have been merely written off as stress, for she had a very stressful position, or related to her pregnancy, which was in the first trimester. Her doctor measured her total T4. The figure came up within the normal range. The doctor sent her on her way with mild reprimands to slow down, watch her diet, and exercise more.

Eventually, Rebecca came to see me. Upon testing her total and free T4 levels, I determined that her free T4 was low, but her total T4 appeared falsely normal because she had increased levels of TBG protein in her blood. In her case, the excess TBG was a result of her being pregnant. Subsequent testing showed a low free T4 and a high TSH. Rebecca was treated with thyroid hormone and had a normal pregnancy. Unfortunately, however, her child is showing developmental delay and lower than average intelligence, not uncommon problems for children of women with untreated thyroid deficiency.

Hypothyroidism in pregnancy is a serious issue. It is estimated that 2.5 percent of pregnant women have some form of hypothyroidism. However, the symptoms of hypothyroidism may overlap those of simply being pregnant and the diagnosis may be missed. Hypothyroidism is associated with an increased risk of pregnancy complications. Moreover, as in the case of Rebecca, a 1999 study published in the *New England Journal of Medicine* showed that women with mild thyroid deficiency during their pregnancy had children with subsequent developmental and intelligence defects.

NORMAL TESTS, LOW THYROID FUNCTION

Do you have symptoms of hypothyroidism, but have been told that your thyroid test is normal? This is a common situation. There are several conditions that result in low thyroid function despite normal thyroid tests—including both TSH and T4 tests. Each of these conditions can cause hypothyroid symptoms, most notably low metabolism and weight gain.

Presubclinical Hypothyroidism

As noted in Figure 7.3 showing the natural history of thyroid disease, the first thing that indicates a dysfunctional thyroid is not reduced T4 levels, but heightened TSH levels. If your TSH is normally at the low end of the normal range—like it is for the majority of us—then doubling, tripling, or even quadrupling of the level (e.g., from 1 mIU/mL to 4 mIU/mL) may be highly significant and indicative of low thyroid function.

Please note that normal range for all these tests depends on the laboratory. However, the normal range for TSH is generally 0.5 mIU/mL to 5.5 mIU/mL. In other words, 5 mIU/mL is considered normal—but for most people normal is around 1.0 mIU/mL. This means your TSH can increase 500 percent and still be considered normal! If you have symptoms of hypothyroidism and a TSH test at the upper range of normal, you may have presubclinical hypothyroidism.

The only way to know if you really have presubclinical hypothyroidism is to wait until you develop full-blown hypothyroidism. Only in very rare circumstances do I recommend taking thyroid hormone for a presubclinical condition. The symptoms of hypothyroidism are the same as those for many other conditions including menopause, chronic fatigue syndrome, depression, and growth hormone deficiency. Recently a study was done to determine if treatment with thyroid hormone could improve the symptoms of hypothyroidism in people with normal thyroid function tests. The results, published in the *British Medical Journal* in 2001, proved that thyroid hormone was no more effective than placebo for relieving symptoms.

Sick Euthyroid Syndrome

When the body is under stress—and stress can be caused by major life-cycle events such as a death in the family, or seemingly innocuous physical changes such as those brought on by a crash diet—one possibility is the production of reverse T3, created when the wrong iodine is removed from the T4 hormone. Reverse T3, you'll remember, is completely inert. Stress also causes the brain to shut down production of TRH and TSH so that the body cannot compensate for low thyroid hormone levels.

The name given to this cycle is *sick euthyroid syndrome*. The "eu-" prefix to "thyroid" is from the Greek for "good" or "well," so "sick euthyroid syndrome" implies that the thyroid is well but the rest of the body is sick. Low thyroid levels are thought to try to put the body at a lower level of metabolism in order to protect it from whatever illness or stress it is experiencing. It's all a natural biological adaptation to stress.

Dieting may not seem like a stressful situation on the surface, certainly not compared to being wounded in battle or undergoing the breakup of a long-term relationship. But the upshot is the same: All the body knows is that something has changed. One day it had plenty of food; the next day it's starving. It reacts by slowing metabolism, and as the regulator of metabolism, the thyroid and its hormones act as leaders in this slowdown.

Interestingly, sick euthyroid syndrome often happens in conjunction with mild thyroid failure. I see this all the time among my patients. The person has mild thyroid failure but the TSH test, pushed and pulled in opposite directions, ends up normal. The result: normal thyroid hormone levels and normal TSH with symptoms of hypothyroidism. It is a situation frequently missed by doctors. Patients are severely symptomatic but are told nothing is wrong.

Regardless of how the problem starts, doctors often miss it. The standard requirement of hypothyroidism is a high production of TSH. In the case of sick euthyroid syndrome and its related conversion problems, the opposite happens: TSH production is low or nonexistent. The pituitary gland also may not sense a T3 deficiency because T4 levels are normal. The normal T4 levels fool the pituitary gland into thinking that everything is just fine, when in reality the body is deficient in T3, the active hormone.

Doctors rarely test for active T3 (total triiodothyronine or free triiodothyronine levels) or reverse T3, which is the key to indicating these conditions. Even some endocrinologists, who are quite familiar with sick euthyroid syndrome and conversion problems, are convinced it occurs only in very sick patients—such as those on life support.

Let me emphasize: You don't have to be sick to have these conditions. Stress of any type, including mental stress, minor illness, or crash dieting, can definitely produce these problems, though to a lesser degree than the conditions suffered by critically ill patients. In this setting, treatment with T4 alone—traditional therapy—may not be effective because it cannot be converted to active hormone. Thus, T4/T3 combination therapy may be indicated, something I will discuss later in this chapter.

Central Hypothyroidism

In rare cases—about 1 in 20,000 people—hypothyroidism is not caused by failure of the thyroid gland but instead by failure of the pituitary gland or hypothalamus. The most common cause of this is a pituitary gland tumor. Other causes of central hypothyroidism include head trauma, brain tumors, problems with blood flow to the pituitary gland, tuberculosis, syphilis and other infections, and other diseases such as hemochromatosis and sarcoidosis. Sometimes a tumor in the pituitary gland causes an abnormal and nonfunctional form of TSH to be made. Through all of this, TSH level may be normal, while free T4 is low normal or obviously low. Though central hypothyroidism is rare, the diagnosis should not be overlooked—particularly since it may involve a brain tumor. Early in the disease, all testing may be normal. The first indication may be something as simple as weight gain. The TRH stimulation test may be helpful in diagnosing central hypothyroidism.

Thyroid Hormone Resistance

Complete thyroid hormone resistance is an extremely rare condition: There have been only about 600 cases reported to date. In thyroid hormone resistance, the thyroid gland is perfectly normal. The problem is in every cell of the body—each of which contains the thyroid hormone receptor and binding sites for the hormone receptor complex to bind to DNA and turn genes on and off. It is described as "reduced tissue responsiveness" to thyroid hormone. The actual problem is caused by a genetic defect in the gene that makes a component of the thyroid hormone receptor, so proper binding cannot occur.

Individuals with thyroid hormone resistance typically have mild symptoms of hypothyroidism and an enlarged thyroid gland. In reality, the TSH test is normal but T4 and T3 levels may be elevated. The reason: There is enough thyroid hormone around, but it is not working properly. Thyroid hormone resistance typically runs in families. It is rarely diagnosed, and cases of "partial" thyroid hormone resistance may escape diagnosis altogether. One tip-off to thyroid hormone resistance may be a failure to lose weight or improve when treated for low thyroid, despite increasing dosages of medication.

Unpredictable Thyroiditis

Thyroiditis is a temporary inflammation of the thyroid gland caused by antibodies or infection. Symptoms, and abnormal blood tests, can come and go. Sometimes the flow of antibodies and the autoimmune attack on the thyroid is unpredictable. Antibody levels can wax and wane, resulting in alternating periods of hyper- and hypothyroidism. This antibody flux is related to stress in your life, so relieving the stress tends to make the problem better. Thyroiditis can be caused by a virus. Some patients report a flu-like illness that occurred a few weeks prior to the onset of symptoms.

The catch: The thyroid tests are abnormal only if you measure them at the right time. At other times, the testing is normal, but the hormones are only transiently in the normal range, on their way to being higher or lower. Thyroiditis can make the neck swollen or tender, but this symptom doesn't always occur. Because of the effect hypo- and hyper-thyroidism have on mental health, patients with thyroiditis are commonly misdiagnosed as having bipolar disorder—popularly known as manic-depression.

Rhonda's Story

Rhonda, a bank teller, started experiencing mood swings. One week she was down in the dumps and could hardly get out of bed, the next week she was agitated and sleepless. Rhonda was told she had bipolar disorder and started taking the medication **lithium**. *This is when her problems really began. The mood swings became more and more violent until she found herself contemplating suicide. Ultimately we discovered that she did not have bipolar disorder at all. She had thyroiditis. Her thyroid gland had become inflamed and would periodically release bursts of thyroid hormone into her system. These periods were followed by episodes of low thyroid hormone. The swings in thyroid hormone were causing her moods to go on a roller-coaster ride. The lithium Rhonda took made her thyroid problems worse. Eventually, her thyroid shut down altogether (not uncommon), and she was placed on a stable prescription of thyroid hormones. The mood swings vanished.*

WILSON'S SYNDROME

In the early 1990s a Florida physician, Dr. E. Denis Wilson, theorized that many of the symptoms of hypothyroidism were caused by low levels of thyroid hormone, despite normal thyroid tests. He reported that his patients had dramatic improvements when treated with thyroid hormone, most notably, T3. He called this condition "Wilson's syndrome." Dr. Wilson popularized his theory with an expensive advertising campaign. He subsequently received complaints to the Florida medical licensing board and was forced to pay a $10,000 fine and to stop practicing medicine for 6 months.

Despite this, Wilson's Syndrome and T3 therapy have gained tremendous popularity among physicians that practice alternative medicine and antiaging medicine. It is interesting to note that the American Thyroid Association confirms that there is no scientific evidence for Wilson's syndrome and does not recognize its existence.

TREATMENT OPTIONS FOR HYPOTHYROIDISM

If there's a positive aspect about hypothyroidism, it is that it is easily treatable. There are several highly regarded forms of thyroid hormone designed to treat hypothyroidism with a minimum of side effects. Those pharmaceuticals—coupled with a proper diet—help thyroid patients today live a full, normal life. The main goal of therapy is to restore thyroid hormone levels to normal. This means that you must have periodic blood tests to make sure all your levels remain in the "normal range."

Levothyroxine (Levothroid, Levoxyl, Synthroid, and Generics)

For many patients with hypothyroidism, levothyroxine is the ideal medication to treat their condition. One small pill a day is able to completely cure the condition. Levothyroxine is synthetic T4, the hormone that must be converted to active T3 and provides the base of the thyroid cycle. The vast majority of physicians prescribe levothyroxine as the replacement medication of choice. However, if you have a conversion problem—such as that brought on by stress or poor diet—then your body may have trouble converting levothyroxine into an active form of the hormone.

I do feel that brand-name levothyroxine—Synthroid, Levothroid, or Levoxyl—offers an advantage over generics. The quality control for the branded versions is much better than it is for generics. Since the cost between brand name and generic is only a few dollars each month, I recommend you avoid the generic version of thyroid hormone.

Several medications, medical conditions, and minerals interfere with levothyroxine efficacy and absorption. Among them are cholestryamine (Questran), iron supplements or vitamins with iron, calcium supplements, Maalox, Mylanta, or other aluminum-containing antacids, soybeans and soy products, bowel problems in which the pill is not absorbed completely, forgetfulness (the pill must be taken every day), and heat damage (the pills are damaged by heat, so they should not be kept in a car or near a stove). Estrogen-containing medications can affect levels as well. Food can affect the absorption of thyroxine through the intestines. *For best results, thyroxine should be taken on an empty stomach.*

Liothyronine (Cytomel)

In my experience, at least one-half of patients with hypothyroidism do not feel well on standard levothyroxine therapy. This is because levothyroxine provides the body only with T4 and depends on the body's ability to convert T4 to T3. As discussed earlier, many people have problems with this process. Because of this, many (but not all) endocrinologists add liothyronine, a synthetic form of triiodothyronine (T3), to levothyroxine (T4). (T3, you'll recall, is the more active form of thyroid hormone.) This cutting-edge treatment has yielded terrific results, but it is still controversial among endocrinologists.

In 1999, a study in the *New England Journal of Medicine* reported the "Effects of Thyroxine as Compared with Thyroxine plus Triiodothyronine in Patients with Hypothyroidism." The protocol of this study was to reduce the dose of levothyroxine by 50 micrograms per day and replace it with a single daily dose of 12.5 micrograms of triiodothyronine. Patients reported improvements as a result of adding T3.

The body is supposed to be able to produce T3 from T4, but for patients with conversion problems from illness, nutritional deficiencies, or stress, this process can be weakened. Many patients on T4-only regimens cannot produce adequate amounts of necessary T3, producing symptoms such as weight gain and fatigue—signs that active thyroid hormone is low, even though blood tests may show that T4 and TSH levels are normal. Many people who take levothyroxine alone continue to suffer from metabolism problems, including weight gain (or, at least, little weight loss), dry skin, and fatigue. Many of these symptoms improve with T3 therapy. For many patients, it also provides them with new energy and a new lease on life.

There are limitations to this therapy, of course. The exact dose of T3 is controversial. As mentioned earlier, the thyroid gland makes about 20 percent T3 and 80 percent T4; however, most physicians feel that this does not translate to thyroid hormone medication dosing. I recommend that the dose of T3 should not exceed 10 percent of the total thyroid hormone dosage. Many people are successful using the substitution schedule used in the *New England Journal of Medicine* article (replace 50 micrograms of T4 with 12.5 micrograms of T3). Contrary to this article, however, I recommend that the T3 be taken two or three times a day. T3 is short acting, so its effectiveness wanes if it is not taken multiple times per day. A long-acting version of T3 is currently under development. Some pharmacies can also make their own version of time-released T3; however, the quality control of time-released T3 varies from pharmacy to pharmacy (see below).

Liotrix (Thyrolar)

Liotrix is a synthetic mixture of liothyronine (T3) and levothyroxine (T4) that is available in a single tablet. Available in different strengths, the ratio of T3 to T4 in this fixed combination tablet is 1:4 (e.g., 1 microgram of T3 for every 4 micrograms of T4). Many doctors feel that the percentage of T3 is too high. Another problem with liotrix is that it requires refrigeration.

Desiccated Thyroid (Armour Thyroid and generics)

Some patients prefer the natural thyroid hormone, known as Armour Thyroid—the hormone made of dried cow or pig thyroid—which already contains both T4 and T3. Unfortunately, these pills' quality and potency varies widely from tablet to tablet, and T3 levels in particular vary along with the pills. Because of the health risks associated with high levels of T3, it is easier—and safer—to use synthetic thyroid hormones.

Sustained-Release T3

Sustained-release T3, custom-made by compounding pharmacists has shown promise as the "perfect" method of taking T3. This is because the T3 that is in Cytomel, Thyrolar, and Armour Thyroid is very short acting. The majority of the T3 from these products is out of your system after a few hours. Sustained-release T3 is in special capsules that provide a slow release of the hormone into your system over 12 to 24 hours. The problem with sustained-release T3 is the same as with all products made by compounding pharmacists: Quality control varies widely. In March 2001, officials from the Georgia Drugs and Narcotics Agency became concerned when several patients who had their T3 filled at a Georgia compounding pharmacy were hospitalized for a condition known as thyrotoxicosis (life-threatening high thyroid levels). It was thought that pills might have contained 100 times the prescribed dose of T3.

Several pharmaceutical companies have expressed interest in developing a standardized version of long-acting T3. Until this option is available, I recommend that you be extremely cautious using custom-compounded T3.

Thyroid Hormone Abuse

There are some people who adhere to the philosophy "If a little is good for me, then more must be better." Maybe that's the case with some things, but with thyroid hormone it is a prescription for disaster. Unfortunately, since thyroid hormone is usually recommended for people suffering from weight gain caused by hypothyroidism (and that's key—it's not simply weight gain), some patients will increase their dosage on their own, thinking that taking more hormone will speed their metabolism and help them lose weight even faster.

Let me emphasize: *This is extremely dangerous.*

First of all, the "benefits" (if you want to call them that) are short-term at best: yes, metabolism may pick up. Yes, this may help shed a few pounds. But the body is as ill equipped to handle what becomes a "forced hyperthyroidism" as it is to handle hypothyroidism. Increased dosages will blow blood pressure sky high, cause the heart to fibrillate and function poorly, weaken muscle tissues, and bring on thinning of the bones (osteoporosis).

Think of those stories you've heard about popping diet pills. The active ingredient in many diet pills is caffeine. Why? Because caffeine keeps you hopped up. Caffeine helps get rid of water weight by forcing you to go to the bathroom a dozen times a day. Caffeine deadens your appetite. In the short-term, you'll lose weight, but at what cost? You won't be able to sleep. Your sex drive will become nil. You won't be able to concentrate, much less think. And, all the time, your body systems are becoming stressed and weakened.

Thyroid hormone is a serious matter. Endocrinologists painstakingly work to find exactly the right dosage for their patients, tweaking the daily regimen by as little as 12 micrograms—that's 12 millionths of a gram, or .000012 gram—and having patients come in regularly for blood tests to make sure that dosage is still correct. Like any other drug, thyroid hormone is not to be abused. The results can be calamitous.

Estrogen and Thyroid Hormone

If you take thyroid hormone and either start or stop taking any type of estrogen medication, your thyroid hormone levels will be affected. This includes starting or stopping HRT or birth control pills. If you become pregnant, you will have much higher estrogen levels, which can also influence your thyroid hormone levels. Estrogen increases TBG levels, soaking up free thyroid hormone. The result is that you need more thyroid hormone to get the job done. If you have a change in your estrogen status, you should have your thyroid levels monitored carefully.

DIET AND LIFESTYLE FOR A HEALTHY THYROID

A balanced, nutritious diet is important for people with hypothyroidism. A proper diet not only helps you lose weight; it also promotes optimal thyroid function, psychological well-being, and physical health. Along with diet principles discussed in previous chapters, I also recommend the following:

Lots of Fruits and Vegetables

Fruits and vegetables act as antioxidants. Among the best-known antioxidants are beta-carotene, vitamin A, and vitamin C. Antioxidants promote the binding of what are called *free radicals*—oxygen-rich substances in the body that damage cells and hinder the immune system. Remember, immune system attack is the cause of hypothyroidism. Antioxidants clear toxins from the body and are even thought to help ward against cancer.

Foods High in Selenium and Zinc

Selenium and zinc function as antioxidants. Moreover, selenium has a dual role—besides its antioxidizing properties, it helps convert T4 to T3. Lack of selenium and zinc can reduce levels of active T3 by preventing its conversion from T4. Although selenium and zinc supplements are available from most health-food stores, I recommend that you increase your consumption of these vital minerals by eating the proper foods. Foods high in selenium include whole grains, tuna, halibut, mushrooms, oatmeal, wheat germ, and sunflower seeds.

Because selenium is also needed for survival of bacteria, persons infected with a bacterial illness often find themselves with a selenium deficiency—and get a double whammy because the bacteria, growing fat and happy off all the selenium they're diverting, also produce substances detrimental to the production of thyroid hormone.

However, too much selenium can be as damaging as too little. Among the side effects of too much selenium: abdominal pain, nerve damage, and diarrhea. It is estimated that 50 milligrams a day is enough to keep your thyroid healthy and provide a decent amount of antioxidant activity.

Table 7.1
FOODS HIGH IN SELENIUM

Halibut
Mushrooms
Oatmeal
Sunflower seeds
Tuna
Wheat germ
Whole grains

Table 7.2
FOODS HIGH IN ZINC

Beef
Herring
Maple syrup
Sunflower seeds
Turkey
Wheat bran

Diets low in zinc have been found to promote damage to the thyroid gland. Down's syndrome children are usually low in zinc, and many are hypothyroid as well. Obese people have the same problem. A diet featuring a proper level of this trace mineral can help assuage the problems caused by thyroid dysfunction. Foods high in zinc include beef, herring, maple syrup, turkey, wheat bran, and sunflower seeds.

Don't Eat Raw "Goitrogens"

Goitrogens are a class of foods that block thyroid function. They include cabbage, brussels sprouts, turnips, rutabaga, kohlrabi, radishes, cauliflower, cassava, millet and kale. These vegetables are only considered a problem when consumed raw. *Cooking minimizes the goitrogenic potential of these foods.*

Table 7.3
GOITROGENS

Brussels sprouts
Cabbage
Cassava
Cauliflower
Kale
Kohlrabi
Millet
Radishes
Rutabaga
Turnips

Don't Eat Too Much Soy

Soy products have many health benefits. Soy is a healthy source of protein. Soy also contains natural estrogen-like compounds (see Chapter 6). When it comes to the thyroid, however, too much soy can cause problems. Studies have shown that overconsumption of soy products blocks the absorption and action of thyroid hormone and may even induce autoimmune thyroid disease. The estrogen-like effect of soy also increases binding proteins in the blood, lowering free thyroid hormone levels. Soy menopause products that contain isoflavones can also cause thyroid problems.

Exercise

Regular exercise is a critical element in maintaining a healthy metabolism. Hypothyroidism makes people tired, less energetic, and less motivated to exercise. Try to exercise during a time in the day when your energy levels are at their peak.

Reduce Stress

As noted earlier, stress can cause improper processing of thyroid hormone, causing the condition of sick euthyroid syndrome. Stress reduction can improve thyroid hormone processing, increase metabolism, and help you lose weight.

Avoid Antibacterial Products

Antibacterial products, from dishwashing liquids to bar soap and toothpaste, have become very popular in the last few years, promising cleaner skin and less risk of infection. But many of these products contain a chemical called Triclosan—and Triclosan has been shown to interfere with thyroid hormone metabolism. My recommendation is to avoid antibacterials at all costs. The "regular" versions of the products usually do an excellent job of killing microbes to start with—and without any ill effects.

Beware of "Thyroid Support Formulas"

These products, which usually come as dietary supplements, promise to "supply the nutritional needs of the thyroid" and contain iodine (in the form of kelp, bugleweed, or bladderwrack), vitamins, minerals, and tyrosine. Tyrosine, you'll remember, is the backbone of the thyroid hormone molecule. It's all well and good, but I'm not sure it has much effect—you get vitamins and minerals from a balanced diet (or, if need be, supplements), and you get tyrosine from protein.

CHAPTER EIGHT

CORTISOL, STRESS, AND THE ADRENAL GLAND

ADRENAL GLAND STEROIDS AND YOUR WEIGHT

As you've read this book, you've seen the way the body, its glands, and its organs function based on feedback. Produce too much of a particular hormone and metabolism goes haywire; the metabolism problems, in turn, change the amounts of other hormones going through the body; and those hormone levels, in turn, throw off other body functions.

The body is a versatile mechanism, and it can handle a multitude of variations in diet, exercise, stress, and weight—for a time. But it remains a machine that must remain within certain norms—it must be continually well tuned—or problems result, problems that tend to cause other problems.

In the case of adrenal gland hormones, the body can create a vicious circle. Too much adrenal steroids will make you fat. Being fat makes your adrenal gland produce more adrenal gland hormones.

The problems with cortisol excess are very similar to Syndrome X, and the insulin resistance syndrome discussed in Chapter 3. The principal adrenal gland hormone, **cortisol**, controls body fat in both amount and distribution. Cortisol also controls your muscles—their bulk and strength.

WHAT IS CORTISOL?

Let's start with two definitions:

- **Steroid**: A generic term for any hormone with the classic four-ring structure. Steroids include cortisol, androgens, estrogens, progesterone, and others.

- **Glucocorticoids** or **corticosteroids**: A specific class of steroids that have a major role in the control of glucose and other nutrients. Glucocorticoid hormones include cortisol, cortisone, and many medications. Corticosteroids are not to be confused with anabolic steroids or androgenic steroids, discussed in Chapter 4. Corticosteroids are made primarily from the adrenal gland and, in many ways, have the opposite actions of anabolic steroids. *Corticosteroids promote fat accumulation and muscle loss.* Nevertheless, everybody needs some corticosteroids.

Remember: All of our hormones are carefully balanced. Corticosteroids are beneficial for life, and when balanced with the other hormones in our bodies, they contribute positively to our well-being. But, as always, too much or too little causes trouble. In the case of glucocorticoids, only too much makes you fat. People with cortisol deficiency typically lose weight.

Let me offer a brief word on cortisol deficiency, also known as *Addison's disease*. Addison's disease is usually caused by autoimmune destruction of the adrenal gland. (A famous sufferer: John F. Kennedy.) Usually, Addison's disease is slow and smoldering: people feel tired and sick, lose weight, and may have belly pain. But, sometimes, an infection of the adrenal gland can cause a more sudden and more complete loss of glucocorticoids. This is a bad situation.

Marcia's Story
Marcia, an 18-year-old high school senior, went to spring break in Mexico. While there, she got sick but decided to wait until she got home to go to the doctor. On the plane ride back, she fell seriously ill and broke out in a rash. Her blood pressure was dangerously low; her stomach hurt. Upon landing, she was immediately taken to a hospital, but it was too late. She died 2 days later.

Marcia had contracted an infection known as meningo-coccemia, an ailment that attacks adrenal glands, destroys them, and causes loss of glucocorticoids and rapid death. Although it is a rare condition, I have seen several other cases of meningococcemia in my career as an endocrinologist. Every one has had the same sad outcome.

There are a number of medications containing glucocorticoids. They come in all forms: pills, creams, eye drops, nasal sprays, gels, lung inhalers, and injections. You've probably heard of the most common—prednisone and cortisone—and the terms people use when they're taking them: "on cortisone" or "on steroids."

Although necessary to treat many diseases, these medications have horrible side effects. They flood the body with extra corticosteroids and induce what doctors call a "disease state," in which diseases like *Cushing's syndrome* can suddenly take root. (The induced version is called iatrogenic Cushing's syndrome.)

Natural forms of Cushing's syndrome are less common, but do occur. In natural CS, a much more serious, medical overproduction of cortisol causes the weight gain; as I will detail later, excess fat can also raise cortisol levels. Cushing's syndrome is really a catch-all term to describe a variety of different hormone-producing tumors that all lead to cortisol excess.

THE ADRENAL GLANDS

The adrenal glands are triangular-shaped glands located on top of each kidney, and—as with the kidney and many other organs—there are two of them. And, also like the kidney, you need only one to survive.

Five major classes of hormones are produced by the adrenal gland—three types of steroid hormones and two types of nonsteroid hormones, epinephrine (adrenaline) and norepinephrine (noradrenaline).

The adrenal gland is really two organs rolled into one. The outer portion of the adrenal gland, known as the *adrenal cortex*, is responsible for making steroid hormones like cortisol, DHEA and aldosterone. The adrenal cortex has three layers: the *zona glomerulosa*, which produces cortisol; the *zona fasciculata*, which produces aldosterone; and the *zona reticularis*, which produces aldosterone and DHEA.

Aldosterone is an example of what's known as a *mineralocorticoid*, a type of steroid hormone that controls the body's minerals. Aldosterone can act like cortisol a little bit, but its main function is to regulate the body's salt and water balance. It also plays a major role in controlling blood pressure; aldosterone-producing tumors cause very high blood pressure. In addition, some cancers of the adrenal gland can produce too much glucocorticoid and too much mineralocorticoid. Still, aldosterone has little to do with your weight.

The middle part of the adrenal gland is called the *adrenal medulla*. It's like a separate organ. The adrenal medulla, as previously noted, produces epinephrine and norepinephrine, which are considered stress hormones. As with aldosterone, excessive production of adrenaline can cause high blood pressure, and that excessive production can often be brought on by a tumor.

YOUR BRAIN CONTROLS YOUR ADRENAL GLANDS

How does cortisol work? It interacts directly with your genes, the same as other steroid hormones. Glucocorticoids bind to the glucocorticoid receptor inside the cell, and this entire complex binds to DNA, turning genes on and off. Think about what was described in Chapter 1, the lock-and-key design for hormone-receptor interactions.

The brain and the pituitary gland control the adrenal glands, just as they do the thyroid, testicles, and ovaries (see Figure 8.1). The brain sends signals through a region known as the hypothalamus, the most important part of the brain for regulating hunger, weight and metabolism. The hypothalamus produces a hormone called corticotropin-releasing hormone, or CRH for short. CRH stimulates the pituitary gland to release its hormone, adrenocorticotrophic hormone (ACTH), which, in turn, tells the adrenal gland to make glucocorticoids. Normally, when cortisol levels go up, a signal is sent to the brain to ease up on CRH and ACTH production. This careful balance ensures that you have the right amount of glucocorticoids.

But what is the right amount? It depends. Glucocorticoid levels fluctuate throughout the day. They surge early in the morning and gradually fall throughout the day, hitting a low sometime around 4 P.M. This is why timing is critical when a blood test is done.

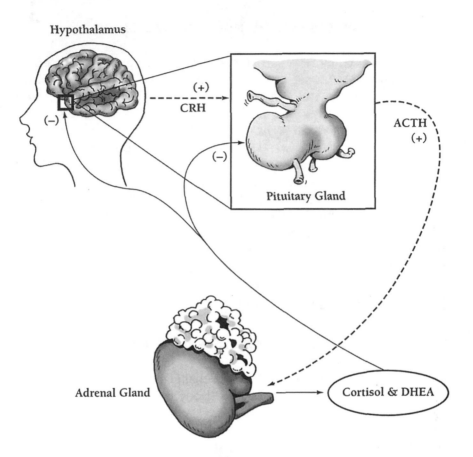

Figure 8.1
GLUCOCORTICOID ENDOCRINOLOGY:
HORMONE FEEDBACK LOOPS

Higher centers in the brain send signals to the hypothalamus, which produces corticotropin-releasing hormone (CRH). CRH stimulates the pituitary gland to make adrenocorticotrophic hormone (ACTH). ACTH stimulates the adrenal glands to produce cortisol and DHEA. Cortisol and DHEA "feed back" to the hypothalamus and pituitary gland, slowing ACTH production. Positive "feedback" is denoted by +, and negative "feedback" is denoted by – .

THE ADRENAL GLANDS AND YOUR MOOD

There is a strong link between glucocorticoids and mood. Most people who are depressed have very high cortisol levels, though the reason isn't exactly known; it is thought that maybe the brain is very stressed by depression. Whatever the reason, people who are depressed frequently have many of the signs of cortisol excess.

Cortisol excess can cause depression, severe mood swings, or even euphoria, as well as anxiety and insomnia. In some cases, involving tumors or excessively high doses of medication, cortisol excess has even been known to cause psychosis with wild hallucinations. Glucocorticoids influence the release of brain chemicals (aka neurotransmitters) such as serotonin and norepinephrine, and cortisol excess disrupts the delicate balance between the pituitary gland and the adrenal glands. Almost any psychiatric illness, even mild ones, may result in cortisol excess; and, as just noted, the reverse can occur as well. The body's fine balance works both ways.

STRESS AND THE ADRENAL GLANDS

Given that the main function of the adrenal gland is to make stress hormones, they work overtime when the body believes it is under stress. Remember, stress comes in many forms: A crash diet causes one kind of stress, while a tight deadline at work causes another kind. Constant worrying or physical exertion is also stress. Any one of these can cause the adrenal glands to kick into overdrive.

The most immediate kind of overdrive is the "fight-or-flight" response. The main hormone the adrenal glands produce under stress is adrenaline, which makes your heart beat faster and revs up your body. Adrenaline is a counterinsulin hormone, so insulin levels go up when there's lots of adrenaline around. Under normal conditions, adrenaline levels are spiked: they happen, the body responds, and then things get back to normal. For a short time, you may want something to calm your nerves (food, alcohol, whatever), but when the spike wears off, body systems return to normal. So adrenaline, overall, has little effect on your weight.

But the body is also producing cortisol when it's under stress. These hormones tend to stick around, and they can cause symptoms that eventually lead to weight gain.

As I noted at the beginning of the chapter, it's all part of a vicious circle. Higher cortisol production because of stress leads to weight gain. Weight gain leads to more stress—whether it's from a crash diet to lose the weight, or stress on organs to handle the weight, or simply the need to maintain the weight because the body's gotten used to it, or even something psychological almost wholly unrelated to the weight gain. It's all stress, and it all causes more cortisol to be produced.

As the *Journal of the American Medical Association* noted in 1999, "Chronic stress . . . that evokes prolonged distress can influence cardiovascular, immune and endocrine function, and these alterations are sufficient to enhance a variety of health threats." *People under chronic stress have shorter lives.*

Stress causes heart attacks, that's a common fact. But we tend to overlook the hormonal reasons for this: High stress leads to high cortisol. High cortisol leads to insulin resistance. Insulin resistance often leads to coronary artery disease. The heart attack is the final straw.

Now, we all have some stress in our lives. For the most part, the body can handle cortisol surges caused by stress. But if there's too much stress, the body can't keep up with the detrimental effects of the stress hormone surges.

GLUCOCORTICOID MEDICATIONS

There are many, many types of glucocorticoid medications used to treat a number of conditions, including inflammatory bowel disease, lupus, asthma, sarcoidosis, arthritis, kidney disease, and liver disease. These medications, because of their immune suppression ability, are used frequently in organ transplant patients (and not without the Cushing's side effects). Even some types of cancer may in part be treated with glucocorticoids.

Prednisone is one of the most frequently used glucocorticoid medications, but there are many more. These medications are mostly synthetic versions of the glucocorticoids your adrenal glands naturally make.

Because these medications are so frequently prescribed, patients and even physicians forget about the serious side effects. Let me remind you, the side effects of these medications can be as serious as having Cushing's syndrome. If you take any of these medications—

especially the pills—on a daily basis, you should be closely monitored by your physician. You should work with your physician to get on the lowest possible dose of steroids and should work on a plan to try to taper the steroids even further. In my career, I have had very few patients who could not eventually stop taking steroid medications. Many doctors think it is too dangerous to stop the steroids, but I believe it is more dangerous to continue taking them.

A note to patients: If you have been taking steroids for more than 30 days, your body is dependent on them; some would say addicted. If you stop taking them abruptly, you might face serious medical consequences. Your adrenal glands have turned off their steroid production. Your steroid dose must be slowly tapered. Most endocrinologists will tell you that you need to take about as many days to taper the steroids as you have been taking them. For example, if you have been taking corticosteroids for a year, you should slowly decrease your dose over the course of one year before completely discontinuing the medications. I do not recommend that you do this by yourself; this requires careful monitoring by an endocrinologist.

EFFECTS OF EXCESS GLUCOCORTICOIDS

What do glucocorticoids do? First of all, they're necessary for life. Without them, you would die. But in excessive amounts, glucocorticoids have several negative effects as well:

Fat buildup
Glucocorticoids increase the amount of fat in your body and in a particular distribution. Remember the different body shapes discussed in Chapter 3: apple and pear, gut and butt. Glucocorticoids cause fat buildup in the belly, chest and face like the apple shape—the worst type of "metabolically evil" fat. This fat buildup can cause many of the symptoms of insulin resistance and Syndrome X.

Increased appetite
Anyone who has ever taken a steroid medication can tell you they can never get enough to eat. Think of our discussion of the brain and the adrenal glands. The hypothalamus is a part of the brain responsible for appetite. Glucocorticoids tickle the hypothalamus, making you ravenous.

Muscle breakdown

Once the muscles break down, the next steps are muscle weakness, slowed metabolism, and insulin resistance. For this reason, the hormones involved are known as *catabolic hormones* because they break down muscle tissue. Androgens are called *anabolic hormones*; they build muscle up. Catabolic, of course, is the opposite.

Normally, there is a basic amount of muscle breakdown and regeneration that always occurs. The body can use muscle for fuel. If you stress or starve yourself, or eat a diet too low in calories (such as many of the fad/crash diets that guarantee rapid weight loss), glucocorticoid levels will rise, breaking down muscle protein to produce amino acids (the building blocks of protein). These, in turn, can be converted by the liver into glucose to use as fuel. In other words, the stress of starvation causes the body to break down its own muscle to be used as fuel.

If cortisol levels go too high, huge amounts of muscle are broken down, a big load of amino acids go to the liver, and huge amounts of glucose are produced, a process known as *gluconeogenesis*. The high glucose levels in the blood increase insulin levels and can lead to insulin resistance and diabetes.

Proper dieting does not stress the body: Cortisol levels remain low, and fat is broken down instead of muscle.

There are other side effects of muscle wasting. Your metabolism slows. You feel weak and tired. You don't want to exercise, even though it would be good for you (and probably help take off some of that stress naturally).

This is why you should not go on a crash diet. The body senses that it is starving, gets stressed, and releases glucocorticoids, leading to this muscle breakdown. (High stress levels of any type can also do this.) Next, weak muscles, insulin resistance, and slowed metabolism. If you follow my eating guidelines while dieting, the body is not as stressed, and fat is broken down instead of muscle.

Glucocorticoids can also lead to breakdown of other tissues, such as bone and skin. Bone loss can lead to osteoporosis, and skin breakdown can lead to easy bruising, stretch marks, or thin skin with a ruddy appearance.

Then there are the hormonal imbalances. As I noted in Chapter 7, strict dieting causes low thyroid action and slowed metabolism. And you're never just affecting one hormone; the hormones become a series of falling dominoes, each trying to rectify the body's situation as best it knows, each causing more problems down the line.

Immune suppression

Glucocorticoids keep the immune system in check. They have potent anti-inflammatory properties but also interact with white blood cells to suppress the immune system. This is why people under a lot of stress tend to get sick: The immune system has been weakened by stress via glucocorticoids. And yet doctors prescribe glucocorticoids such as cortisone or prednisone to treat medical disorders caused by immune system overactivity. Glucocorticoids are also used to treat severe allergies. It's a difficult balance. We will discuss how to cope with glucocorticoid medications (if you must take them) later in the chapter.

Upset stomach, ulcers, gastroesophageal reflux disease (GERD), increased stomach acid production

Have you ever been really upset and ended up with an upset stomach? Here's why: Excess glucocorticoids crank up stomach acid production, leading to upset stomach and possible stomach ulcers. And that's why stress causes stomach ulcers.

Bloating and fluid retention

Earlier, we briefly discussed aldosterone and its fluid retention properties. Glucocorticoids have some overlap with the actions of mineralocorticoids. They will stimulate the glucocorticoid receptor very well, but also stimulate the mineralocorticoid receptor to some extent. The result is salt, water retention and bloating. Excess mineralocorticoid activity can also make blood potassium drop—leading to cramping and muscle weakness.

CUSHING'S SYNDROME

It's hard to talk about cortisol without talking about Cushing's Syndrome. Here's the story: Cushing's syndrome (CS) is a medical/hormonal condition resulting in excess glucocorticoids. It's not caused by stress; it's caused by a tumor. Another ailment with the appearance of CS, iatrogenic CS, is not caused by a tumor, but by steroid medications.

Both can be severe and devastating.

Tamika's Story

*Tamika was a 40-year-old woman. She'd had two children,
was a stay-at-home mother, and wasn't much into exercise.
So, when she started gaining weight, she mostly disregarded
it—even though her face became round and moonlike, her
belly got big with purple stretch marks, and her arms and legs
became skinny. She felt lousy and tired all the time. Just signs
of becoming old and fat, she thought.*

*Eventually, she stopped having menses and went to visit
her doctor. His initial recommendation: diet and exercise.
These had little effect, and she went back. Blood tests determined she had diabetes and high blood pressure, and further
investigation indicated a microscopic tumor in her pituitary
gland. The tumor was removed; to give you an idea of how
small it was, it was removed through her nose. With the tumor
removed, Tamika's diet and exercise started having the proper
effect, and her body returned to normal.*

Tamika was lucky; not all people are. Another patient of mine, discussed in Chapter 5, began having similar symptoms. However, along
with the weight gain and fatigue, she also grew hair on her face. It
turned out she had a very large cancer of the adrenal gland. Despite
extensive surgery and chemotherapy, she died 2 years later. The length
of her life was a remarkable feat in itself; she had been expected to survive only 6 months.

Please note that, although the symptoms were similar, these
women had different conditions. Adrenal gland cancer is a cause of
CS, but most of the time CS isn't cancer at all, but rather a benign,
hormone-producing tumor that is frequently successfully removed
surgically.

If these cases sound like insulin resistance, that's because—in one
way—they are. Glucocorticoids such as cortisol are known as "counter-insulin hormones." They work against the actions of insulin, thus
creating the need for higher insulin levels and the components of
Syndrome X.

Cushing's syndrome is called a "syndrome" because it describes
many conditions that all result in cortisol excess.

The main causes of CS are

- Pituitary gland tumor (also known as Cushing's disease).
- Adrenal gland tumor.
- Various other cancers that produce ACTH (known as ectopic ACTH-producing tumors). These tumors are most common in the lung.
- Steroid medications (iatrogenic CS).

Seth's Story

Seth was a 48-year-old man who had to take daily steroids because of his severe asthma. The steroids made him fat and gave him a number of the symptoms listed earlier in this chapter. He followed our suggested diet, lessened the stress in his life, and started exercising, all of which contributed to him losing weight and feeling better and healthier.

Unfortunately, the steroids had taken their toll. One day, Seth developed severe back pain. He had suffered a compression fracture of the vertebra, a telltale sign of osteoporosis.

Incidentally, many dogs and cats are given steroids to help with allergies. They can get all the same problems as humans.

About Cushing's Syndrome

Cushing's syndrome was named after a famous Boston neurosurgeon, Harvey Cushing, who first described the condition. He discovered the most common cause of the syndrome was a small tumor in the pituitary gland. Cushing's syndrome caused by a pituitary tumor is called "Cushing's disease." Other cortisol-excess conditions are "syndromes"; only the pituitary-caused one is the "disease."

Cushing's syndrome is fairly rare: About 1 in 1,000 people have it. But not everyone has been diagnosed. Women are four times as likely to develop Cushing's compared to men, and some overweight people have Cushing's, but don't know it.

SYMPTOMS OF CUSHING'S SYNDROME

Could you have Cushing's? I've provided a list of both major and minor symptoms below. Though most overweight people have a few of these symptoms, this does not mean you have Cushing's syndrome. However, if you have many of the symptoms or have one of the serious symptoms, you should ask your doctor to check you for Cushing's.

Muscle weakness/wasting
This becomes very pronounced. You may have trouble sitting up from a chair and may need to use your arms to help you up. The thigh muscles are particularly affected: This is known as *proximal muscle weakness* (*proximal* means "close"; and the muscles close in are affected more than the distal, or far, muscles like the lower leg). Arms and legs look thin due to this muscle wasting, despite weight gain.

Excessive weight gain in a short period of time
Many people gain huge amounts of weight, but others gain a small amount. Regardless of the pace of weight gain, the **body-fat distribution** is noticeable. It particularly builds up in the belly, leading to a big belly. Other places the weight gain is noticeable are the face (makes the face round and moon-like), the hollow space over the collarbones (which becomes filled in with fat), and the back of the neck or between the shoulder blades (where a fat pad can develop, known as a buffalo hump). Doctors refer to the below appearance as "Cushingoid." Some overweight people just appear Cushingoid, but if you do look like this, see your doctor. Other Cushingoid features are thin arms and legs, red face, striae (see below), and thin skin with bruises.

Stretch marks, aka striae
Many overweight people have striae, especially women who have been pregnant, but simply being overweight can cause striae. The striae to become concerned about are those that are wide (more than ½ inch), or purple or red in coloration, all of which can indicate Cushing's syndrome.

Insulin resistance and/or diabetes
Again, just being overweight can cause insulin resistance or diabetes, and most people with insulin resistance or diabetes do *not* have Cushing's syndrome. Despite this, these conditions are common in

Cushing's syndrome. Sometimes, the insulin resistance is so severe that the there is *acanthosis nigricans,* which I discussed in Chapter 3. Insulin resistance occurs because of muscle breakdown. That breakdown leads to a large amount of amino acids sent to the liver, which are then turned into glucose.

If you are overweight and have insulin resistance or diabetes, you are unlikely to have Cushing's syndrome unless you have some of the other features. However, if you do have any of the other features, such as the particular body-fat distribution, high blood pressure, or striae, you should be checked by your physician for Cushing's.

High blood pressure

We talked of mineralcorticoids earlier in this chapter. In Cushing's syndrome, very high glucocorticoid levels lead to cross-reactivity with the receptor. In that case, both glucocorticoid and mineralocorticoid receptors are stimulated. Though high blood pressure and obesity alone are unlikely to be Cushing's syndrome, they could be, and your doctor should check to make sure either way.

Infections

Glucocorticoids lower your immune system. In the case of CS, the very high levels of glucocorticoids can lead to severe immune suppression and multiple infections. Common infections include yeast infections of the vagina and/or mouth, bladder infections, and sinus infections. It is not uncommon for someone with CS to come down with exotic infections typically seen in AIDS patients.

Thinning of the bones (osteoporosis) or fractures

Glucocorticoids are notorious for this. In Chapter 6, we talked about how women are at particular risk for osteoporosis. Osteoporosis in Cushing's is similar to postmenopausal osteoporosis, but it tends to be more severe.

Kidney stones

When the bones thin, calcium is lost. Where does it go? The kidneys. Calcium in kidneys is what forms kidney stones.

Effects of male hormones

Sometimes, adrenal gland overactivity leads to production of multiple hormones, including male hormones. You'll recall the discussions of hirsutism and other effects of male hormones in Chapter 4, Androgens. Severe hair growth is known as *virilization* and may be associated with balding (in a pattern similar to a man), increased sex drive, deepening of the voice, and growth of the clitoris into what may resemble a small penis. Virilization in either sex is a worrisome sign for adrenal gland cancer. Men may have excessive hair growth and/or increased sex drive.

Menstrual irregularities
The excess male hormones present in CS can also cause menstrual irregularities. This is, in fact, one of the most common symptoms of CS.

Skin problems
Thin skin, easy bruising, poor wound healing, and acne are the most common of these. The reason: Glucocorticoids have potent effects on the skin. Thinning of the skin can cause the face to appear red or ruddy, a condition known as *plethora*. If you are older, thin skin is normal. However, *if you are young and your skin suddenly becomes very thin, this is a warning sign*.

Mental Problems
In the early stages of CS, mental changes may be a dead giveaway that your weight gain is more than just overeating. Patients with CS report feeling depressed or agitated, as well as having poor sleep, poor sex drive, poor memory and an inability to concentrate.

TESTING FOR CUSHING'S SYNDROME

Although there are many causes of Cushing's syndrome, the initial testing is the same for all forms. The first set of testing is to determine if you have an overproduction of cortisol. If so, your endocrinologist will do additional tests to determine which type of Cushing's you may have.

Cautions about Testing for Cushing's Syndrome
- Testing for CS is one of the most controversial subjects in the field of endocrinology. Experts have heated arguments about testing protocols.
- Testing is still crude. Tests that are easy to perform usually give unreliable results. The more reliable tests usually require you to

take medication (sometimes for days) or even receive injections of very expensive medications prior to blood testing. These "stimulation" and "suppression" tests require up-to-date endocrinologists, because protocols frequently change.

- Many people are inappropriately tested for Cushing's with a simple blood cortisol test. Because cortisol levels in your blood will fluctuate (see section on hormone fluxes in Chapter 4 and refer to diurnal rhythms above), a simple blood test alone is rarely helpful. Unless the doctor draws your blood at a specific time (see below), serum cortisol is useless.

- Many people with symptoms suggestive of Cushing's are not tested by their doctor. If you think you have it, ask your doctor to test you.

- **An elevated test does not mean you definitely have Cushing's.** Confirmatory tests are almost always needed. Do not get overly concerned that you have adrenal gland cancer or some other horrific problem. Your levels are most likely elevated because of excess weight or other stressors.

- On the other hand, a normal test does not always mean you are OK. Sometimes, cortisol is produced episodically and can be missed on initial testing. If you have symptoms that are very suggestive of Cushing's but have a normal test, ask your doctor to repeat the test. I have had patients who had negative testing the first two tries, but on the third were positive and subsequently were found to have tumors.

- A rare variant of Cushing's exists that is known as ***Food-induced Cushing's***. Since Cushing's is rare enough, this variant is really, really rare. In food-induced Cushing's, the body's hormone/receptor system gets "cross-wired" and one of the hormones produced by the body when it detects food in the stomach, known as gastrointestinal peptide, or GIP, stimulates the adrenal gland to produce corticosteroids. This can be detected only if you are tested right after you eat.

Serum cortisol level

One of the best tests for Cushing's is of the blood cortisol level, but ***timing is everything!*** Some doctors get confused about when to draw the blood. The key to interpreting blood cortisol levels is the fact that *people with CS lose their diurnal cortisol rhythms* (see Figure 8.2). Their levels are high all day and all night long. So, if you test in the morning when everyone has a high level, the test is useless. Late in the day, cortisol tends to drop in people without CS, but stays at the same level in those with CS. So a "normal" in the morning is "high" in the evening.

Because of this fact, a cortisol level drawn at midnight can be very valuable. Unfortunately, it is very inconvenient—to say the least—for most people to get a blood test at midnight. Most doctor's offices are closed—for that matter, most offices of any sort are closed. However, some persuasive endocrinologists can coax your local emergency-room doctor to give you the royal in-and-out treatment.

A new test to accurately measure cortisol levels in saliva is now available. The **midnight salivary cortisol test** is an alternative to a midnight blood test. It turns out that saliva is an excellent bodily fluid from which to measure hormones. And cortisol levels in the saliva tend to be extremely useful for sorting out who has CS from those with pseudo-Cushing's. Many physicians are not yet performing salivary cortisol measurements; however, I expect this to become a popular test in the future.

24-hour urine free cortisol

This is currently the standard screening test for Cushing's. You have to collect all your urine in a container over a 24-hour period. If cortisol is produced in excess, it is spilled out the kidneys in the urine and can be measured.

The urine free cortisol test, or UFC, is a very good screening test … unless you are stressed, depressed, drink heavily, or are overweight. In those cases, your UFC can be elevated up to 4 times the upper limits of normal (normal is usually below 90 micrograms per 24 hours, depending on the lab doing the measurement) and still be in the pseudo-Cushing's range (a measurement less than 360 micrograms per 24 hours can still be pseudo-Cushing's). If it is greater than 4 times the upper limits of normal, you definitely have CS and your endocrinologist should initiate further "localization" testing, such as blood work and MRI or CT scans of adrenal and pituitary glands, looking for a tumor.

Sometimes, doctors measure another hormone in the urine known as "17-ketosteroids," but I feel this is unnecessary. To me, *simply put, all tests with "17" in the name are worthless tests.* (An exception is the 17-hydroxyprogesterone test for congenital adrenal hyperplasia, which was discussed in Chapter 5.)

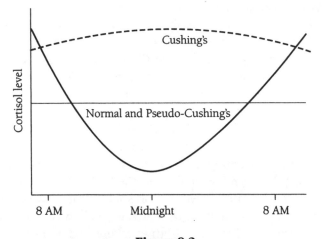

Figure 8.2
DIURNAL CORTISOL FLUXES

In normal people, and in those with pseudo-Cushing's, cortisol levels vary
throughout the day. The peak is usually around 8 A.M., the nadir is around midnight. Patients with Cushing's syndrome lose diurnal rhythms, and, cortisol levels stay constant and high throughout the day.

Suppression testing

A test known as a *1 mg dexamethasone suppression test* is a fairly good
way of ruling out Cushing's. You must take a tablet of a potent glucocorticoid known as dexamethasone at midnight the night before your
test. At 8 A.M. the next day, blood is collected and measured for cortisol. Normally the synthetic glucocorticoid (dexamethasone) will suppress your adrenal gland's production of cortisol. However, in
Cushing's, corticosteroid production goes unchecked. (Remember feedback loops: In this case, they're gone.)

Why do we use dexamethasone and not prednisone or some other
corticosteroid medication? Most corticosteroid medications are detected
on blood testing, thus invalidating the test. Dexamethasone, however
is not detected, so the cortisol measured is all from your body.

Doctors keep lowering the acceptable cortisol limit for this test. In
the past, if your morning cortisol level was less than 5 micrograms per
deciliter, you were considered normal. Now, this number is going
down as doctors are detecting subtler and subtler cases of CS. Some

doctors now consider 3.5 mcg/dL as the cutoff. Unfortunately, this test has the same limitations as the urine test. If you are stressed, depressed, drink heavily, or are overweight, the test is *not* valid.

I HAVE A POSITIVE TEST FOR CUSHING'S...WHAT DO I DO NOW?

Most people with positive tests actually do *not* have Cushing's. As discussed above, just being overweight can cause you to produce excess cortisol in levels high enough to make your test abnormal. Stress— mental and emotional—and heavy drinking can also do this. If you have a positive test, your endocrinologist must do further testing to determine if you have true Cushing's or pseudo-Cushing's syndrome.

What if confirmatory tests are positive?
You probably have Cushing's. Now your endocrinologist needs to find out where the excess cortisol is coming from. At this point, your doctor will do more blood tests as well as imaging studies such as CT or MRI scans to determine the type and location of your cortisol-producing tumor. If your tumor is found (usually in the pituitary gland or adrenal gland, but sometimes in the lung or other organs), it should be removed surgically.

What if confirmatory tests are negative?
You probably still have cortisol excess, but the cause is not a tumor. The cause is stress! It's either the stress your fat is putting on your body, or some other physical or emotional stress in your life. (That includes the stress of drinking a lot of alcohol.) And don't forget—if you have the serious symptoms of CS (see above), ask your doctor to retest you.

PSEUDO-CUSHING'S SYNDROME

The term *pseudo-Cushing's* has been given to the condition that has all the appearances of Cushing's but without the physical presence of a tumor. Many people with this disorder are overweight and have many of the features of Cushing's as described above, most notably the central obesity, moon-shaped face, diabetes, and high blood pressure. Here's where the body feedback loops come into play once again:

Cortisol makes you fat, there is no doubt about that, and being fat makes you have too much cortisol. The vicious cycle goes around and comes around.

Fat is what throws everything off. Too much fat produces hormonal disregulation and, finally, cortisol excess. The thing is, fat is an endocrine organ itself. It is a gland, and it makes hormones just like any other gland. The major hormone made by fat cells is leptin, (see Chapter 10), but fat cells produce many other substances. One in particular, called *inflammatory cytokines*, revs up the immune system, prompting the adrenal gland to pump out more corticosteroids to calm it down. The process plays havoc on fat cells. The result: more cortisol, more fat, and more inflammatory cytokines. It's another vicious cycle.

In order to be successful in losing weight, you have to get your cortisol levels down. For starters, this means getting rid of your stress.

BALANCE YOUR DIET TO LOWER YOUR CORTISOL

Though I hope you're learning a lot about your body, your hormones, and the way every body system interacts, you may have bought this book simply for its dietary recommendations. That's OK; our eating suggestions will help you lose weight and offer recommendations on how to cut stress and be healthier in your daily life.

This begins with cutting your cortisol. By lowering insulin resistance and balancing your hormones, cortisol levels should decline. Moreover, diets low in carbohydrates and sodium help prevent bloating and fluid retention.

One of the many things cortisol excess does is make people hungrier. By following the diet recommended in this book, hunger will be reduced. Your insulin will stop surging, and you will be able to use your calories to give you increased energy instead of having those calories turn into fat.

Among our recommendations:

- *Eat small, frequent meals (nibbling/grazing).*
- *Maintain a low-salt diet.* Because of the side effects mentioned above—bloating and high blood pressure—a low-salt diet will help you. Salt makes you retain water. Salt also helps deprive bones of calcium. Avoid added salt as much as possible, and have your blood pressure checked regularly.

- *Watch your glycemic index.* Keep those insulin levels down. (See Chapter 3)
- *Make sure you get enough chromium.* Chromium deficiency causes insulin resistance. See Chapter 3 for more on chromium.
- *Cut down on alcohol.* Heavy alcohol use makes the adrenal gland overreact and may induce pseudo-Cushing's syndrome.
- *Cut down on stress.* This may be the hardest one of all. Many people use food as a way of coping with stress. Food is enjoyable; food is comfortable. When in a stressful situation, whether it be emotional or physical, it's natural to want food. It may not make the stress go away, but it seems to ease the mind, if only for a few minutes, and so much of stress is in the mind.

Unfortunately, you can't eat without consuming calories and nutrients, however empty. Here comes that vicious cycle again: You get stressed, you eat, you gain weight, you feel more stressed, you eat again.

You have to break the cycle. Find new stress-reduction techniques. Work out a few times a week. Take a walk. Practice relaxation. Think of food for its nutritional value, not for its ability to make you feel good. When you relieve stress by means other than eating, you take a double step closer toward balancing your hormones. Not only do your cortisol levels drop, but insulin doesn't spike—one of the major sparks to those cycles.

Here are a few simple ways of reducing stress:

- *Exercise.* Exercise helps your body better handle stress by improving cardiovascular and musculoskeletal systems. Exercise improves insulin resistance. If your body is healthier, it will be better able to withstand the physical drain of stress. But note: The best type of exercise for lowering cortisol is slow and steady. Extreme exercise, such as marathon running, can actually raise your cortisol.

  If you have real CS, or are taking steroid medications, you should exercise with caution. Your muscles have become weakened from the excess steroids and are susceptible to a condition known as *rhabdomyolysis* (literally, death of the muscle).
- *Practice positive self-talk and improve your self-esteem.* Tell yourself that you can do it. You talk to yourself every day. Think about what you are saying. Are you hard on yourself? Do you give up

easily? You control how you talk to yourself. Tell yourself that you are in control. As you see results, it will be easier and easier to give yourself mental rewards. Don't worry about failure. Remind yourself that this is not an easy road, but you can do it.

- *Meditation, yoga, and massage.* All are excellent ways of handling stress. Meditation relaxes your mind. Yoga combines meditative techniques with stretching, one of the most overlooked parts of exercise. And massage works the muscles, loosening the knots and freeing the toxins that have collected during stressful times. For all of these methods—in fact, for all forms of exercise and stress reduction, period—drink lots of water.

- *Time with friends and family.* Your friends and family are your greatest support. Let them know what is going on with your life. If you are trying to lose a meaningful amount of weight, involve them in the process. You will receive support up front, but will also get ongoing congratulations every time they see that you have lost more weight.

- *Alcohol.* As mentioned, heavy drinking raises your cortisol. Avoid heavy drinking at all costs. Drinking in moderation (1 or 2 drinks per day) may be a good stress reliever, but don't overdo it. Drinking in moderation should not raise your cortisol, but it can raise your estrogen (see Chapter 6).

- *Herbals.* Several herbals have been touted as stress relievers. Be careful with herbals: With many, their claims remain unproven. Some herbal preparations can react with prescription medications, producing toxic effects.

- *Medications.* SSRI medications such as Prozac, Zoloft, Paxil, and Celexa, originally used only for depression, are now widely prescribed for anxiety. For some, these medications may be helpful. Older medications available for stress and anxiety include a class of drugs known as *benzodiazepines,* such as Xanax, Ativan, and Valium. These drugs tend to be addictive. Unless you have a true anxiety disorder, diagnosed by a psychiatrist, I do not recommend these medications. It is all too easy for us to pop a pill instead of facing the real issues in our life.

GROWTH HORMONE

WHAT IS GH?

Growth hormone (GH) was once the province of pediatricians and pediatric endocrinologists. If your child was small for his or her age, these professionals would prescribe GH to make the child taller. It worked like a charm.

Today, we are seeing GH in a new light. GH is increasingly being recognized as an important hormone for *all* ages. *Growth hormone deficiency* (GHD) is now recognized as an adult disease. And, treatment with GH has a number of benefits: It reduces the amount of fat in the body and increases muscle mass; it improves heart function and exercise performance; it improves mood and the sense of well-being; it strengthens bones; and it helps wounds heal faster. This chapter will examine the ways that GHD can make you lose muscle and gain fat, and how the addition of GH can reverse that trend.

First a caution: GH is *not* a cure-all. Excesses of GH can cause a number of problems, most notably insulin resistance, diabetes, high blood pressure, carpal tunnel syndrome, breast enlargement, and even cancer.

But you don't necessarily need GH—in a pharmaceutical form—to improve your health. Your body makes GH naturally, and by following a good diet, exercising, and cutting your fat intake, your GH levels will naturally improve and help do some of the work in improving your metabolism.

Growth hormone is so named because it makes children grow. But it's much more than that. It's an anabolic hormone—a muscle builder—but not a steroid. GH and testosterone have similar effects on body composition, decreasing fat and increasing muscle mass.

GH has a different structure than the four-ring chemical structure of a steroid. It's known as a *peptide hormone*, and unlike steroids—which are made from cholesterol—GH (and all peptide hormones) are made from amino acids, the building blocks of protein. Peptide hormones cannot be taken by mouth, because they'll be digested like food. Rather, like insulin, peptide hormones must be injected.

During childhood, GH—combined with your genetics—determines your height. Children who do not make GH are very short. Until a few years ago GH, made from human pituitary gland extracts, was given to short children to make them grow. Unfortunately, a rare and fatal brain disease known as Crutzfeldt-Jakob disease (similar to mad cow disease) was linked to natural GH. In 1981, a synthetic GH was developed, and this is the kind that's used today.

Although GH can influence many different types of cells in your body, the main target of GH is the liver. GH tells the liver (and other organs) to produce a second hormone known as **insulin-like growth factor-1** or **IGF-1**, a hormone called that because its chemical structure is similar to that of insulin. (IGF-1 is also known as **somatomedin C**.) IGF-1 is extremely important; in fact, most of what we consider the action of GH is mostly the action of IGF-1.

BODY WEIGHT, BODY FAT, AND GH

Low GH levels can make you gain weight. And studies are beginning to show that treatment with GH helps you lose *fat*, but to lose *weight* you must optimize GH with proper diet, sleep, and exercise. GH, whether produced naturally or taken as an injection, has potent muscle-building and fat-burning effects. GH improves your mood and gives you more energy, so you feel like exercising.

If you suffer from growth hormone deficiency (GHD), your body will have several indications of obesity and related problems. First of all, GHD is associated with central obesity—fat around the belly. This is the "metabolically evil" type of fat that is associated with insulin resistance, type 2 diabetes, high cholesterol, heart disease, and strokes.

Second, GHD causes Syndrome X, just as excess cortisol and insulin do (see Chapter 3). And, finally, there is what's called "obesity-related hyposomatotropism." This is another example of the vicious cycles created when the body is out of hormonal balance.

One study (Shalet et al., 1998) noted: "Morbid obesity is accompanied by suppression of GH release, which may resolve spontaneously with weight loss. In fact, distinction between the two is not possible with any degree of certainty at the present time."

So, being overweight lowers GH levels; having lower GH levels makes it easier to gain weight. Central obesity also contributes to weight gain, because it lowers GH levels. In fact, *the fat cell itself* lowers GH levels. In other words, obesity itself can cause severe GHD.

And the problem gets worse as you get older. Just as fat lowers your GH levels, so does aging. Talk about vicious cycles.

Scientists suspect that the obesity-GH link may be due to another hormone, leptin (see Chapter 10). Others believe the problem lies deeper in the brain. And still others blame insulin or free fatty acids as the culprit for lowering GH in obese people.

Studies have shown, however, that enhancing GH levels can help you lose that extra fat around the middle—and keep it off. Moreover, removing that extra fat around the middle will also improve your insulin levels.

How does GH do it? GH helps you lose fat by making the fat burnable as fuel. The byproduct of this change is more energy. It works because fat cells have GH and IGF-1 receptors. The stimulation of these receptors causes fat cells to break down fat. The process, called *lipolysis*, was discussed in Chapter 4. GH also counters the effects of insulin. It's an interesting contradiction, actually. Insulin promotes fat accumulation, but GH promotes fat breakdown.

But here's where GH can be dangerous. Because it counters the effects of insulin (like cortisol), taking GH can cause diabetes in some people. However, since it helps improve insulin resistance as well, there may be the opposite effect. The upshot is that some people who take GH may get diabetes, others will not. All the more reason to make sure that if you take GH, you should be closely monitored by a physician experienced in its use.

Remember this book's theme: Hormonal balance is key. GH is an important addition to the fight against obesity, but more is not necessarily better.

THE BRAIN AND GROWTH HORMONE

As with other hormones produced by the pituitary gland, GH is a hormone strongly influenced by feedback (see Chapter 1). When the body reports the need for more GH, the pituitary springs into action. Similarly, when the pituitary notices a rise or fall in the level of GH, it takes steps to regulate its production. Once again, the brain influences the hormone and the hormone influences the brain.

Special cells in the pituitary gland called *somatotrophs* make GH. Signals come from the brain by way of the hypothalamus, and it is a hormone made by the hypothalamus, called **growth hormone releasing hormone (GHRH)**, that stimulates the pituitary gland to make GH (see Figure 9.1).

A second hypothalamic hormone, **somatostatin**, inhibits pituitary gland production of GH. Interestingly, medications that mimic somatostatin cause dramatic weight loss in some people (see Chapter 10). Obviously, GH does not act by itself, but rather in concert with many hormones.

How does the system work? The pituitary gland secretes GH in a pulsatile manner. Like other hormones, it's secreted according to the diurnal rhythms of the body. **GH secretion is greatest while you sleep.**

GH has effects throughout the body, but the liver is the major target. Both GH and IGF-1 feed back to the hypothalamus, signaling proper (or improper) levels—a delicate regulatory system. Food also influences the pituitary gland and its production of GH (see the section on GH and insulin below).

But GH isn't just a hormone for the body. As we have discussed, GH (or lack of it) can have **potent effects on your mind**. GH deficiency (GHD) is associated with a decreased sense of well-being, poor energy, and mood swings. Adding GH to a regimen, on the other hand, can have beneficial effects: Memory may improve, as can your mood, sense of well-being, and energy level.

And GH can help you sleep better. This trait has the circular effect of helping your GH levels surge, since GH is produced while you sleep. Healthy sleep leads to a rise in GH levels; poor sleep can lead to a decline. Continued trends of either one can continue to boost or deplete GH levels, and the cycle will keep on going.

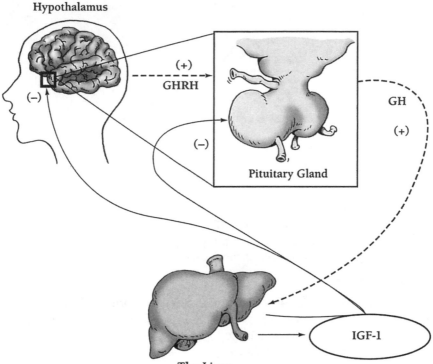

Figure 9.1
GROWTH HORMONE ENDOCRINOLOGY: HORMONE FEEDBACK LOOPS
Higher centers in the brain send signals to the hypothalamus, which produces
pulses of growth-hormone-releasing hormone (GHRH). GHRH pulses stimulate the pituitary gland to make growth hormone (GH). GH stimulates the liver
to produce insulin-like growth factor-1 (IGF-1). IGF-1 "feeds back" to the
hypothalamus and pituitary gland, slowing GH production. Positive "feedback"
is denoted by + and negative "feedback" is denoted by –.

AGING AND GROWTH HORMONE: SOMATOPAUSE

The problem of declining GH gets worse as you get older. As you
might expect, GH levels peak during puberty and slowly fall throughout the rest of your life. By age 30 to 40, levels are half of what they
were during puberty (see Figure 9.2). This natural decline in GH levels
is known as **somatopause**.

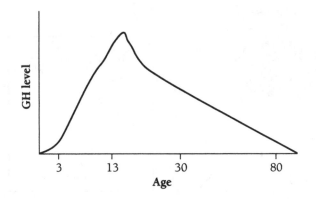

Figure 9.2
GH DECLINE WITH AGE
Growth hormone levels peak during puberty and then decline throughout life.
By age 30 to 40, levels are half of their pubertal peak.

In the past, this drop was considered normal. But now—as
research has revealed with other hormones—doctors are realizing it
may not be so. According to a 1999 article in the *New England Journal
of Medicine,* "There is evidence that GH deficiency in adults is delete-
rious, increasing the risk of death from cardiovascular disease."

Many antiaging physicians now advocate GH supplementation in
older individuals. The goal is to restore GH levels to the level of a 30- to
40-year-old. However, you don't restore those levels by "loading up" on
GH; in fact, the key is to take very low doses of the hormone. The higher doses of GH are used for people with overt GH deficiency (usually
caused by a pituitary gland tumor).

But why? If a little works well, wouldn't a lot work better? Not necessarily.

In somatopause, higher doses can cause a whole new set of problems. It's never easy in endocrinology; a fine balance is always necessary.

But that's not to downplay the great impact of GH. The substance
is increasingly being used as an antiaging hormone because it appears
to reverse some of the effects of aging.

And improvements in body composition are not the only benefit.
Restoring youthful levels of GH can improve skin tone, reverse hair
graying and make internal organs grow longer. It can actually—just as
the advertisements say—make you look younger. And feel younger

too: GH can improve your sex life, and—in a twist that seems worthy of a science fiction novel (or, perhaps, one of those cheesy ads in an adult magazine) make a man's penis or a woman's clitoris larger. The changes can be so dramatic that GH has been referred to as "hormonal plastic surgery."

Justin's Story

Justin, an advertising consultant, was starting to feel his age. At 62, he had spent 35 years in an industry—advertising—known for creating stooped shoulders and acid-filled stomachs. At 59, he had left the agency where he'd worked for many years to start a consulting firm—a way to keep his hand in the business, he figured, while pondering retirement. Still, he didn't want to go into retirement the way he felt: worn out, sallow, with a hand tremor and a general fatigue about life.

He heard about the effects of GH and saw an endocrinologist for a GH stimulation test. Justin was found, indeed, to have GHD, and was started on low-dose GH injections. After a few months of therapy he began to notice a difference, he said.

"My hand stopped shaking—that was the first good sign," he recalled. "But better than that was the energy. I felt lively and creative, the way I felt when I was in my 20s and first getting into advertising." His sex life also improved, he noted. Never a man with a powerful libido, he still found that his sexual potency had improved and that he enjoyed sex more. He reports that his wife strongly approves of him taking the hormone.

STRESS AND GH: GH RESISTANCE

As we've seen so many times, stress can disrupt hormonal balance in a manner as to promote weight gain. Stress can be physical, emotional, or caused by diseases such as hypothyroidism, diabetes, liver disease, kidney disease, AIDS, or severe burns. The excess fat in our bodies can also cause physical (and hormonal) stress on the body. When stress affects GH and GH receptors, you can have a multitude of problems. Stress can lead to sleep problems. Since GH is made when you sleep, sleeping less means less GH. Even without sleep problems, stress can have a direct effect on your brain and pituitary gland, causing less

GH production. Stress also causes damage to GH receptors and GH resistance. Damaged GH receptors mean that the GH does not function properly. This is similar to insulin resistance, discussed in Chapter 3. The difference with GH resistance is that unlike what happens with insulin, the body cannot compensate with heightened GH levels. The pituitary gland is already too pooped out to keep up with the demand.

The most severe form of GH resistance is known as *Laron's syndrome*. This genetic condition is caused by a severe mutation of the GH receptors. GH levels are very high, but IGF-1 levels are low (the GH receptor in the liver doesn't work and IGF-1 cannot be made). The result is a human of very short stature, one that cannot be helped by treatment with GH. Fortunately, we now know enough to treat these children with IGF-1, bypassing the GH receptor entirely.

AIDS is a condition associated with high-level GH resistance. Because of this, doctors are now treating AIDS patients with megadoses of GH, attempting to overcome this resistance. GH therapy improves muscle mass and muscle strength, but studies have not yet shown that it will prolong life. There is also very limited information on long-term safety and proper dosing for GH in AIDS patients.

GROWTH HORMONE AND INSULIN

So far I've concentrated on the positive effects of GH. As I noted before, it would seem like this is *the* wonder drug, the hormone to have if you want to lose weight.

But as we've seen before, hormonal balance is critical. If GH levels are not perfect, insulin is adversely affected. Abnormal GH levels, whether high or low, can cause insulin resistance. GH is a counter-insulin hormone and, when high, can cause the body to boost insulin production in order to compensate. Low GH causes low muscle mass and high fat mass, another setup for insulin resistance. Then there's outright GH deficiency, which causes insulin resistance and the vicious cycles of Syndrome X and other weight-gaining conditions.

So either way, too high or too low, abnormal GH levels cause insulin resistance.

Insulin and GH have a push-and-pull relationship. When you eat, insulin is released from your pancreas a few hours later, but there's a surge of GH to help suppress the insulin surge. If you have a decent-sized meal, then don't eat for 4 to 6 hours, you can temporarily raise your GH levels. A good way to take advantage of this is to have a big meal and then eat nothing for 4 to 6 hours. Then hit the weight room for an intense workout. A strenuous workout at this time makes GH levels surge even higher, stimulating muscle growth.

But this runs counter to the way the best diets work, which is through the concept of grazing—several small meals eaten over the course of a day. That's one reason high GH levels can cause diabetes. And diabetes, of course, drops you into a cycle where—if you're not careful—you may eat so as to make insulin levels peak and then plunge, as opposed to carefully maintaining them throughout the day.

So, you have to be careful. Near-perfect GH levels are needed to help balance insulin.

GROWTH HORMONE DEFICIENCY (GHD)

There are many causes of GHD. Pituitary gland problems cause the most severe form, but even stress can cause decreases in GH levels. (You'll recall that cortisol rises and testosterone and thyroid fall in response to stress.) Emotional deprivation and other forms of stress can lower GH levels; as I've noted before, stress—because of its effects on a variety of hormones—is one of the many causes of weight gain (see Chapter 1).

Stress disrupts your body's hormonal balance, slowing your metabolism and halting progress toward weight loss.

The classic form of GHD is childhood GHD. Children born with GHD do not grow, and pediatric endocrinologists use GH to restore normal growth.

If untreated, these children will remain short. They are considered "midgets"—not a term used in polite conversation anymore—because their body proportions are normal. Most, however, take on a pudgy appearance—keep in mind the GH effect on fat and muscle—so that many resemble cherubs.

In the past, patients stopped taking GH when they achieved a normal height. Now most endocrinologists advocate lifelong treatment with GH, though the dosages decrease after adult height is achieved.

As with all hormonal conditions, severe, moderate and mild forms exist. The most severe cases of adult-onset GHD—90 percent, in fact—are usually caused by a tumor in the pituitary gland. Patients with pituitary tumors can be deficient in many hormones, but GHD is the most common hormonal deficiency. Despite this, many of these patients are not offered the opportunity for GH replacement

I have one patient—we'll call her Danielle—who suffered from a pituitary gland tumor. Danielle underwent surgery and everything appeared to be going well. All of her hormones were replaced properly—except the GH.

Danielle didn't feel "right." She told her doctor that she felt weak and enervated and was gaining weight. The doctor didn't think much of it—after all, the tumor was gone and Danielle was obviously healthy, if not lively.

But then Danielle fell and broke her wrist. Upon examination, she was found to have osteoporosis. At that point, tests indicated that her GH levels were extremely low. She was put on GH injections. Not only did her bone heal, but she could now resume a normal life.

Pituitary gland tumors may sound terrible—and, not to downplay them, they are—but most of them are benign (noncancerous) growths, not malignant. The main reason they cause problems is because they get bigger. Sometimes the pituitary gland tumor compresses the normal gland, and this compression can cause a hormone deficiency. Sometimes the tumor itself makes too much of a particular hormone; for example, too much GH causes acromegaly (see below), while too much ACTH causes Cushing's disease (see Chapter 8).

Sometimes GH levels are OK until the tumor is removed. (Surgery through the nose—transsphenoidal—is the treatment of choice for most pituitary tumors, in case you were wondering.) GH levels tend to fall after the pituitary gland has been operated on.

Who's at risk for GHD? People who have had a head injury, any type of brain tumor, or radiation to the head. The diseases hemochromatosis (discussed in Chapter 4), sarcoidosis, and histiocytosis can also damage the pituitary gland and can cause GHD.

Sometimes patients with pituitary tumors have multiple hormone deficiencies including growth hormone, thyroid (TSH), sex hormones (LH and FSH), and cortisol (ACTH). This is known as *panhypopituitarism.*

Less frequently, the back of the pituitary is damaged. This part of the gland (the posterior pituitary gland) produces a hormone known as vasopressin, aka antidiuretic hormone. This hormone prevents you from urinating too much. Without it, you may urinate up to 5 gallons (yes, *5 gallons*) each day. This is called diabetes insipidus (DI), as opposed to the more common type of diabetes, which is called diabetes mellitus.

Another cause of GHD is simple aging. As we age, we lose lean body mass and gain fat. GH declines are partially responsible for this. Advocates of GH as an anti-aging hormone claim that restoring GH levels to those of a 30- to 40-year-old will reverse the muscle loss/fat gain cycle.

Other physical declines associated with aging may also be due to GHD. These include osteoporosis, wrinkling skin, and decline in kidney function. Psychological aspects of GHD include low energy, mood swings, depression, and social isolation.

SYMPTOMS OF ADULT GHD

The symptoms of adult GHD are very vague and often ignored. They may be mistaken for other hormonal imbalances. Among the indicators are:

- *Weight gain/unfavorable body composition.* As we have discussed, this is a major component of GHD. GHD makes you lose muscle and gain fat, especially "metabolically evil" fat around the middle.
- *Poor general health*
- *Depression/lack of a sense of well-being*
- *Lack of energy/fatigue*
- *Social isolation—loss of zest for life*
- *Reduced capacity for exercise*
- *Difficulties with sex life*
- *Emotional irritability*
- *Poor memory*
- *Difficulty relating to others*

GHD AND YOUR HEART

Studies have shown that patients with severe GHD (from pituitary gland problems) have **twice** the risk of dying from heart disease. A GH imbalance of *any type* can cause heart problems. GH increases the thickness of the heart's walls and affects its function. If there's a deficiency, it can cause a condition known as *dilated cardiomyopathy*—the heart gets big, floppy, and weak. The condition usually leads to heart failure.

GHD is associated with premature atherosclerosis and with decreased HDL (good) cholesterol and increased LDL (bad) cholesterol. Of course, it's well known that high cholesterol is a cause of coronary artery disease and heart attacks. Restoring youthful GH levels can improve the cholesterol profile.

But balance, again, is important. GH excess can cause heart problems as easily as GHD can: The heart gets very big and thick and has trouble pumping (part of the phenomenon called *acromegaly*—see below). **Heart disease is the number-one cause of death in patients with growth hormone excess.**

Testing for GHD

There are a handful of ways you can be tested for GHD:

- *Growth hormone levels.* This is not a good test. The hormone levels fluctuate greatly. Even a level of zero could be normal.
- *Insulin-like growth factor-1 (IGF-1) levels.* A low IGF-1 level is very suggestive of GHD. But here the problem is interpretation: who says what level is low? A normal IGF-1 level, in fact, is seen in many patients with severe GHD. For this reason, if you have symptoms of GHD and a normal IGF-1 level, you should still proceed with GH stimulation testing (see below). Most endocrinologists feel that IFG-1 levels should be compared to age-adjusted normal values. Anti-aging doctors believe that they should be compared to the nomal values of a 30 to 40 year old. Anything less is GHD.

  Either way, IGF-1 levels should be monitored at least once every 6 months for those people who take GH.

- *Binding proteins*. There has been a lot of interest in measuring one of these proteins, **insulin-like growth factor binding protein-3 (IGFBP-3),** as a way of diagnosing GHD. At this time, however, this test is mostly used in research settings.
- *Stimulation tests* (also known as *provocative testing*). This is the best and most accurate way of testing for GHD. The classic stimulation test is known as the insulin tolerance test. Here, a patient is given a large dose of insulin. The blood sugar drops to dangerous levels, which somehow provokes GH to be released. (GH, you'll recall, is an anti-insulin hormone.) The insulin tolerance test is *best* in terms of diagnosing GHD, but *worst* in terms of risk and hassle factor. Now, GH secretagogues (medications that stimulate GH secretion from the pituitary gland), such as **GHRH, arginine, clonidine, glucagon,** and **levodopa,** can be administered to patients to stimulate GH secretion. Usually, a baseline sample of blood is obtained, and then the secretagogue is administered. Repeat samples of blood are drawn every 30 minutes or so for the next couple of hours. All of the stimulated GH levels must be less than 5 mg/L in order to diagnose GHD. In children, however, GH levels less than 10 may be abnormal.

Treatment of GHD

In 1996, GH therapy was approved for treatment of adult GHD. Despite this, treatment is still debated among endocrinologists. Most, however, agree that GHD should probably be treated. Studies as long as 10 years have been published demonstrating that long-term treatment with GH is both *safe* and *effective.*

GH is given as a daily injection, though some patients take it less often. GH comes as a powder that must be mixed with water or in a premixed form. Injection devices can be different: Some companies use a "pen" injection method, which can be easier to use than standard injection. The Genotropin MiniQuick is a prefilled and premeasured syringe of GH that is the most hassle-free. Unlike other types of GH, this formulation of GH does not require refrigeration. This is because the device keeps the powder and the liquid separate. When ready to inject, the two are automatically mixed with a twist of the syringe.

Aside from these types of convenience factors, all brands of GH are essentially equal. Table 9.1 lists the types and brand names of GH.

The goals of GH therapy are to lose fat, gain muscle (restore normal body composition), improve muscle and heart function, normalize cholesterol, increase energy, and improve quality of life.

You should use GH only under the supervision of a qualified endocrinologist.

How much is the right amount?

Studies have reported a *highly variable response* to dosing of GH. In the past, dosing of GH was based on body weight. Today, most doctors start with a low dose and slowly increase the dose according to side effects and your response to therapy. This is known as "individualized dose titration." There are many reasons why each individual responds so differently to similar doses of GH. Your dose will depend on the magnitude of your deficiency and the level of GH resistance. If you have a pituitary gland disorder, your dose will be higher than if you have a somatopause-related decline. Stress and illness cause GH resistance, and higher doses may be required to overcome this resistance. Some people will respond to very low doses of GH, but others require much higher doses. I usually have patients start on a dose of 0.2 mg at bedtime for a couple of months, then increase to 0.4 mg. (GH can also be measured in IU, or international units. 1 mg = 3 IU.) The dose can be further increased every few months. Most patients with adult GHD rarely need more than 1.6 mg of GH per day.

Bodybuilders and patients with AIDS may take doses of GH as high as 6 mg per day. Taking mega-doses of GH is similar to taking mega-doses of steroids (such as testosterone). The high dose is considered *pharmacologic*, meaning that the dose is higher than the body would produce on its own. Standard doses are intended to *replace* a deficiency. This is called a *physiologic* dose. In the case of AIDS, the mega-dose is intended to stimulate muscle growth to overcome AIDS wasting syndrome.

To closely mimic your diurnal rhythms, I recommend you take your injection at bedtime. It may take as long as 6 months to even begin to notice an effect.

How high do you go?

This is a controversial area. No one can even agree on the perfect way of monitoring GH therapy. Most doctors will follow IGF-1 levels as a

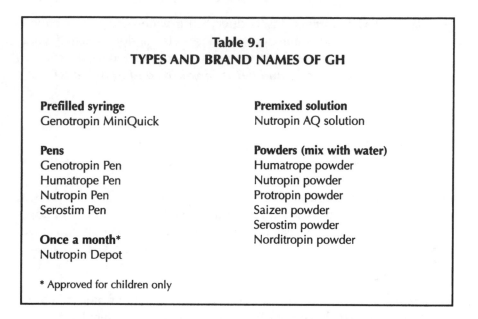

Table 9.1
TYPES AND BRAND NAMES OF GH

Prefilled syringe
Genotropin MiniQuick

Premixed solution
Nutropin AQ solution

Pens
Genotropin Pen
Humatrope Pen
Nutropin Pen
Serostim Pen

Powders (mix with water)
Humatrope powder
Nutropin powder
Protropin powder
Saizen powder
Serostim powder

Once a month*
Nutropin Depot

Norditropin powder

* Approved for children only

marker of therapy. Traditional endocrinologists treat to raise IGF-1 levels to "normal for age." Different ages have different normal values; the older you are, the lower the "normal" value. Other physicians recommend treating to a level considered normal for a 30 to 40 year-old, regardless of age.

Hate shots?
GH is now entering an age of new technologies. A needle-free GH injector device, known as Cool.Click, is now approved for use. A long-acting GH injection is now available which requires only one shot a month. This form of GH, known as Nutropin Depot, is approved only for use in children at this time. And we have the technology to create a GH patch. It's not yet available, but in the future, you may be able to slap one on, just like other hormone patches.

SIDE EFFECTS OF GH TREATMENT

Interestingly, side effects occur more frequently in older patients and heavier patients. The most common side effect of GH therapy is fluid retention.

- *Bloating and edema.* This is due to the water and salt retention caused by GH. It seems to be a dose-related side effect. If your dose of GH is lowered, this symptom should subside.
- *Muscle and joint aches and pains (myalgias and arthralgias).*
- *Headache.*
- *Blurred vision.*
- *Carpal tunnel syndrome.* This is due to swelling in the wrist. A nerve to the hand gets pinched off, causing symptoms of hand pain and numbness. It's also dose-related; if the dose is lowered, things should get better
- *Blood sugar problems/diabetes.* As mentioned earlier, GH has a variable effect with insulin. Abnormal GH, whether high or low, can cause insulin resistance or even diabetes. You should have your blood sugar checked periodically if you take GH. (Diabetes and GH are also related to acromegaly, discussed near the end of the chapter.)
- *High blood pressure.* This is also a result of salt and water retention. If you take GH have your blood pressure checked regularly.
- *Breast enlargement.* Almost 10 percent of men and women have reported breast enlargement from GH.
- *Cancer risk.* Any substance that causes cells to grow has the potential of causing cancer. Increased IGF-1 levels have been linked to prostate cancer in men, and GH has been shown to cause cancer in laboratory animals. Patients with GH excess (see the section on acromegaly) do have increased risk of certain forms of cancer (including breast, prostate, and colon cancer). However, thus far, GH therapy in replacement doses has not been linked to cancer. Some researchers even argue that GH may *prevent* certain forms of cancer. The bottom line: The question remains unanswered.
- *Other risks.* A 1999 study published in the *New England Journal of Medicine* investigated the use of GH in critically ill patients in an intensive care unit. The study had to be stopped prematurely because patients on GH were dropping dead. Obviously, GH is not appropriate in all situations. Also, because of careful studies like this one, we are learning when to use and when not to use GH.

GH therapy does have other "side effects." Foremost among them is the cost. Full replacement doses can cost up to $20,000 per year. Children with true GHD and AIDS patients need the highest doses. In many cases, this is covered by insurance, and insurance companies will pay for treatment of adult GHD if proper stimulation testing has been done. But lower doses of GH, used for somatopause, may still cost several thousand dollars per year and may not be covered by insurance. Several of the manufacturers of GH have programs that will help you work with your insurance company. Because of the high cost, many insurance companies will raise your insurance premiums (sometimes double or triple) after you start taking GH.

Minimizing Side Effects of GH Treatment

Instead of jumping whole-hog on the GH bandwagon, you may want to consider alternative forms of therapy, such as diet, exercise, and other types of GH releasers.

If you take GH, your physician should keep your IGF-1 level no higher than that of a 30- to 40-year-old and should help you to balance your other hormones (thyroid, testosterone, estrogen, insulin, etc.). Many side effects of GH therapy are temporary and get better with time.

But, despite GH's promise, there's no guarantee. The field is still very new, and much, much more research needs to be done. Although there are many promising studies, not all studies show that GH helps. Despite these warnings, GH is frequently abused, particularly among athletes and bodybuilders. It is almost impossible to test for GH in athletes, and the only ones who get caught are those who are found to have the vials on them. Athletes claim that GH enhances their performance, but there is not much scientific evidence. Moreover, the majority of Americans frown on its use as unsportsmanlike. Endocrinologists agree that the use of GH by bodybuilders and athletes with normal GH and IGF-1 levels is *dangerous*.

How to Optimize Your Body's Natural GH: Alternatives to Growth Hormone

There are several ways of tapping into your body's natural supply of this mostly beneficial hormone.

Diet and GH

Remember, the more body fat you have, the lower your GH levels. And, as you lose fat, your GH levels will surge, helping you lose more fat. *Crash diets, however, lower your GH levels.*

The **hormonal health diet** (Chapter 11) is the ideal diet for enhancing GH levels, with one exception: the nibbling concept that keeps insulin levels low. Unfortunately, this diet also can keep GH levels low. To really boost your GH levels, you should eat 3 meals a day with 4 to 6 hours of fasting between each meal. I do not recommend this, however, if you are also trying to fight insulin resistance. If insulin resistance and GHD are both issues, I recommend you use the frequent small meals as recommended in Chapter 11. If you want to maximize GH levels and insulin resistance is not an issue, the "feast-fast cycle" may give you an additional advantage.

Protein is key to making the weight loss/GH gain cycle work. Protein is used to build muscle. If you raise your GH levels, but are not eating enough protein, you won't see much good—you have to provide your body with all the tools. Eat the right amount of protein. Extra protein is easily converted into fat and stored in fat cells.

Low-fat diets work best. High-fat diets block the release of GH.

You should also eat low-glycemic-index carbohydrates. They keep insulin levels low, and insulin blocks GH actions and makes you fat.

Finally, drink lots of water. I cannot emphasize this enough. Drink at least eight 8-ounce glasses a day. Water is a major component of muscle. Without enough water, you can become dehydrated and your muscles suffer.

GH Use in the Livestock Industry

As we have discussed, hormones are increasingly being used in animals as a means of boosting muscle mass—and profits. We really don't know if the GH given to animals has any effects on humans who consume the animals. GH is a peptide hormone, and if not destroyed by cooking, the GH is likely destroyed by digestion. Furthermore, as mentioned, animal GH does not work in humans. Unlike other animal hormones (refer to Premarin in Chapter 6), GH is very species-specific. So the GH in the meat you eat probably has little effect on your body.

Exercise

Exercise is very important to lowering weight and raising GH levels. The best kinds of workouts for GH are strenuous ones. Intensive exercise can make GH levels surge.

Once you start exercising, GH will help you keep exercising, making your muscles stronger. The more you exercise, the stronger you get. This has long been a truism, but few realize GH's role.

Sleep

Remember, GH is released when you sleep. If you don't sleep well, you won't produce enough GH.

GROWTH HORMONE SECRETAGOGUES

These medications and nutraceutical products stimulate the pituitary gland to make GH. GH secretagogues fall into two categories: those used in a research setting and for stimulating, and those sold as nutritional supplements.

Growth-hormone-releasing hormone (GHRH) has been approved only as a research tool and is used in GH stimulation testing. In experimental settings, it has restored normal GH levels. In the future, GHRH may be used as an alternative to GH—but for GHRH to work, the pituitary gland must be normal. Growth-hormone-releasing proteins (GHRP), MK-677 and Hexarelin, are GH-releasing agents used in experimental settings.

Over-the-Counter GH Releasers

Several amino acids, when taken in high enough doses, will stimulate your pituitary gland to make GH. They're touted as a "natural" way of enhancing GH levels. Amino acids can cost less than $1 per day, and they're available in most health-food stores and drug stores.

- *Arginine.* When I test patients for GHD, I give them an intravenous infusion of arginine. It's an extremely potent GH releaser that works by blocking **somatostatin** release. You'll remember that somatostatin inhibits GH release. There are side effects, such as upset stomach or nausea. There's also no agreed-upon dosage.

- *Ornithine.* This has a very similar chemical structure to arginine. Half the dose of ornithine gives the same results as arginine, but it costs twice as much—and watch out, it can cause diarrhea.
- *OKG (L-ornithine alpha ketoglutarate).* This is not exactly an amino acid, but it has a similar structure. This potent GH releaser has been used in France to rebuild body tissue after surgery, trauma, and burns.
- *Combination amino acid products.* The above amino acids are often combined in "GH booster" or "GH stacker" products that you may see in health-food stores or over the Internet. Sometimes the amino acids **lysine, glycine,** and **glutamine** may be added. These combination products have potent abilities to raise your GH levels. They're referred to as "stacking" amino acids, but unfortunately, most have not been carefully studied. Side effects can be severe. Research continues to determine the perfect combination of amino acids.

GHB (Gamma Hydroxybutyrate)

This is an extremely potent stimulator of GH. It's similar in structure to a brain chemical known as GABA (gamma-aminobutyric acid). Its primary side effect is induction of deep sleep—sometimes so deep that the person cannot be aroused. Obviously, this is not a side effect to be taken lightly.

There was a 34-year-old bodybuilder, in terrific shape, who was found in a deep sleep, practically comatose, in his house. He was finally admitted to the hospital because he could not be aroused. Turns out he had taken a big dose of GHB. There is a happy ending to the story: He slept for 3 days, finally woke up, and felt fine.

But I wouldn't encourage everyone to try it. In fact, I don't recommend GHB at all; I believe it's dangerous, for the reasons cited above, and would sooner try another course of action if GH stimulation is needed.

Prescription Medications

I do not recommend that you take these medications to raise your GH levels. However, if you are taking these medications for other reasons, you should know they may be raising your GH levels as a side effect.

- *Levodopa (Sinemet)*. This medication, used to treat Parkinson's disease, resembles the brain chemical **dopamine**. It's often used to test for GHD, and it's a very potent releaser of GH.
- *Ergoloid mesylates (Hydergine)*. In the past, Hydergine was widely used in an attempt to improve memory in older people. It's rarely used today. You may have heard it referred to as a "smart drug," but for some it's not all that smart: It can cause headache and insomnia.
- *Clonidine (Catapres)*. Clonidine is a widely used high blood pressure medication, available in both pill and patch forms. It's another potent stimulator of GH, and—like GHB—can make you sleepy.

  (There's a reason some of these GH releasers make you sleepy: GH, you'll recall, is released when you sleep. These medications are simply helping along what comes naturally, though in much more potent form than body processes.)
- *Phenytoin (Dilantin)*. Phenytoin, a commonly used medication, is used to prevent seizures. GH stimulation is merely incidental.

Forget the secretagogues, give me the good stuff:
- *IGF-1*. This is the final product of all the GH secretagogues. GHRH is at the top of the process, and IGF-1 is the last—and arguably the most important—catalyst to GH production. And, since it's the substance that seems to do all the work, it seems like the logical solution to avoid all that other stuff and just take IGF-1.

  Well, bodybuilders have already started using IGF-1 and claim it works. Studies do show that it does increase muscle and reduce fat, as well as build bone and nerves. It's also used in children who have a defective GH receptor. They have lots of GH, but it doesn't work.

  My own feeling is that IGF-1, though more research needs to be done, may be the ideal hormone in solving many of the problems we've discussed in this chapter and in this book. It's more potent than GH and appears to have fewer side effects. And, although GH may cause diabetes, IGF-1 appears to *improve* diabetes. It improves blood glucose and lowers insulin levels. In fact, it's actually being investigated as a treatment for diabetes.

  This could be at least part of the solution we've been looking for to solve many hormonal problems, including obesity. Keep in mind it's *not* a magic bullet—diet and exercise remain paramount—but it can certainly boost the effects of a balanced life.

ACROMEGALY, GIGANTISM, AND GH EXCESS

For most of this chapter, we've talked about how GH makes bones and cartilage grow. But there is a dark side to this growth: Sometimes the pituitary gland develops a tumor that produces excessive amounts of GH. This condition is known as **acromegaly**.

What effects does this have? You've probably seen someone with acromegaly in the *Guinness Book of World Records* or on a professional wrestling show. If a child develops a GH-producing pituitary tumor before puberty, he will become a "giant," a condition given the rather obvious name **gigantism**. Today, most of these children are diagnosed and treated.

Victims of gigantism don't usually grow up to be basketball players or Herculean strongmen. Gigantism provides them with a whole new set of problems, particularly skeletal and muscular conditions. The human body isn't usually meant to be 8 feet tall. For those who develop a problem with GH excess after puberty, after growth has ceased, it's even worse.

Then there's acromegaly, the condition caused by GH excess in adults. People with acromegaly end up with very large hands and feet—the name itself means "big extremity"—and a variety of problems, listed below. Interestingly, acromegaly can mimic insulin resistance and Syndrome X. Why? When produced in high levels, GH directly works against insulin, creating insulin resistance.

Sandra's Story
It started slowly. One day, Sandra—a 50-year-old homemaker in Miami, Florida—put on her shoes and noticed that they didn't fit correctly. It was as if her feet had grown a half-size or so, almost overnight. As time went on, though, she realized her feet had grown—and so had her hands. Her health started deteriorating. Her blood pressure shot up and she developed diabetes.

One day she went to the dentist for a checkup. The dentist took x-rays and posted them on a light board for Sandra to look at. "The spaces between your teeth," he said, using the handle of a dental mirror as a pointer, "are growing larger."

It all started coming together. Sandra told him about her feet and her hands. The dentist referred her to an endocrinologist, who diagnosed acromegaly. He booked Sandra into surgery to remove the pituitary tumor that had caused all the trouble. Within months after the surgery, Sandra was feeling better. Her hands, feet, and spaces between her teeth, however, remained enlarged.

Features of GH Excess (Acromegaly)

- *Weight gain.* Both GH deficiency and excess are associated with weight gain.
- *Diabetes.* GH is an anti-insulin hormone and, at high levels, causes insulin resistance that can lead to diabetes.
- *Change in appearance.* Besides the growth of the hands and feet, acromegaly causes the brow to thicken, the nose to broaden, the jaw to protrude, the teeth to space out, the tongue to grow, and the forehead to gain a large, deep furrowing. Andre the Giant, who had acromegaly, had a number of these features.
- *High blood pressure.*
- *High cholesterol.*
- *Acanthosis nigricans.* This is a skin condition that causes a dark velvet-like skin rash on the neck, armpits, face, and knuckles (see Chapter 3).
- *Heart disease.* In the case of acromegaly, the heart gets big and thick. High cholesterol levels lead to an increased risk of heart attack; in fact, the leading killer among people with acromegaly is heart attack.
- *Growth of hands and feet.*
- *Carpal tunnel syndrome.* This pain of the wrist joint is particularly common.
- *Arthritis.*
- *Risk of cancer.* Several types of cancer, most notably colon cancer, happen more often in people with acromegaly.
- *Skin tags.* These tiny growths of excess skin are often seen in patients with acromegaly. Interestingly, the greater the number of skin tags, the greater the risk of colon cancer.

Treatment Options for Acromegaly

What can you do if you have acromegaly? Fortunately, it's not irreversible. Surgery, radiation, and medication are all options, and all have been known to control—or even solve—the problem. Most patients opt for surgery right away, but new and more effective medications are being developed.

CHAPTER TEN

HUNGER HORMONES AND THE FUTURE OF WEIGHT LOSS

HUNGER AND APPETITE

THE MOST COMMON HORMONAL DISORDER IS NOT HYPOTHYROIDISM, NOT DIA-BETES, NOT ESTROGEN DECLINE. **The most common hormonal disorder is obesity.**

Now, if you've read this book this far, this comes as no surprise to you. Everything I've talked about comes back to obesity. A lack or overabundance of certain hormones causes changes in metabolism. Those changes either prompt the body to start putting on weight immediately or start a boomerang effect that will cause it to put on weight soon enough. Either way, the end result is a weight problem—and that weight problem can lead to a whole host of other problems.

You'd think the endocrinology community would be aware of this. In fact, just the opposite is true. For years, the endocrinology community has ignored obesity. For the most part, in fact, endocrinologists haven't seen the forest for the trees. They treat the individual hormonal problems contributing to obesity, or caused by obesity, but they don't treat the obesity itself.

It's only recently that new discoveries have opened endocrinologists' eyes. Most neuroscientists agree that hunger originates in a portion of the brain called the hypothalamus. As I've noted elsewhere in this book, the hypothalamus is the part of the brain that controls the pituitary gland—the master gland—and thus many of our hormones.

But studying how the hypothalamus affects hunger—the "science of hunger"—is only beginning. It's a fairly wide-open field.

There are certain things known about hunger and the hypothalamus. One is the idea of "satiety," the concept that you eat until you're satisfied. In the hypothalamus, there is a sector called the ventromedial hypothalamus; it's nicknamed the **satiety center**. Hormones that influence satiety include **serotonin, somatostatin, bombesin,** and **cholecystokinin**. **Leptin**, a newly discovered hormone produced by fat cells, is known as a "satiety factor" because of its potent effects on appetite.

Satiety has both physiological and psychological implications. During times of satiety, hunger is at a minimum. Yet some people never feel satisfied. They never reach satiety. For some, this may be a hormonal disorder.

Other hormones have also been linked to quelling appetite. These hormones, known as cytokines, cause extreme loss of appetite and wasting from diseases such as cancer and AIDS. Cytokines have powerful abilities to fight cancer and infections, but for some reason can eliminate hunger. Needless to say, these dread diseases are not recommended ways of losing weight.

If the satiety center portion of the hypothalamus is damaged, it can lead to an uncontrollable appetite. Physicians have spent decades of research focused on satiety centers and "satiety factors"—hypothetical hormones that make the brain feel full—in attempts to help control appetite without killing it off altogether.

Another part of the hypothalamus, related to the satiety center, is the **hunger center**—the lateral hypothalamus. This part of the hypothalamus produces hunger. If this region is damaged, there is no hunger. Scientists theorize that the condition *anorexia nervosa* may be linked to damage to this brain region.

Ultimately, hormones trigger hunger, uniting your brain, glands, and your appetite.

THE EVOLUTION OF HUNGER

Our hormone mechanisms are deeply evolved. They have developed to cope with times of famine, to make the most of the nutrients we consume (recall the thrifty gene hypothesis, discussed in Chapter 3), and to make sure we respond to food in our vicinity.

However, today, with abundant sources of high-calorie food all around, our antiquated hormone/hunger mechanism works against us. For example, if you are overweight, your body does not need food. In fact, depending on how overweight your are, you could go without eating for weeks to months without harming your body. Your body fights against this, though, causing you to be hungry hours after you just ate. Or what about when you were hungry for that dessert? Your body just consumed a healthy meal, and all of a sudden you're hungry for dessert! Why? Well, that's just millions of years of evolution working against you.

Our senses, our organs, our very being demand that we search for—and eat—food. Consider:

- *Taste and smell.* Imagine walking down the street, smelling freshly baked bread. Suddenly, you are hungry. Smelling or anticipating the taste of delicious food can really turn on the hunger centers of the brain. And if you eat a little good food (an appetizer, for example), you get hungrier! Similarly, if it smells and tastes bad, you lose your appetite.
- *Appearance of food.* Just looking at good food makes you hungry.
- *Variety.* Variety makes us hungry. This may be why you get hungry for dessert even though your stomach is bursting. This also explains the success of many fad diets. These diets frequently have very limited food choices. The monotony of the diet somehow reduces appetite. This is also why meal replacement products such as bars and shakes can be so successful.
- *Stomach distention.* Distention of the stomach sends powerful hormonal signals to the brain, inducing satiety. Foods high in fiber, which distend the stomach without adding a lot of calories, can greatly improve satiety. Refer to Chapter 2 for more information on fiber.
- *The "set point."* Many scientists believe in the concept of a set point. Think of it as a "natural resting point for your body weight." Each of us has a somewhat predetermined body weight. If you become heavier than your set point, appetite is turned off and you lose weight. If your weight drops below the set point, you get hungry and gain weight. I believe that the set point does exist to an extent; however, if you follow our eating suggestions and exercise regularly, you can lower your set point so that your body now feels comfortable at a lower weight.
- *The fat cell is a smart cell.* It knows and regulates your body weight.

Your body tends to want stability. If your weight drifts above your set point, appetite tends to go down and you shed a few pounds. If you lose weight, the opposite occurs: Your metabolism slows and hunger increases as your body craves to get back to the set weight.

The concept of a set point is not new and not unique to humans. Animals tend to have their own set points. But you can change a set point with a delicious diet. Take the family dog, for example: If he gets dog food only, he'll be lean and trim. But start adding those table scraps, and Rover starts to plump up—particularly if he's not getting much exercise.

What is new regarding set points is research on brain control of the set point by means of the newly discovered hormone *leptin*. After all, the brain affects behavior, physical activity, cravings, hunger ... *and* produces potent hormones.

The set-point concept also brings back the concept of satiety. Satiety hormones (also known as satiety factors) are the key regulators of body weight. They send a "stop eating" signal to the brain.

The upshot of all this is simple: Don't be a victim of your set point. You can change your set point. As you achieve a new, healthy weight, and balance your hormones, you can achieve a new set point.

This chapter will discuss the most recent breakthroughs in this area. However, as you will see, there is a great deal more to discover. This area of endocrinology is really in its infancy.

METABOLISM, BODY HEAT, AND THE FAT CELL

In Chapter 3, I talked about free fatty acids, lipotoxicity, PPAR receptors and fat cells, all of which contribute to insulin resistance and, therefore, obesity. The bottom line: Fat cells contribute to insulin resistance by releasing toxic fatty acids into the bloodstream.

That's not the only function of fat, however. Fat is important for regulating body temperature and metabolism as well as the production of important hunger hormones. When your body is in the storage mode, fat cells grow, storing your excess calories for the future—making you fat, in other words. When your body is in the fat-burning mode, fat is burned as fuel instead of being stored.

The production of body heat—produced through fat burning or other method—is called **thermogenesis**. It's a major indicator of metabolism. If you think of food as fuel—and that's what it is at bottom, the fuel to keep your body running, just as gasoline keeps your car running—you can do one of two things with it: burn it or store it. If you store it, it's stored as fat.

Meanwhile, through complex brain-hormone interactions, the body controls its own body temperature. (A fever is an extreme example of this.) A higher body temperature—increased thermogenesis—raises metabolism. The hormones that raise metabolism, in fact, do so mainly by increasing thermogenesis. Low body temperature means lowered metabolism; we've seen this is an indicator of low thyroid function.

BAT AND WAT

There are two types of fat: brown fat and white fat. Most thermogenesis occurs in brown fat tissue (also known as brown adipose tissue, or BAT). BAT produces a specialized blood protein known as *thermogenin* that allows for the production of body heat.

BAT is controlled by nerves and stress hormones. The stress hormones epinephrine and norepinepherine, released from nerve cells and the adrenal gland, activate BAT, increasing thermogenesis. A special receptor for these hormones is found only in BAT. It is called a β-**3 receptor**. (Other tissues in the body have β-1 and/or β-2 receptors.) Stimulation of the β-3 receptor increases metabolism. It does this by increasing thermogenesis (heat production) and lipolysis (fat breakdown). And the hormones epinephrine and norepinephrine work by stimulating b-receptors.

Since the only place β-3 receptors are located is in BAT, this makes it the ideal target for a metabolic enhancement drug. Theoretically, there should be very few side effects, because only the β-3 receptor is being affected. This would likely be the magic drug we've all waited for. And, indeed, several major pharmaceutical companies (including Merck and Pfizer) are investigating β-3 receptor stimulator medications as a way of enhancing metabolism and helping with weight loss.

Unfortunately, these medications are not as great as they seem. It turns out that the original β-3 research was done on mice. And, as we continue to have to remind ourselves, mice are different from humans. Humans do have β-3 receptors, but we lose most of them within the first 6 months of our lives. After that, there just aren't many β-3 receptors at all.

So, early studies of β-3 medications on humans have been, as expected, disappointing. Newer compounds still under investigation do hold promise, but no one knows if these medications will really work.

White adipose tissue (WAT) is quite different than BAT. WAT produces hormones. Yes, WAT is a hormone-producing gland just like the thyroid gland or the adrenal gland. The two most important hormones made by WAT are leptin and resistin.

BAT DYSFUNCTION

Just as healthy BAT can be part of the cycle to help lose weight, dysfunctional BAT can get in the way. And, ironically—or perhaps not so ironically, considering the constant feedback loops of the body—obesity can cause BAT dysfunction. If you are very overweight, your brown fat tissue cannot produce heat properly, so your metabolism is lowered and it becomes even harder to lose weight, ad infinitum.

Fat cells also produce a substance known as **tumor necrosis factor** (TNF). Obese humans have very high levels of TNF. This substance is known to cause insulin resistance and increased cortisol levels. This may explain why being overweight causes insulin resistance and pseudo-Cushing's. TNF in high levels is toxic to the body and may be associated with other complications of obesity, such as low estrogen and testosterone levels, and may even be linked to heart disease and strokes.

WHAT ARE HUNGER HORMONES?

To an extent, most hormones can influence your appetite. Insulin, thyroid hormone, estrogen, progesterone, and cortisol—all have potent effects on appetite. We have discussed these in great detail because there is much more known about them.

But there are hundreds of other hormones that also affect appetite, and, unlike those listed above, they're not necessarily made by traditional glands. In fact, one of the biggest hormone producers in the body is the … fat cell. Yes, the same little piece of the puzzle that collects and reproduces and causes so much of our misery also makes hormones. Until recently, the fat cell was thought of as an innocent bystander in the obesity saga, but now we know better. The fat cell turns out to be one of the biggest hormone producers in the body. It is the perpetrator, not the victim.

Other hunger hormones are produced by other parts of the body central to digestion and food storage. The intestines also produce potent hunger hormones, influenced by the foods you eat. These hormones, known as *gut peptides*, have effects on hunger and satiety. Our knowledge of these hormones is limited, but growing every day.

HORMONES, METABOLISM, AND GENETICS

For the vast majority of us, both genes and environment control body weight. In some cases, however, severe genetic obesity can be caused by a variety of genetic mutations.

How do genetics and environment combine? The Pima Indians, who we talked about in Chapter 3, are a good example. As humans have developed, food has become easier to come by, cheaper, bigger, more calorie-rich, and fattier. Combine this with the invention of the car and now the computer, and exercise and physical expenditure has come to an all-time low.

So the genes that allowed your great-great-grandfather to be lean are working against you. If you were to adopt the diet and activity level of someone 200 or 300 years ago, you would likely lose weight. Genes and environment thrive on one another.

Much of evolution has favored fat storage. Now evolution is working against us.

LEPTIN: THE SATIETY FACTOR WE'VE BEEN SEARCHING FOR?

Leptin is, simply, one of the most significant discoveries in the history of the science of obesity.

A mutant strain of mice, known as *ob/ob* (a genetic term for a double mutation of a gene resulting in obesity), was found to have a syndrome of obesity and related complications very similar to Syndrome X in humans. The *ob/ob* mouse was hungry all the time and had high insulin levels, increased body fat, high cortisol levels, low thyroid levels, and high blood sugar. In addition, these mice had low body temperature, indicating low metabolism.

Scientists believed that the *ob/ob* mouse lacked a satiety factor—a hormone, still undiscovered, they called "leptin." To prove this theory, in the 1970s a scientist named D.L. Coleman performed some odd experiments—animal rights activists would cringe—that are now considered classics of the genre. These studies, known as *parabiosis* experiments, sought to prove the existence of leptin.

Parabiosis is not the kind of thing we perform on humans. Two creatures, in this case the mice, are surgically joined right down to their circulation, like artificial Siamese twins. Hormones made in one mouse, therefore, could be transferred to the other mouse.

When a fat *ob/ob* mouse was united with a lean mouse, a startling thing happened. The mutant obese mouse lost weight! The theory that these obese mice lacked a blood-born factor that shut off appetite in the brain was strengthened. But it would take many years before the actual gene for leptin (known as the *ob* gene) would be cloned, and its hormone product, leptin, was discovered.

That finally happened in 1995. The obesity gene was cloned, and leptin (initially known as the ob protein) made prime time. Researchers demonstrated that they could make the *ob/ob* mouse lose weight by injecting it with the missing hormone. This critical study was direct evidence that leptin regulates body weight and body fat. Since this time, obesity has been viewed as a hormonal disorder.

The discovery of the leptin system is one of the most important medical breakthroughs in developing a new understanding of obesity.

So, what is leptin? Leptin is a traditional hormone, though produced by fat cells, in that it is secreted into the bloodstream, travels throughout the body, and binds with a receptor in the traditional lock-and-key fashion to turn on and off genes. Unlike many of the previous hormones discussed in this book, it is not controlled by the pituitary gland. Leptin does, however, control both the pituitary gland and the hypothalamus.

And what makes leptin? White adipose tissue (WAT). Brown adipose tissue (BAT) is responsible for heat production, while WAT is responsible for hormone production.

Leptin is the key to registering satiety. It is the hormone that signals the brain that the stomach is full. It's the hormone that acts on the brain to regulate appetite and energy expenditure. Because of this, scientists have referred to leptin as an **adipostatic hormone** (adipo = fat).

Leptin is similar to many hormones:

- As with all hormones, leptin has a receptor—actually, several different types of receptors.
- As with most hormones, mutations of the leptin receptor cause leptin resistance and result in obesity.
- To help leptin work properly, the body needs zinc, the same mineral that helps insulin work properly.
- Interestingly, leptin also helps control body temperature.

The main target of leptin is the hypothalamus, where it finds lots of leptin receptors, the place that regulates food intake and body weight. Scientists have linked the hypothalamus to body weight for many years, but the discovery of leptin, a hormone produced by fat cells, acting directly on the hypothalamus was a huge breakthrough. It quieted skeptics who had claimed that obesity is simply a matter of weak willpower. Among endocrinologists, there's no longer an argument: **Obesity is a hormonal disorder.**

There has been a tremendous amount of research on leptin in the past several years, and the more that's discovered, the more complicated leptin becomes. It seems that leptin is involved in all aspects of life. It even has a role in puberty: Scientists have known that puberty occurs when a boy or a girl accumulates a certain percentage of body fat. Heavier children tend to have puberty at a younger age. And leptin plays an important role in deciding when that will begin.

As an endocrinologist, I find it amazing that this hormone, with such tremendous importance, was only recently discovered. Given the speed at which news travels in the modern scientific world, there are now countless numbers of scientists jumping on the leptin bandwagon doing their own research—and more power to them. I just wonder how many other yet undiscovered hormones there are—likely thousands.

LEPTIN DEFICIENCY

Although very rare, in some humans leptin deficiency—just like that of the *ob/ob* mouse—has been discovered. These were among the first people to receive injections of leptin.

Studies have shown that injections of genetically engineered leptin (similar to the way that insulin, GH, and other hormones are manufactured) can make very obese individuals with leptin deficiency lose weight. In fact, they can lose lots of weight. These individuals are still being treated with leptin and are still losing weight.

There is a suggestion that with time, the leptin will lose its effect. However, doctors keep cranking up the dosage and the weight keeps falling off, without any special diets or exercise. Leptin alone has made them shed the pounds.

But though the results are quite dramatic, leptin deficiency *appears* to be very rare, and most obese individuals should not expect such dramatic results. It may not be as rare as doctors think, however. Thousands of people have been tested, but millions have not. We have no idea if, perhaps, *partial* leptin deficiency exists. If so, this may be even more common.

And though leptin deficiency is rare, **leptin resistance** is quite common. But at this time, testing for leptin levels is not widely available. Most testing is done at research centers, not doctor's offices, and the process has yet to become routine.

FAT MICE AND FAT HUMANS: INSIGHTS FROM LEPTIN RESEARCH

Studies in obese mice who do *not* make leptin have consistently shown that injections of leptin allow them to lose weight, raise metabolism, and eventually achieve a normal body weight. But the way leptin works in humans turns out to be more complex than the way it works in mice.

After the initial excitement of making fat mice thin, researchers, hoping for similar results, turned their attentions to obese humans. But, contrary to mice, the vast majority of obese humans have *high* leptin levels. This is known as **hyperleptinemia** (hyper = high, + emia = in the blood). And the fatter humans are, the higher the leptin levels.

The view on what to do, then, is mixed. Some researchers believe that injecting obese humans with leptin would do more harm than good. Other scientists have taken an opposing view, deciding to treat overweight humans who have leptin resistance with very high doses of leptin.

This concept may seem innovative, but it's not so new. For example, I've mentioned the best way to treat type 2 diabetes is to improve insulin resistance—with diet, exercise, and medications. But if that can't get insulin levels down, what do doctors do? They prescribe insulin. They take the attitude of "if you can't beat them, join them." Even though insulin levels are already high, insulin injections are needed to get the insulin levels high enough to overcome the resistance.

So, when it comes to leptin, why not try the same strategy? Maybe obesity in humans, some researchers think, is caused by leptin resistance.

This has parallels in the mouse world. Another strain of obese mice, known as *db/db*, is resistant to leptin. This is due to a problem with the receptor for leptin. The *db/db* mouse is identical to the *ob/ob* mouse, but instead of *low* leptin levels, the *db/db* mouse has very *high* leptin levels—just like obese humans. And all because the *db/db* mouse has a dysfunctional, mutated leptin receptor.

Humans cause their own leptin resistance by becoming overweight. The obesity actually *causes* the receptor to become dysfunctional, something known as an *acquired defect*. But—when it comes to losing weight, at least—this is a good thing. The leptin resistance in humans is reversible, whereas—because the mice are born with it—in the *db/db* mouse it is not.

So obesity causes leptin resistance. The fatter you are, the higher your leptin levels, and the higher your levels, the greater your resistance. It all makes sense: the more fat cells, the more leptin they can make. When you lose weight, leptin levels plunge. It's all another vicious cycle.

Studies are now under way where obese people, who already have high levels of leptin, are being given large doses of the hormone. Initial results are modest: Those on the highest doses lost about 16 pounds over 6 months. These results are very preliminary, and much more research is needed. Another problem is that the injections tend to be very painful. This makes it difficult to administer appropriate doses of leptin.

Scientists are hypothesizing one reason for the modest results may be that the leptin, though injected, is not getting into the brain. Early studies have shown this is true in mice. Somehow, obesity causes a problem with leptin entering the brain.

Some scientists have proposed administering leptin directly into the brain. This is pretty drastic but has been very successful in mice. However, I recommend you try the **Hormonal Health Diet** in Chapter 11 before you start injecting leptin—or anything else—into your brain.

You will continue to hear about leptin. New types of leptin, medications that mimic leptin (and are small enough to enter the brain), and medications that enhance the action of leptin are all under development. And several companies are developing medications known as leptin promoters that entice the body to make more of its own leptin. The promoter actually binds to DNA near the leptin gene, cranking up the gene's production of leptin. Unlike leptin, this medication will be available in pill form and will not have to be injected.

Ways to Enhance Your Leptin

- Lose weight. Break the vicious cycle. Weight loss markedly improves the ability of leptin to enter the brain and function properly.
- Improve insulin resistance. Insulin resistance and leptin resistance go together. Follow our insulin-reduction strategies and leptin actions will be improved.
- Lower cortisol levels. High cortisol inhibits leptin effect. Reduce stress in your life as discussed in Chapter 8.
- Enhance your growth hormone levels. Recall that leptin resistance can lower your GH levels. As GH levels rise, leptin action is improved. As leptin action improves, GH rises. (See Chapter 9.)
- Get plenty of zinc. This mineral regulates leptin and helps it work properly. Foods high in zinc include oysters, beef, wheat germ, lima beans, and dairy products.
- Do not smoke. Smoking lowers leptin levels. Yet another reason to quit.

THYROID HORMONE AND LEPTIN

We've seen before that stress and improper dieting harm the endocrine system in several ways, forcing up production of some hormones, bringing down the production of others, until the body is completely out of whack and desperately trying to cope with what it perceives is a drastic situation. Thyroid hormone is one of those that suffers a drop in production, particularly the active T3 form of the hormone.

Table 10.1
FOODS HIGH IN ZINC

Beef
Dairy products
Lima beans
Oysters
Wheat germ

Stress and crash diets also make leptin levels drop. It's the falling leptin levels, in fact, that are the key regulator of the thyroid levels. Leptin does this by controlling the cells in the hypothalamus that produce TRH. Remember, TRH stimulates TSH, which stimulates the thyroid gland to produce its hormone.

Interestingly, under normal condition low thyroid levels signal the production of more thyroid hormone. However, during crash dieting, low leptin levels prevent this from occurring. In other words, low leptin levels are more important than low thyroid hormone levels in the regulation of TRH.

Experiments in mice have shown that leptin injections can prevent the fall in thyroid that occurs as a result of starvation or strict dieting. Leptin administration similarly prevents the drop in other hormones that occur with strict dieting, including gonadotropins (brain sex hormones), estrogen, and testosterone.

Meanwhile, α-MSH stimulates thyroid hormone release, while AgRP inhibits thyroid hormone release.

So the focus has been on the key actions of leptin and α-MSH. With their effect of raising thyroid hormone levels, metabolism is enhanced and the body burns more fuel more effectively. It's a major area of research today. Unfortunately, most of the work has only been done in rodents, but early conclusions are promising.

OTHER FAT-CELL HORMONES

Leptin is just one of a multitude of hormones made by fat cells. White adipose tissue is glandular tissue, secreting hormone just like any other gland.

Resistin

This is a newly discovered hormone made by WAT, the same type of fat tissue that makes leptin. The more fat you have, the more resistin you make. The name describes this hormone appropriately because resistin causes insulin resistance. Resistin works in concert with other chemical messengers such as tumor necrosis factor and free fatty acids (see Chapter 3) to do its dirty work. Researchers are now working on medications that can neutralize resistin as a possible treatment for obesity, diabetes, and insulin resistance (known as *resistin antagonists*).

Adiponectin

Another hormone produced by fat, adiponectin is known as a cytokine hormone (similar to leptin and tumor necrosis factor) and is thought to play a role in obesity, insulin resistance, and diabetes. Studies have shown that low levels of adiponectin are closely related to body weight and degree of insulin resistance.

NEUROHORMONAL FACTORS RELATED TO LEPTIN

Pro-opiomelanocortin (POMC)

If you have red hair, listen up.

POMC, or melanocortin, is a special hormone made by the pituitary gland. It is known as a "prohormone" because, by itself, it doesn't do much. Leptin stimulates the pituitary gland to pump out POMC. Special enzymes break apart POMC into a variety of hormones, each having its own special activity (see Figure 10.1).

Mice with a mutated POMC gene are very fat. They also have a dirty-blond coat. That's because one of the POMC hormones gives pigment to skin and hair and, without it—with the mutated version—you get a dirty-blond or red hair appearance. These mice also have adrenal gland problems. ACTH, the pituitary hormone that stimulates the adrenal gland, also comes from the breakup of POMC.

Treatment of these mice with α-MSH—discussed next—helped them lose weight. In addition, the blonde hairs went away.

Humans with POMC mutations have also recently been identified. Just like the mice, these individuals are obese and have light skin and

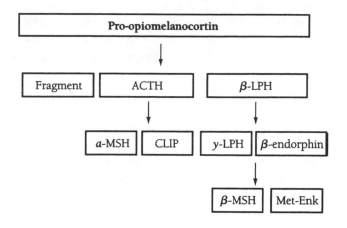

Figure 10.1
PRO-OPIOMELANOCORTIN AND ITS ACTIVE FRAGMENTS
Pro-opiomelanocortin (POMC) is a large "precursor" hormone produced by the pituitary gland. This inactive hormone is broken apart by special enzymes into several active hormones including adrenocorticotrophic hormone (ACTH), alpha- and beta-melanocyte stimulating hormone (MSH), and endorphins.

red hair. So, although it's very rare, if you are very overweight and have light skin and red hair, you may have a POMC mutation causing your obesity.

Although not yet tried in humans, injections of α-MSH may help those with POMC mutations lose weight.

Alpha-Melanocyte Stimulating Hormone (α-MSH)

α-MSH is one of the hormones produced when POMC is broken apart. Leptin stimulates the POMC gene, which enhances production of α-MSH.

α-MSH is key to understanding obesity. It induces satiety and tells fat cells to quit storing fat. α-MSH also has its own special receptor known as the melanocortin-4 (MCR-4) receptor.

Scientists have found that the interaction between α-MSH and its receptor is vital in keeping a normal body weight. MCR-4 receptors are located on TRH-producing cells in the hypothalamus (see below).

Although the study of α-MSH and MCR-4 is still in its infancy, chemical compounds are in development that act like α-MSH and stimulate MCR-4. These compounds, known as MCR-4 agonists, suppress appetite and are being studied by pharmaceutical companies as potential weight-loss medications.

Agouti-Related Protein (AgRP)

This protein blocks the actions of α-MSH, enhancing appetite and causing weight gain. It works by blocking the MCR-4 receptor—the opposite of α-MSH. The result is that too much AgRP makes you fat.

Usually AgRP presents little threat to us. Under normal conditions, the body only has only a low level of AgRP production, mostly in the skin. But the agouti mouse, from which the protein takes its name, has a genetic mutation causing it to have very high AgRP levels throughout the body, not just in its skin. Thus the α-MSH does not function properly, and the mouse becomes very fat. Studies have also shown that levels of AgRP are increased in obese humans as well.

Again, the study of this hormone is just getting started. But pharmaceutical companies are investigating ways of using our knowledge of AgRP to develop new weight-loss medications.

Melanin Concentrating Hormone (MCH)

MCH, yet another hormone made by the brain—this time in the lateral hypothalamus—is a hormone that is critical in the regulation of appetite and metabolism. It is a peptide hormone, like other brain hormones.

When there is leptin resistance—the leptin doesn't work properly—or leptin deficiency, MCH production goes up, stimulating appetite. But the real news is that the same thing happens with crash dieting. MCH rises, increasing your appetite. It's yet another reason to avoid these diets.

Mice with a mutated MCH gene have been studied, and they're very lean—they just don't eat much. But mice with high MCH levels are very hungry, and very fat.

Research is at hand on MCH and its corresponding receptor. The MCH receptor, in fact, has been recently cloned. The MCH receptor is located in parts of the brain that control functions such as taste, smell, appetite, and feeding urges. Together, these brain regions coordinate to regulate food intake and body weight.

Medications that block the MCH receptor are potentially an excellent approach for development of new weight-loss medications. If you can block the actions of MCH, appetite goes down.

Neuropeptide Y

Neuropeptide Y (NPY) is among the most abundant brain chemicals. Leptin's most powerful actions take place in the brain, affecting NPY. Leptin works in the hypothalamus by keeping NPY levels low.

NPY is a potent stimulator of appetite. In a normal situation, leptin suppresses NPY, keeping levels low. But if leptin resistance develops (or, rarely, leptin deficiency), NPY levels rise, unchecked, making you ravenous.

Neuropeptide Y also has more complex actions on the hypothalamus and other areas of the brain, promoting accumulation of body fat and slowing metabolism.

The worst effect may be that when you go on a crash diet, neuropeptide Y levels skyrocket, working against you. It can also stimulate your body to produce excess cortisol—causing all the problems of this condition discussed in Chapter 8.

In particular, NPY increases production of the hypothalamic hormone corticotropin-releasing hormone (CRH), which stimulates the pituitary gland to make ACTH, which then stimulates the adrenal gland to make too much cortisol.

A more gradual weight loss, as we suggest, keeps neuropeptide Y levels low.

Neuropeptide Y is not the only brain hormone linked to leptin, and in fact animals that lack neuropeptide Y are of normal weight.

At least five pharmaceutical companies are working on medications to block NPY (NPY inhibitors) as potential weight-loss medications.

MORE BRAIN CHEMICALS AND HORMONES

Serotonin

You're probably quite familiar with this substance, since its discovery has led to a greater understanding of depression and an entire class of what are known as *SSRI (selective serotonin reuptake inhibitors)*—antidepressant drugs such as Prozac, Paxil, Celexa, Remeron, and Zoloft. Not officially a hormone, serotonin is a brain chemical known as a neurotransmitter that helps regulate hunger and appetite. It's made from the amino acid tryptophan, and because of serotonin's importance in regulating hunger and appetite, tryptophan is known as an essential amino acid.

Reactive hypoglycemia and carbohydrate cravings are also linked to serotonin. This fits in with commonsensical notions of depression and fatigue, since many people "treat" their problem by eating, and usually eating sweets. You'll recall the information about carbohydrate cravings in Chapter 2. You feel bad, you have low energy, you grab some sweets to make it go away—which an initial sugar rush does. But then the spike subsides, even plunges, and it's back on the roller coaster.

Some people do not produce enough serotonin. This can be caused by stress, high carbohydrate diets, and weight gain around the middle. Serotonin problems can interfere with mood (causing depression or anxiety), sleep (reducing GH production), weight, and even the menstrual cycle. Low serotonin levels have been linked to depression, anxiety, and PMS. SSRIs are now used to treat all of these conditions.

But SSRIs also have an interesting side effect: They can influence your weight, causing either weight *loss* or weight *gain*. In my clinical practice, I have seen that Prozac and Zoloft commonly cause weight loss (in the first 6 months only) but that Paxil and Remeron usually cause weight gain. But I have seen the opposite occur with all of them! And these drugs aren't too different from prescription diet pills such as Phen-Fen. And, of course, even some people gained weight on these medications. The point is that serotonin has powerful influences on your weight, but it is not the *only* factor.

The antidepressant medication venlafaxine (Effexor) and the weight-loss medication sibutramine (Meridia) work by increasing levels of both serotonin and norepinephrine. This combination approach seems to both decrease hunger and increase satiety. Patients who take sibutramine tend to lose about 25 pounds in 6 months. If the medication is discontinued, however, the weight is regained. The antidepressant medication bupropion (Wellbutrin, Zyban) affects both the norepinephrine and dopamine systems and also causes weight loss. Sibutramine also increases dopamine. So, it seems that serotonin, norepinephrine, and dopamine are all interrelated when it comes to regulating weight.

Currently, a "designer" serotonin medication is under development. This medication works by stimulating only a special serotonin receptor known as serotonin receptor 2c. Research shows that the 2c receptor is the one that is most important when it comes to influencing hunger and appetite. Early reports claim that the medication works better than available medications and with fewer side effects.

St. John's wort is a nutraceutical that affects the serotonin system in a way similar to SSRIs. It has been promoted as an herbal treatment for both depression and obesity. Studies on St. John's wort have not been consistent. It appears that St. John's wort is not very effective for weight loss.

Gamma-Aminobutyric Acid (GABA)

GABA is a potent brain chemical that is affected by several prescription medications. Benzodiazepine medications such as Xanax, Valium, and Librium relieve anxiety and make you sleepy by stimulating the receptor for GABA. This class of medications has also been reported to promote *weight gain*. A medication called topiramate (Topamax), indicated for the treatment of epilepsy, has a slightly different effect on the GABA receptor. Unlike benzodiazapines, topiramate causes *weight loss*. Although not yet approved for the treatment of weight loss, studies are under way.

Urocortin

Another hormone that may be developed as a diet drug in the future, urocortin is a brain hormone released when the body is stressed. In animals, it's been shown to reduce appetite and cause weight loss.

Melatonin

Melatonin is made by a poorly understood gland in the brain known as the pineal gland. (Interesting bit of trivia: Because we don't understand what, exactly, the pineal gland does, in years past it was thought to be the "seat of the soul.") Though many doctors think melatonin can help with weight loss, I'm not among them. Recent evidence even suggests that melatonin may cause weight *gain*.

PANCREATIC HORMONES

The main hormone made by the pancreas is insulin. But it's not the only one. The pancreas, you may recall, is really two organs rolled into one. The *exocrine pancreas* makes digestive enzymes that are secreted into the gut. The *endocrine pancreas* is found in specialized islands of cells, known as the islets of Langerhans, and produces hormones that are secreted into the blood. Different cells in the islets produce different hormones.

Three other important pancreatic hormones are glucagon, somatostatin, and amylin. Each, like insulin, is closely related to the food you eat, and each affects your appetite.

Glucagon

Glucagon is a peptide hormone made in the pancreas, alongside insulin, in the islets of Langerhans. It's a digestive hormone, released when food—particularly protein—leaves the stomach and enters the small intestine.

It helps perform a wide variety of tasks: It slows the exit of food from the stomach, making you feel full; acts to raise blood sugar; and tells the liver to pump out glucose.

Glucagon is also known as a counter-insulin hormone. Diabetics who are prone to insulin reactions carry a syringe of glucagon. If they have severe low blood sugar, a shot of glucagon will make their blood sugar shoot right up.

Rare cases exist of tumors of glucagon-producing cells, known as **glucagonoma**. In these cases, the extremely high glucagon levels created by the tumors cause diabetes. The condition is accompanied by an itchy red, sandpaper-like rash. And yes, though this is very, very rare, I bring it up because it's not rare if you're the one who has it. If you have diabetes and an itchy red rash, visit your endocrinologist and ask to have your glucagon levels tested. He may look at you funny at first, but be persistent.

Authors such as Barry Sears agree that glucagon is the counterpart to insulin. In *The Zone*, Sears claims that "optimal glucagon-to-insulin balance is the portal to the zone." But Sears is only partially correct: Although glucagon does have activities opposite insulin, it's one of a number of counter-insulin hormones, including cortisol, GH, and epinephrine. You can't look at glucagon and insulin in a vacuum.

Here are two steps to balance glucagon and insulin:

- Follow our eating suggestions.
- Increase intake of vegetable protein, especially soy protein. Vegetable proteins favor glucagon production over insulin production—so if you are making too much insulin, vegetable proteins may help. The down side is that increased glucagon levels could suppress GLP-1 levels (see below), negating the effect; the lowered insulin means less hunger, but increased glucagon means lower GLP-1 and increased hunger. It's a wash.

Somatostatin

In Chapter 9, somatostatin was discussed as a hormone that lowers GH levels. Higher GH levels aid in weight loss, so this was not necessarily conducive to weight loss. Somatostatin is primarily produced by the hypothalamus, but it's also created in the islets of Langerhans in the pancreas, just like insulin and glucagon. Again, it's a hormone that blocks other hormones—in this case, the secretion of its sister pancreatic hormones, insulin and glucagon. It shuts down β-cells, the pancreatic cells responsible for insulin secretion.

But in certain situations, somatostatin may also help with weight loss, despite its counterproductive effects on GH. One of these situations is that of **hypothalamic obesity**, a condition in which a brain injury or certain brain tumors cause obesity by damaging satiety centers in the ventromedial hypothalamus. Hypothalamic obesity is perhaps the most difficult form of obesity to treat. Insulin levels are very high, but not because of insulin resistance, something known as *primary insulin hypersecretion (PIH) syndrome*. Scientists hypothesize that damage to the hypothalamus may increase nerve signals to the pancreas, boosting insulin levels and causing extreme hunger. The high insulin levels also cause nutrients to be stored as fat, instead of being burned as energy.

Somatostatin injections in these patients dramatically lower insulin levels. Once the insulin levels go down, weight is lost and leptin levels also go down. Carbohydrate cravings are dramatically reduced.

There's also a long-acting form of somatostatin, known as **Octreotide**, which causes dramatic weight loss in some obese patients with hypothalamic obesity.

This treatment does not work for everyone, and even those with hypothalamic obesity don't all respond. For some reason, whites tend to have higher response rates than other racial groups. But the interesting thing is that for those in which the treatment does work, it really works well. People lose a great deal of weight and without going on a special diet or exercising. Long-term studies are ongoing.

Amylin

Little is known about amylin—another pancreatic hormone—but early studies have shown that it may be a useful agent to treat diabetes and help with weight loss. The synthetic form of the hormone is available in a medication known as Pramlintide. It is being studied as a possible weight-loss medication.

GUT HORMONES

Cholecystokinin (CCK)

Briefly discussed in Chapter 1, CCK is a *gut hormone*—a peptide hormone produced by the small intestine. It's sometimes known as the "feel-full protein." It slows stomach emptying and decreases appetite.

CCK works in several parts of the body, notably in a circular muscle at the bottom of the stomach known as a *sphincter*. CCK tightens the sphincter, and with the sphincter tight, food stays in the stomach. Nerves from the stomach transmit the feeling "I've had enough to eat" to the brain.

CCK also acts directly on the appetite centers of the brain, regulating appetite and making it another satiety hormone, by acting on the nerves of the stomach and intestine, signaling the brain that the stomach is full. Meanwhile, it slows movement of food out of the stomach and into the intestines, making you feel full longer.

CCK has two receptors (like estrogen), named "A" and "B." Mice with mutations for the receptor for CCK-B are overweight, whereas mice with mutations for the receptor for CCK-A are of normal weight. As we have seen, mice models give hints to hormonal causes of obesity.

There's a weight-loss product, **Satietrol**, a dietary supplement made from potatoes, which works by increasing CCK levels before your meal. Satietrol works by slowing the digestion of protein, similar to what the medication Arcarbose does for carbohydrates and Xenical for fat (see Chapter 2). By slowing digestion of protein, the body is tricked into believing that you ate more food than you actually did. Satietrol does its job of slowing the digestion of protein by inhibiting several digestive enzymes. One protein, known as cholecystokinin-releasing peptide (CCK-RP), is pumped out into the gut during a meal. Satietrol prevents the digestion of CCK-RP. Increased CCK-RP means increased CCK, and increased CCK levels means decreased hunger and increased feelings of satiety. Studies in the journal *Obesity Research* have shown that Satietrol does decrease feelings of hunger and does cause modest weight loss of about 1½ pounds per week.

Glucagon-Like Peptide-1 (GLP-1)

A cousin of glucagon, glucagon-like peptide-1 has been gaining lots of attention in the scientific community as a possible cure for obesity and diabetes. Several companies are currently investigating the use of this hormone as a cure, in fact.

GLP-1, produced by the gut, controls insulin secretion and feeding behavior. Like CCK, GLP-1 slows emptying of the stomach and reduces hunger.

Incidentally, another hormone, known as **gastric inhibitory polypeptide (GIP),** is secreted alongside GLP-1. GIP is also thought to play a role in hunger and satiety, but less is known about this gut hormone. Recall that in the rare condition of food-induced Cushing's, the GIP and cortisol systems get cross-wired so that GIP stimulates the ACTH receptors in the adrenal gland, resulting in high cortisol levels after every meal (see Chapter 8). High glucagon levels block the secretion of GLP-1.

Many studies on GLP-1 have been performed in animals, but humans have not yet been tested. Early studies are promising, though.

GLP-1 also increases insulin secretion, and for this reason, GLP-1 has been also investigated as a potential treatment for diabetes. It sounds like the ideal drug for diabetes, since it lowers blood sugar (by increasing insulin) but also helps you lose weight—not what you'd expect from something that raises insulin levels.

With this new twist—GLP-1 increases insulin and causes weight loss—a lot of diet-book authors would be at a loss.

Because GLP-1 is a peptide, it cannot be taken in pill form or the stomach will simply digest it. It must be injected.

Medications that act like GLP-1, known as GLP-1 receptor agonists (one of which is called exendin-4), have been shown to cause weight loss in rats. Exendin-4 is made from the venom of the gila monster, a reptile native to deserts in Arizona. This medication is much more potent than GLP-1.

The GLP-1 agonist medications are potent stimulators of the satiety centers. Look for exendin-4 studies on humans sometime in the future.

BLOOD PROTEINS: ARE THEY HORMONES?

Uncoupling Proteins, aka Thermogenins

Yet another area being hotly investigated by drug companies, thermogenins are made by brown fat tissue (BAT) and are responsible for thermogenesis. The more uncoupling proteins in your system, the higher your metabolism.

There are three types of uncoupling proteins: the prosaically named UCP-1, UCP-2, and UCP-3. UCP-2 and UCP-3 are most promising for weight loss, but so far research has been limited to mice.

Scientists have been working on ways to increase uncoupling proteins as a form of increasing metabolism and causing weight loss. There are also medications under development mimicking UCPs that could be injected and would speed metabolism.

More research is needed in this field. Researchers estimate that it will be at least 10 years before a UCP-like drug is available for weight loss.

Wnt-10b

This unusual-sounding blood protein was recently discovered to be involved with fat formation. It is thought to be a hormone, but very little is known about Wnt-10b. Researchers have discovered that the Wnt-10 protein prevents fat-precursor cells (known as pre-adipocytes) from developing into full-fledged fat cells (adipocytes). Blocking Wnt-10b's actions results in increased fat and even turns muscle into fat. In the future, medications that mimic or enhance Wnt-10b may be an effective way to cause weight loss.

CHAPTER ELEVEN

LOSING WEIGHT
NOW

THERE'S A CHEESY OLD SONG CALLED "IN THE YEAR 2525." In one verse the singers describe that all the food and nutrients you require will be "in the pill that you took today." It's doubtful that eating a simple pill will make you overweight.

Meanwhile, just in the last few pages, you've read about all the wonderful hormones being discovered by scientists and doctors, and similar medications being researched by pharmaceutical companies. The year 2525 may be a few hundred years off, and scientists may not succeed in putting a day's worth of food in a tiny pill, but it is quite conceivable that by 2020—or even 2010—all you will need to do to lose weight is pop a pill or inject a substance into your skin.

Eat without regret! Lose weight without dieting!

Yes, it is a very real possibility.

But not realistic for the way we live. To be honest, you could take pills now that would help you lose weight quickly. You see ads for them all the time. But these pills, often related to amphetamines, may have terrible side effects. They make your heart race, give you headaches, make you feel nauseous. The side effects are a drastic price to pay for a quick fix. In the worst cases, they can take years off your life.

That's why we come here, to the old tried and true: diet and exercise.

The human body is a machine that was designed to move. If we walked as much as we should, if we did the occasional labor to firm up the muscles in our arms and our stomachs, we wouldn't be in the bind we are today. Yes, we are a fast-paced society, and a fast-paced society has little time for walking, lifting, and preparing well-balanced meals. Instead, we go full blast in our heads all day long, pop in a microwavable dinner when we get home, then veg out in front of the TV set. I do it too. It's hard not to.

But it's worth a try to move toward a healthier lifestyle. Often the most rewarding things in life are not the easiest. They take a little effort. But they're well worth it when they're done—when you've established the habits that will take you to the next level.

On the following pages are eating suggestions and menus for a better, healthier life. They're not restricted to heaps of vegetables and endless sessions of sit-ups; as I've discussed throughout *Hormonal Balance*, cutting stress is as important to losing weight as cutting calories.

MAKE IT A HABIT

Changing your lifestyle for the better requires commitment to that change until it has become a habit, a way of life, and no longer a burden. Just like the habit of getting up in the morning and the systematic way that we prepare for work, so too will the habit of an improved diet and exercise become as automatic. The key to success is that the change becomes a habit!

GOAL SETTING

For every action you take, there must be a plan for guidance and a goal to define your achievement. You must determine how much weight loss is appropriate and how you will achieve it. Obviously that will require change in eating habits and exercise.

You should start with short-term goals and long-term goals. Short-term goals allow you to be successful in the short run. The last thing you want is to be overwhelmed by goals that seem too lofty to aspire to.

These goals are vital to your success:

- **Put your goals in writing.** Writing down your goals will help you keep them in mind. Keep your list on the refrigerator or on the bathroom mirror. Continually review and update your goals.

- **Set a date for the completion of each goal.** Setting a date will help you to stay focused and motivated.
- **Keep a food diary.** This will help you see the frequency of eating, the foods you eat, and the quantities. Analysis of this record keeping will allow you to make more specific changes. Use your food diary to help you with grocery shopping and meal planning.
- **Set exercise goals.** Be specific about the kind of exercise you will engage in. Determine your short-term goal for duration of exercise and a long-term goal that will be necessary for you to achieve your weight loss.
- **Change your behavior.** This will be one of your biggest challenges. To be successful you must, in some way, change your behavior. You became overweight by engaging in specific behaviors, which will require change. Perhaps you worked late into the evening, didn't have time to exercise, and ate fast food on the way home. You may now need to consider exercising in the morning before work, for example. To overcome a fast-food attraction, you may have to prepare meals and snacks at home to take to school or work.

Setting Goals for Your Weight

How much weight should you lose? This is a difficult decision. Many of us will have difficulty achieving a "normal" body weight. This does not mean that some weight loss will not be beneficial. In fact, many scientific studies have shown that weight loss as little as 5 to 10 percent of your initial body weight will help regulate hormones and improve medical problems caused by obesity such as diabetes, high blood pressure, and arthritis. For others, this seemingly small amount of weight loss is not enough. We strive to have a "normal" weight. But what is normal?

Standardizing Height and Weight: Body Mass Index (BMI)

BMI, or body mass index, is the new standard for adjusting weight for height, assigning a numerical value to this ratio. BMI is a widely used standard to determine if you fall in the healthy (or "normal") range or if you are overweight or obese. BMI is defined as body weight in kilograms

divided by the square of height in meters (kg/m²). This is a complicated metric formula that is easily converted to pounds and inches. You
can calculate your own BMI by using the following formula:

$$\text{BMI} = \frac{\text{(weight in pounds)} \times 703}{\text{(height in inches)} \times \text{(height in inches)}}$$

For example, if you weigh 180 pounds and are 5 feet, 6 inches,

$$\text{BMI} = (180 \times 703)/(66 \times 66) = \mathbf{29}$$

A normal or healthy BMI range is between 18.5 kg/m² and 25
kg/m². BMI values greater than 25 kg/m² are good indicators of
degrees of excess fat and health risks. Overweight is defined as a BMI
between 25 and 29.9, and obesity is defined as a BMI greater than 30.
Table 11.1 lists BMI and weight categories.

Table 11.1

BMI	Weight Category
<18.4	Underweight
18.5–24.9	Normal
25–29.9	Overweight
30–34.9	Class I Obesity
35–39.9	Class II Obesity
40–59.9	Class III Obesity
>60	Super Obesity

BMI is now the standard used by scientists and doctors to study
weight and health risk. The higher your BMI, the higher your risk of
medical problems and death.

BEYOND THE BMI

The body mass index is a ratio of weight and height. Other factors such
as body frame, waistline, and body composition are not part of the BMI—
but are important variables to consider when measuring health risk.

Waist circumference is a measure of fat in the belly, which is more dangerous than other types of fat (see Chapter 3). The waist circumference is an excellent way of determining if you have *central obesity*. Men with a waist circumference greater than 40 inches and women with a waist circumference greater than 35 inches have central obesity. The waist circumference has replaced an older measure, known as the waist-to-hip ratio, as a better indicator of central obesity.

Do you have central obesity?

Men: A waistline of more than 40 inches.

Women: A waistline of more than 35 inches.

Body-fat analysis helps you to determine how much of your weight is lean tissue (muscle, blood, and bone) and how much is fat. There are many methods of measuring body composition, or your percentage of body fat, including underwater weighing, CT scanning, ultrasound, bioimpedance analysis (BIA), body calipers, and DEXA. Each of these methods has advantages and disadvantages. In general, tests that are easy to perform, such as bioimpedance analysis and body calipers, are less accurate (but easier and cheaper) than underwater weighing, CT scanning, and DEXA (Dual Energy x-ray Analysis). Despite this, I believe that bioimpedance analysis or body calipers are excellent ways of keeping track of body fat.

Body-fat analysis can be useful when you hit a plateau. Because lean tissue is denser than bone, it is possible to lose body fat and maintain your weight. Although your weight is the same, you are leaner and your clothes will be looser.

SET SHORT-TERM GOALS

These should be goals that you can realize in a short period of time. They are, however, stepping-stones to the long-term goal of improved eating and exercise with subsequent total weight loss desired. Write your goals down and keep them visible.

For example, your goal for weight loss may be 30 pounds. To remain positive and enthusiastic about the feat at hand, set a short-term goal of a 3- to 5- pound loss in 1 month. If you currently exercise sporadically, then a good short-term goal is to exercise 3 times a week for 15 to 30 minutes. However, your long-term goal may be to exercise 5 times per week for a sufficient time that will burn a minimum number of calories.

SET LONG-TERM GOALS

Long-term goals are the end results of your daily efforts. They can be achieved only by the culmination of your daily commitments. They cannot be achieved without the short-term goals and plans. An excellent mid-range goal is a 10 to 15 percent reduction from your starting body weight (e.g., 20 to 30 pounds for a 200-pound individual). An appropriate long-term goal is achievement of a normal body weight (BMI less than 25). Other goals may be to wear a smaller pants or dress size or to improve medical problems (such as high blood pressure, arthritis, and diabetes). After you reach your long-term goals, don't quit. Continually update and revise your goals.

SET GOALS FOR EXERCISE

Planned Exercise

If you've never exercised before, then be sure to get clearance from your medical doctor.

However, if you have exercised recently but without any commitment, then set a realistic short-term goal that is achievable. For example, "I will exercise 4 times per week for 15 minutes." The long-term goal is to exercise sufficiently to burn a specific number of calories each week.

Regular exercise is the key to maintaining lost weight. **Remember: Weight loss without exercise is temporary.**

Increase Daily Activities

Formal exercise is not the only way you can burn calories. Any type of activity, from shopping to gardening, can burn calories. One of the reasons that obesity has reached epidemic proportions is that modern technology has almost eliminated the need to move your body. The car, telephone, elevator, electric garage-door opener, and television with remote control are all contributors to this phenomenon. You can get rid of some of these "conveniences" and burn extra calories.

The following are recommendations by the American College of Sports Medicine:

- Walk up stairs instead of taking the elevator or the escalator.
- Park your car a little farther away from your destination and walk the extra distance.
- Take a short walk around the block.
- Play actively with the kids.
- Mow the lawn.

HAVE REALISTIC EXPECTATIONS

Your weight-loss results will depend on whether you are a novice or a veteran at attempting to lose weight. If this is your first attempt at weight loss, you may be more optimistic and a lot more confident in your attempts to succeed than someone who has attempted every diet designed. A positive attitude is critical, as is confidence in your ability to follow the diet plan and make the appropriate food choices as well as portion sizes.

Rate of Weight Loss

Your rate of weight loss will vary considerably, as it is dependent on multiple factors.

1. How do you view this effort in losing weight—as a diet or a lifestyle change?
2. What is your starting weight?

3. What is your weight-loss goal? Is it realistic?
4. Are you very motivated?
5. Are you prepared for changes and new habits?
6. Are you exercising?

Very heavy people often have an extremely rapid initial weight loss. Some of this is water weight. The rate of weight loss usually slows down after a few weeks; this is normal. They will keep losing weight. For those needing to lose 10 pounds, they can expect a 2- to 3- pound weight loss per week. For goal losses of 50 pounds or greater, the initial weight loss may be as much as 5 to 10 pounds the first couple of weeks. A good rule of thumb is that there are 3,500 calories in a pound of fat. If you are at a stable weight and reduce your calories by 500 to 1,000 per day, you will lose 1 to 2 pounds per week.

---

1 pound of fat = 3500 calories

PREPLANNING

Preplanning is a critical element for a successful diet. It will keep you on your diet and will keep you successful. You must have the proper foods around at all times. This means having lots of fresh fruits and vegetables throughout the week.

I recommend shopping once a week from a list. With proper storage and preparation methods, you will have no problem keeping fruits and vegetables fresh and good tasting. Plan on bringing your lunch every day. Prepare snacks in advance.

Don't let lack of preparation make you fail. By having the proper foods available to yourself, you've already won the battle. Eating all these delicious foods is the easy part.

KEEP A FOOD DIARY

The food diary is one of the most helpful ways of accounting to yourself. Keep a small notebook with you at all times. Record everything that you eat. *Awareness is paramount to changing habits.* The food diary will make you very aware of what you eat. It will help you exercise control over eating and is an honest tally of your daily intake.

A few tips on keeping a food diary:

- Record every item eaten.
- Record the amount of each item eaten.
- Record the times you eat during the day.
- Record where you eat and what you are doing.
- Do not wait to record your intake at the end of the day. It will be inaccurate.
- Record immediately after eating.
- Record your emotions.

EATING IN RESTAURANTS

It is easier to be in control of your eating habits when you are the person shopping for the food and preparing it. However, whether it is business or pleasure that takes you away from doing this, you are now faced with the task of maintaining your new habits in unfamiliar surroundings. Eating out can be a great challenge but simplified if you have a plan. Here are some tips:

- Try to select from a menu versus all-you-can-eat buffets.
- Order a green salad with fat-free dressing before your meal.
- Avoid high-fat appetizers.
- Drink water throughout your meal.
- Order sauces and dressings on the side.
- When possible choose dishes that are steamed, poached, boiled, broiled, or grilled.
- Choose red sauces instead of creamed sauces for pasta dishes.
- Avoid filling up on bread before the meal—ask that the breadbasket be removed.
- Choose fresh fruit for dessert or at most share a dessert.
- Avoid alcoholic beverages.

PREPARING TO SHOP

The trip to the grocery store can be the initial link in the chain of events that determines how successful eating habits will be on subsequent days. If the choices made here are according to the diet plan, then the meals prepared and eaten will be too. The following are guidelines to help you adhere to your goals.

- Shop only from a list.
- Do not be tempted by unhealthy items that are shelved conspicuously throughout the grocery store.
- Do not shop when hungry. Shopping on an empty stomach will only lead to compulsive buying and will likely include prepackaged foods that can be consumed fast. Such foods are often laden with fat and salt and are unwise food choices.
- Prepare meals. Prepare as many meals as possible. The time it takes to prepare a meal can often prevent the impulsive, uncontrolled eating that occurs with fast foods.
- Shop as little as possible. The more frequent the trips, the more often the temptations. I recommend that you shop once a week. With the suggestions listed in this section, you will have fresh fruits and vegetables available for the entire week.
- Don't shop for the family favorites. These are likely to be your favorites too.
- Don't be tempted by the store's free food samples as you shop.

PLANNING FOR UNPLANNED EVENTS

Although you may feel that your exercise is now becoming routine, you're adapting well to changed eating habits, and the pounds are gradually being lost, there will always be the unplanned occasion. If your goals have not addressed these events, you will not be adequately prepared for the foods that may be available or the choices you will have to make when the menu includes foods that you ordinarily consider off-limits.

When such events arise, attempt to find out ahead of time the food that is available and make a note of what you will eat. Then, when you arrive at the event, you will be less likely to eat impulsively.

MAINTENANCE: MAKE THIS YOUR LAST DIET

For those in maintenance, you should congratulate yourself. You have made a great commitment and thus far have been successful.

However, the biggest challenge remains: keeping the weight off. Maintenance must be seen as your new way of life, not as a defined period in your life with a starting and stopping point to it. The fact that you have lost your goal weight indicates motivation and success in forming new habits. This is the critical phase, the phase in which you must adhere stringently to your initial goals—this is now your new way of life. It is not the quick fix for a special occasion. You've made the commitment to eat healthy and be more active. Now you need to continue to maintain the same habits that helped you lose your goal weight.

Be sure to revisit your goals frequently to avoid accepting old habits again:

- Eat nutritionally balanced meals.
- Follow the plan. Reassure yourself that your diet plan is an integral part of your weight loss.
- Make a commitment to keep a food diary.
- Your success is always at risk of being threatened by old habits and situations. Before you succumb to your former ways, be prepared to return to the beginning when you first set out on this journey.
- Continue regular exercise.
- For those of you who are not addicted to exercise, remember: **Weight loss without exercise is temporary**.
- Remain positive. A positive attitude will help you through the tough times, always reassuring you that you are making the right choices and changes in your life.
- Be flexible. You will always be changing and adjusting to accommodate your new lifestyle.
- Remain patient.

THE HORMONAL HEALTH DIET

In the pages that follow are eating suggestions and meal plans to help you achieve hormonal balance. *This diet is designed for anyone— whether you want to lose weight, achieve hormonal balance, or do both.* The only variable is portions. If you want to lose weight portions will be smaller than if you want to maintain your weight. If you have a particular hormonal disorder such as **diabetes, insulin resistance, PCOS, menopause,** or **thyroid disease**, this diet is also good for you. The chapters on these disorders have additional eating suggestions.

This diet, like many others, uses "exchanges" as a method of tracking particular food groups. An *exchange* is a term used to describe precise portion sizes of food items within the same category to provide equivalent calories and nutrition, that is, protein, carbohydrate, and fat. For example, one protein exchange will provide 7 grams of protein, one starch exchange will yield 15 grams of carbohydrate, and one fat exchange will yield 5 grams of fat. Exchanges are a method of "portion control." They remind us how much of particular food categories we can have in a day.

The **Hormonal Health Diet** uses the exchange system in a unique way. There are no strict numbers for exchanges. Instead, we provide *minimums* and *maximums* for each exchange. In order to be successful, you must consume at least the minimum of each exchange group and you must not consume above the maximum allowed.

Three exchange categories have unlimited maximums: These are vegetables, fruits, and egg whites. These foods may be consumed in unlimited quantities on this diet.

There is no excuse to be hungry. Whenever you get hungry, you can eat and eat without breaking the diet. The key to success is to stay within the parameters of the diet. Starches (including processed fruits and juices), proteins (other than egg whites), and fats are limited. You must not consume more than the set number of exchanges.

Many of you may believe that this sounds like a crazy fad diet. I assure you it's not. *This is a healthy eating style that will allow you to balance your hormones and achieve a healthy body weight.* With time you will become accustomed to this way of eating and will feel unhealthy if you return to your old eating style.

For those of you who are not accustomed to eating vegetables and fruits, it will be a challenge to get in your minimums. I encourage you to try your best to get in all your vegetable, fruit, and protein exchanges. These foods will fill you up and make you less hungry for the "bad" foods. In addition they will provide the fuel your body needs to maintain a healthy metabolism.

Unlimited Foods	Limited Foods
Vegetables	Starches
Fruits	Milk
Egg whites	Protein (Other than egg whites)
	Fats

The **Hormonal Health Diet** provides for **three meals** and **three snacks** a day. It is important that you have all of these meals. Small, frequent feedings keep hormones in balance and prevent excessive hunger (see Chapter 3). You should try to eat some protein at breakfast and your midmorning snack. This provides energy and quenches hunger later in the day. Lunch and the midafternoon snack should be light. Dinner is protein, starch, and lots of vegetables. A snack at bedtime is important to fuel your metabolism throughout the night.

Although it is important to get all six meals in each day, I cannot overemphasize how important it is to eat breakfast. You've heard it before: Breakfast is the most important meal of the day. This is true. Having breakfast will help you to keep insulin levels (and hunger) low, making you successful (see the plight of the Sumo, Chapter 3).

Exchange Breakdown for the Hormonal Health Diet

Table 1.1 lists the minimum and maximum exchanges for one full day (divided into three meals and three snacks) for both the Weight-Loss Diet and the Weight Maintenance Diet. The range listed is for minimums and maximums. It is important that you follow both minimums and maximums. Be sure to have at least 5 servings of vegetables, 5 servings of fruit, and 6 servings of protein every day. The maximum allowance of vegetables, fruits, and egg whites is unlimited. Remember, if you get hungry, these are the foods you should be eating. The range given is for minimums and maximums.

Table 11.1
MINIMUM AND MAXIMUM EXCHANGES FOR ONE DAY

Food Group	Weight-Loss Diet Exchanges (min-max)	Weight Maintenance Diet Exchanges (min-max)
Vegetables	5–unlimited	5–unlimited
Fruit*	5–unlimited	5–unlimited
Milk	0–3	0–4
Starch	0–4	0–6
Protein**	6–8	6–10
Fat	0–2	0–4

* Maximum for bananas, grapes, and watermelon limited to 5 exchanges per day.
**Maximums do not include egg whites.

CARBOHYDRATE EXCHANGES

Carbohydrates include vegetables, fruits, milk, and starches. As discussed in Chapter 2, not all carbohydrates are created the same. Fruits and vegetables are the best carbohydrates to eat. Carbohydrates that are rapidly digested cause insulin surges and disrupt hormonal balance.

VEGETABLES (MINIMUM: 5; MAXIMUM: UNLIMITED)

One vegetable exchange yields 0–5 grams of carbohydrate, 0–2 grams of protein, zero fat, and 0–25 calories.

An exchange is 1 cup of fresh vegetables or ½ cup cooked. It is very difficult to overeat vegetables. This explains why they are unlimited on the **Hormonal Health Diet**. Besides, all that fiber contributes to early satiety before you can possibly overeat on vegetables! There are a number of vegetables that are not in this group because of their higher carbohydrate content. These "starchy vegetables" are listed in the starch group.

Artichoke	**Cucumber**	**Peppers**
Asparagus	**Eggplant**	**Pumpkin**
Beans	**Greens**	**Radishes**
Beets	**Leeks**	**Spinach**
Broccoli	**Lettuce**	**Sprouts**
Brussels sprouts	**Mushrooms**	**Squash**
Cabbage	**Okra**	**Tomato**
Cauliflower	**Onions**	**Turnips**
Celery	**Pea pods**	**Zucchini**

Vegetable Purchasing, Storage, and Preparation Tips

Artichoke
Artichoke is a flower and should be treated as such. Inspect carefully before purchasing. Artichoke flowers will get brown at the edges as they age. Give the artichoke a gentle squeeze. A fresh artichoke will have tightly packed leaves and will feel firm, but an older artichoke's

leaves spread apart and it feels spongy. Artichoke flowers should be placed in water just like other flowers. Use a small glass for each artichoke. Cut ⅛ inch of the bottom of the artichoke to expose fresh stem and place in the glass of water. To extend storage time, cover the artichoke top with a small plastic bag and use a rubber band to form a seal between the bag and the glass. Artichokes can be steamed whole (40–45 minutes) or in quarters (30–35 minutes) and served with lemon. Remember to remove the "choke" (the purple, fuzzy middle) before eating. To eat, scrape the top of each leaf with your teeth. Save the center "heart" for the end—it's the best part!

Asparagus

Asparagus have a relatively short shelf life and stores may keep them out after they have started to spoil. Look at the "flower" tip of the asparagus. Can you see the individual parts of the flower? Or has the tip started to decay? Asparagus should be stored in water like artichokes. Place a bunch of asparagus in a large plastic cup filled 1/3 with water. Cover the asparagus bunch with a plastic bag and use a rubber band to seal over the cup. Even with proper storage, asparagus tend to spoil quickly. They should be eaten before other vegetables. When ready to eat, gently snap off the lower part of the asparagus stem at its natural breaking point. Do not cut the ends of the asparagus. Asparagus can be eaten raw, blanched, poached, steamed, or stir-fried. Be careful not to overcook. Asparagus should retain a crunch after cooking. Asparagus may also be steamed, then marinated in balsamic vinegar, lemon juice, and spices and served cold.

Beans and Pea Pods

Fresh beans are available in many varieties including green beans (also known as snap beans or string beans), haricots verts, and wax beans. Chinese pea pods and sugar snap peas have similar nutritional value to green beans, but lima beans, peas, and other beans are considered starches (see below). Pre-wash beans and pea pods and keep dry in a zip-lock bag. Eat raw as a snack or in salads or steam, blanch, poach, or stir-fry.

Broccoli and Cauliflower

These vegetables are delicious, inexpensive, and can be kept fresh for a fairly long period of time. Broccoli and cauliflower are flowers and can be stored in a manner similar to artichokes and asparagus, though this takes up a great deal of space. These vegetables also can be pre-processed and kept ready-to-eat. After washing, divide the florets into tennis-ball-sized pieces. Dry well. Store in a zip-lock bag or vegetable bag. Place a paper towel in the bag to absorb any extra moisture. Replace the paper towel every 1–2 days. Broccoli and cauliflower can be kept fresh for 7–10 days in this manner. Pre-processed broccoli and cauliflower florets are also available at most grocery stores, but are considerably more expensive. Soak florets in cold water for 10 minutes before cooking. Broccoli and cauliflower may be eaten raw, steamed, poached, or stir-fried.

Broccoli

Choose heads that have all green and no yellow. Broccoli leaves should not be discarded. They have the highest nutritional content of the entire vegetable. Leaves should be prepared in a manner similar to other greens (see below). Broccoli stems are also a delicious and distinctive part of the vegetable. During pre-processing, separate stems from florets. Peel with potato peeler and eat raw as a crunchy snack or cook like greens.

Cauliflower

This flower comes in white, green, and purple varieties. All three taste about the same. Cauliflower gets a brownish discoloration as it gets older. The discoloration can be easily removed with a sharp knife—the rest of the cauliflower is still good to eat.

Cabbage

Cabbage comes in many varieties, including green and red head cabbage, Savoy cabbage, bok-choi, Chinese cabbage, kale, and Swiss chard. Brussels sprouts are a miniature variety of cabbage. Most cabbage, especially head cabbage, can be stored in the vegetable drawer of your refrigerator for 1–2 weeks. Quarter cabbage heads and steam, or shred and steam, or stir-fry. One pound of raw cabbage cooks down to about 2 cups. *Be careful—eating too much raw cabbage can cause thyroid dysfunction* (see Chapter 7).

Carrots

Some diet experts, who claim that carrots are high in sugar, have maligned this vegetable. I am not one of them. Carrots are low in calories, but high in taste and high on the crunch scale. Many of us need this type of crunch (and carbohydrate) for our snacks. Carrots are available in the large and pre-peeled "baby" variety. Peel carrots using a potato peeler or use them unpeeled, cut into slices. Carrots will store well in the vegetable drawer of your refrigerator for 7–10 days.

Celery and Cucumbers

Celery and cucumbers have little to no calories, but they taste great and are an outstanding snack or salad ingredient. I recommend trying to eat at least 1 bunch of celery and 3 cucumbers each week. Substitute sliced celery and cucumbers for potato chips. Celery can be chopped and added to soups or other vegetable dishes. The darker the celery stalk, the higher the vitamin content. Fresh cucumbers should feel firm and rigid. Grocery stores frequently leave old cucumbers on the shelves. Inspect carefully before buying. Cucumbers should be well washed with soap and water to remove the vegetable oil or wax that is applied by grocery stores. Even better, grow your own. Cucumbers are one of the easiest vegetables to grow from seed. To extend the storage life of cucumbers, wrap in a paper towel and place in a zip-lock bag. Cucumbers can be sliced and marinated with sliced onion, red wine vinegar, or 1–2 tablespoons of table sugar and spices for a delicious cucumber salad.

Eggplant

If you do not regularly eat eggplant, you should start. There are many varieties of eggplant. Each has its own distinctive texture and taste. Eggplant will stay fresh in your vegetable drawer for at least 1 week. The vegetable contains a huge amount of water. When cooking, it is usually necessary to drain excess water from time to time. Eggplant slices can be salted and drained of excess moisture on a rack. It discolors shortly after being cut, but squeezing lemon juice can eliminate this. Eggplant cooks best in stainless steel, pottery, or glass containers, and it can be sautéed, stir-fried, stuffed, baked, or grilled. Eggplant is also an excellent addition to spaghetti sauce.

Greens

There are countless types of greens, including many wild varieties. Common store varieties of greens include spinach, collard greens, turnip greens, mustard greens, and beet greens. Wash greens carefully to remove the grit. Spinach can be eaten raw or lightly steamed. Other greens usually need to be steamed or simmered for 25–40 minutes until tender. Substitute smoked turkey for ham hocks and serve with vinegar.

Leeks and Onions

Leeks and onions are an excellent addition to salads and recipes. Slice leeks in half, marinate in vinegar and spices, and grill. Onions will usually keep in dry storage for 2–3 weeks or in your refrigerator for even longer. Because of their high sugar content, onions must not be cooked with high heat. Lower heat helps prevent discoloration. Raw onion slices are a great addition to a sandwich.

Lettuce

It is a challenge to keep fresh lettuce in your refrigerator for a whole week, but it can be done. Wash the lettuce head using the spray attachment on your sink, carefully keeping the head intact. Dry the head as best as possible and wrap in a towel and place in zip-lock bag or plastic container. Replace towel every 2-3 days. Romaine and iceberg lettuce will store for 7-10 days using this technique. Other varieties of lettuce stay fresh for shorter periods of time. In general the smaller the lettuce leaf, the shorter the shelf life. I recommend using small leaf lettuces early in the week and romaine or iceberg later in the week, thus ensuring a variety of fresh lettuce for the whole week.

Mushrooms

Never use a mushroom that shows any sign of decay. Mushroom decay is full of toxins. The key to keeping mushrooms fresh is keeping them dry and well ventilated. Mushrooms should not be washed until just prior to use. But wash gently—most of the flavor is in the skins. Mushrooms are great raw, steamed or stir-fried and require a very short cooking time.

Okra

This southern favorite is often used in stews where its gooey quality helps thicken the dish. This consistency is often referred to as "gumbo." The smaller the okra pod, the more tender. Okra is great sewed or sautéed with tomatoes, peppers and onions.

Peppers

There are many variety of peppers including sweet, bell, banana, pimento and hot. Peppers will stay fresh for 7-8 days in the vegetable drawer of your refrigerator. Raw peppers are a great snack or salad item. Peppers are also great steamed, stewed, sautéed, stir-fried or stuffed. Hot peppers are a wonderful addition to many recipes.

Radishes and Turnips

These are great raw as a snack. Turnips can be eaten like an apple.

Sprouts

Many types of sprouts are available including bean, alfalfa, radish, sunflower, and broccoli. Most sprouts, except bean sprouts, come still growing. They will usually last for 5–7 days in your refrigerator. Sprouts are a great addition to salads and sandwiches. Bean sprouts are excellent stir-fried.

Squash

The many varieties of squash are perhaps the most versatile of all the vegetables. Summer squashes such as yellow and zucchini are thin-skinned and enjoyable raw or cooked. Avoid buying summer squash that appears tough or if the stem is very dry. Summer squash will store in the vegetable drawer of the refrigerator for about a week. To extend shelf life, wrap summer squash in a paper towel and place in a zip-lock bag. Winter squash, also known as hard squash, include acorn, butternut, pumpkin, and spaghetti squash. Hard squashes will keep for several weeks in your refrigerator. Hard squashes can be steamed, stuffed, or baked and require from 15 to 45 minutes of cooking. Steamed pumpkin with fresh grated nutmeg is a delicious fall treat. Fill acorn squash with cranberries and bake for 45–50 minutes for a beautiful addition to your Thanksgiving table.

Tomatoes

Tomatoes are easy and fun to grow during the summer and taste much better when grown at home. Tomatoes should not be kept in the refrigerator but, rather, on your counter. Most tomatoes require ripening on your kitchen counter for 2–3 days. Buy tomatoes in varying stages of ripeness and eat them as they ripen. Cherry or grape tomatoes usually last for a week when kept on your counter. Green

tomatoes are delicious sautéed or stir-fried with onions. Ripe tomatoes are great raw, stewed, sautéed, or baked. Cut tomatoes into
cubes and marinate with sliced onions, red wine, or balsamic vinegar and spices.

FRUIT (MINIMUM: 5; MAXIMUM: UNLIMITED)

*One fruit exchange yields 15 grams of carbohydrate, zero protein and
fat, and about 60 calories.*

Despite their higher carbohydrate content compared to vegetables,
fruits are unlimited in this plan. Because of their high water and fiber
content, one becomes full easily without overconsumption of calories.
It is also for these reasons that fruit juices and processed fruits are not
unlimited. They are in the starch category. Though not truly a starchy
food, processed fruits are easily consumed in a quantity that rapidly
provides large amounts of calories without the corresponding fullness.
Processed fruits and juices are high in calories and have a very high
glycemic index as discussed in Chapter 2.

Keep plenty of fresh fruit around. Most fruits will last in the fruit
drawer of your refrigerator for a week or so. Mangos, melons, and
pears may be left on the kitchen counter until they ripen (become soft-
er and develop a sweet smell) and then moved to the refrigerator.

The **Hormonal Health Diet** allows for unlimited fruits, with three
exceptions: bananas, grapes, and watermelon. These three fruits,
although very healthy, have a higher glycemic index and can be
overeaten. Bananas, grapes, and watermelon are not off limits. Just
remember, these fruits should be eaten in moderation. Try to have no
more that 5 servings *total* of these three fruits each day.

You must have a **minimum** of 5 fruit exchanges every day. Table
11.2 lists portion sizes that equal 1 fruit exchange.

Table 11.2
FRUIT EXCHANGES

Fruit	Quantity
Apple	1 small
Apricots	4 whole
Banana*	1 small
Blackberries	¾ cup
Blueberries	¾ cup
Cantaloupe	¼ of 6" melon (1 cup, cubed)
Cherries	12
Grapefruit	½
Grapes*	17
Honeydew melon	⅛ of 7" melon (1 cup, cubed)
Kiwi	1
Lemons	2
Limes	2
Mango	½
Nectarine	1
Orange	1 small
Peach	1 medium
Pear	1 small
Pineapple, fresh**	½ cup chopped
Plums	2
Raspberries	1 cup
Strawberries	1¼ cups
Tangerine	2
Watermelon*	4" x ½" or 1¼ cups cubed

* Quantities for bananas, grapes, and watermelon are limited to a maximum of 5 exchanges per day.
** See Starch Exchanges for canned pineapple.

MILK (MINIMUM: 0; MAXIMUM: 3–4)

One milk exchange provides 12 grams of carbohydrate, 8 grams of protein, and variable fat. (Maximum 3 exchanges for weight loss, 4 exchanges for weight maintenance.)

The choice of milk and yogurt will determine the amount of fat. However, this diet plan strongly urges skim and low- or non-fat products. An allergy to milk and lactose intolerance can eliminate this group from the diet. For those of you who fall into this category, there are other options. Soy milk is a great alternative to cow's milk, and there are a large variety of soy products on the market. The protein and carbohydrate content varies greatly, so it is wise to label shop for the product with the most protein and least carbohydrate and fat content. Eden Soy Original and Extra Original both provide 13 grams of carbohydrate, 10 grams of protein, and 5 and 3 grams of fat, respectively. Be aware that some varieties provide as much as 27 grams of carbohydrate, equivalent to almost two carbohydrate exchanges. Table 11.3 lists portion sizes that equal 1 milk exchanges.

By eliminating or restricting milk in the diet, you risk inadequate calcium intake. Most soy milks are fortified with calcium; however, this may not be enough. For more information on calcium, see Chapter 6.

Table 11.3
MILK EXCHANGES

Product	Quantity
Skim milk	1 cup
Skim milk (powdered)	⅓ cup
Yogurt (low-fat or fat-free)	Plain/light sweetened 1 cup
Soy milk (low-fat)	1 cup

STARCH (MINIMUM: 0; MAXIMUM: 4–6)

One starch exchange provides 15 grams of carbohydrate, 3 grams of protein, zero fat (unless prepared with fat), and 80 calories. (Maximum 4 exchanges for weight loss, 6 exchanges for weight maintenance.)

Starch is frequently considered the culprit in failed weight-loss attempts. It is not that starch is bad for you, but of all the macronutrients—starch, protein, and fat—it is the most overeaten. Additionally, starchy foods in meals and snacks are too often accompanied by fat or sugary condiments, such as butter and jellies.

When choosing foods from this group, strive to choose high-fiber, unprocessed varieties. This will add bulk to your diet and consequently provide early satiety. The best starches have a low glycemic index. For more information on good starches and the glycemic index see Chapter 2. Table 11.4 lists portion sizes that equal 1 starch exchange.

Processed Fruit Exchanges

One processed fruit exchange provides 15 to 19 grams of carbohydrate, zero grams of protein and fat, and 60 to 85 calories.

These include dried fruits and juices that are without added sugar. They are a concentrated source of carbohydrates and are limited on this diet owing to the fact that they are easily consumed in large quantities before you get full. For example, one-half glass of orange juice is more quickly consumed compared to a whole fresh orange. Yet both provide the same calories and carbohydrates. Although the nutritional value of processed fruit is slightly less than their fresh source, they remain rich in potassium, many vitamins, and health-protective phytochemicals. Table 11.5 lists portion sizes that equal 1 processed fruit exchange.

PROTEIN (MINIMUM: 6; MAXIMUM: 8–10)

One protein exchange provides 7 grams of protein, zero carbohydrate, and variable fat depending on the cut of meat as well as the choice of meat substitute chosen. (Maximum 8 exchanges for weight loss, 10 exchanges for weight maintenance.)

Table 11.4
STARCH EXCHANGES

Starch	Quantity
Bread: white, wheat French, rye, pumpernickel	1 slice
Bagel	⅓
Biscuit or roll (low-fat)	1 small
Bread crumbs	¼ cup
Breadsticks	1
Bun, hamburger or frankfurter	½
Cooked cereal	½ cup
Puffed cereal	½ cups
Bran cereal	½ cup
Unsweetened, ready-to-eat cereal	¾ cup
Corn	½ cup or 1 small ear
Graham crackers	3″ by 2½″ squares
Oyster crackers	½ cup
Saltine crackers	6
Soda crackers	6
Macaroni noodles (cooked)	½ cup
Matzo	1″ by 5″ square
English muffin	½
Fat-free muffin	1 small
Melba toast	4
Pasta	½ cup
Peas	½ cup
PIta bread	1 small
Popcorn(air popped)	3 cups
White potato	1 small or ½ cup mashed
Sweet potato	½ cup
Pretzels	½ cup
Rice	½ cup
Rice cakes	2
Tortilla, small	1

Table 11.5
PROCESSED FRUIT EXCHANGES

Juices	Quantity	Dried Fruits	Quantity
Apple	½ cup	Apricots	8 halves
Grape	⅓ cup	Apples	4 rings
Grapefruit	½ cup	Dates	3 small
Lemon	½ cup	Figs	3 small
Orange	½ cup	Mango slices	4 strips
Prune	⅓ cup	Peaches	2 halves
		Pears	3 halves
		Prunes	4 medium
		Raisins	2 Tbsp
Other			
Applesauce	½ cup		
Fruit cocktail (unsweetened)	¾ cup		
Pineapple, crushed (in own juice)	½ cup		
Pineapple rings	2		
Jam or jelly, low-sugar	2 tsp		
Syrup, sugar-free	2 Tbsp		

This diet plan recommends very lean and lean meats and meat substitutes. A very lean exchange will provide zero to 1 gram of fat and 35 calories, and a lean exchange will provide 3 grams of fat and 55 calories. Grill, bake, or broil meats in a manner to remove all possible fat. Table 11.6 lists portion sizes that equal 1 protein exchange.

Egg whites are unlimited. Yes, on this diet plan you may have as many egg whites as you want. Egg whites are pure protein, without any fat or carbohydrate. During any weight-loss program, adequate protein eliminates hunger and prevents muscle loss. I recommend an egg white omelet as a delicious way to get in your protein. But egg whites can also be used in recipes in many creative ways.

Table 11.6
PROTEIN EXCHANGES

Meat/Meat Substitute	Quantity (1 oz of the following unless indicated)
Beef	Lean, trimmed of fat Choose round or loin cuts Flank steak, roast (rib, chuck, rump), steak (T-bone, porterhouse, strip, filet), lean ground.
Pork	Fresh ham, Canadian bacon, tenderloin, center loin chop
Poultry	White meat, no skin
Fish	Cod, flounder, grouper, haddock, halibut, trout, tuna, salmon, snapper Canned tuna or salmon in water (¼ cup)
Shellfish	Clams, crab, lobster, scallops, shrimp, imitation shellfish
Game	Buffalo, ostrich, venison
Cheese (non-fat or low-fat)	Less than 3 grams fat per slice
Cottage cheese (low-fat or fat-free)	¼ cup
Egg whites*	Unlimited (2 are equivalent to 1 very lean protein exchange)
Egg substitute* (fat-free)	Unlimited (½ cup is equivalent to 1 very lean protein exchange)
Whole egg	(1 protein and 1 fat)
Lunch meat (fat-free)	1 oz
Soy: Tofu Soy burger	 3 oz (2 protein and ½ starch)
Cooked beans	½ cup (1 protein and 1 starch)

* Egg whites and egg substitutes are unlimited owing to their zero fat content. They contain only protein, which is important during caloric restriction and weight-loss phases.

FAT (MINIMUM: 0; MAXIMUM: 2–4)

One fat exchange provides 5 grams of fat, zero protein and carbohydrate. (Maximum 2 exchanges for weight loss, 4 exchanges for weight maintenance.)

All fats have the same number of calories. See Chapter 2 for more information on types of fat. It is important to realize that even a "good" fat is still fat, providing the same calories as a "bad" or saturated fat. Although unsaturated fats are recommended, they are limited as part of a healthy diet. Table 11.7 lists portion sizes that equal 1 fat exchange.

"FREE FOOD" EXCHANGES—UNLIMITED

The foods in this section do not fit into any of the above exchange categories, but may also be consumed in unlimited quantities on this diet:

Bouillon
Club soda or mineral water
Coffee
Diet soft drinks
Flavoring extracts
Garlic
Gelatin dessert, sugar-free
Herbs, fresh or dried
Mustard
Pepper rings, hot
Pickles
Salsa
Soy sauce
Spices
Sugar substitutes
Tea
Vinegar
Worcestershire sauce

Table 11.7
FAT EXCHANGES

Monounsaturated Fat	Quantity
Oil (canola, olive, peanut)	1/8 tsp
Olives: ripe (black)	8 large
green, stuffed	10 large
Nuts	
almonds, cashews	6
mixed	6
pecans	4 halves
Peanut butter	2 tsp
Sesame seeds	1 Tbsp

Polyunsaturated Fat	Quantity
Margarine: stick, tub or squeeze	1 tsp
Lower fat (30 to 50% veg oil)	1 Tbsp
Mayonnaise (reduced-fat)	2 Tbsp
Nuts, walnuts, English	4 halves
Oil (corn, safflower, soybean)	1 tsp
Salad dressing (reduced-fat)	2 Tbsp
Miracle Whip salad dressing (reduced fat)	1 Tbsp
Seeds: pumpkin, sunflower	1 Tbsp

Saturated Fat	Quantity
Bacon	1 slice
Butter	1 Tbsp
Cheese (regular)	½ ounce
Cream cheese	1 Tbsp
Margarine, fat-free	4 Tbsp
Margarine, reduced-fat	1 tsp
Mayonnaise, fat-free	1 Tbsp
Mayonnaise, reduced-fat	1 tsp
Mayonnaise, regular	1 tsp
Miracle Whip salad dressing (reduced fat)	1 Tbsp
Nuts, walnuts	4 halves
Oil (corn, safflower, soybean)	1 tsp
Salad dressing (reduced-fat)	2 Tbsp
Seeds: pumpkin, sunflower	1 Tbsp
Sour cream, fat-free	1 Tbsp

The Hormonal Health Diet—Breakdown by Exchanges

Here is the technical stuff. Remember, exact numbers aren't always important. These numbers are to be used as a guide to getting in the proper number exchanges. You can use this as a guide to plan your daily meals. The key is sticking to your minimums and maximums and getting in 3 meals and 3 snacks (see Table 11.8). In the pages that follow are easy to follow meal plans and eating suggestions to help you keep on the diet.

Table 11.8
EXCHANGES FOR 3 MEALS AND 3 SNACKS

Meals	Vegetables	Fruit	Milk	Starch	Protein	Fat
Breakfast	0	1	1	1	1	0
Mid-A.M.	0	1	0	1	1	0
Lunch	2	1	0	1	2	1
Mid-P.M.	1	0	0	0	0	0
Supper	2	1	0	1	4	1
Bedtime	0	1	1	0	0	0

Back to Basics

The **Basic Meal Plan** (see Table 11.9) is a simple version of the **Hormonal Health Diet**. It is designed to be

- Easy to plan for (preplanning is key in any diet—see below)
- Easy to prepare
- Easy to follow

The Basic Meal Plan is designed to help you achieve hormonal balance by emphasizing the eating guidelines presented in this book. The diet is on a 3-day rotation schedule. You should follow the days in order, starting again at day 1 after you finish day 3. I suggest you follow this diet for 10 to 14 days before moving on to a diet with more variety such as the 7-day meal plan.

Table 11.9
THE BASIC MEAL PLAN

	Day 1	Day 2	Day 3
Breakfast	Egg white omelet* 1 cup fat-free yogurt ½ cup juice (apple, orange, grapefruit) 1 fruit exchange	2 soy breakfast links (Choose varieties that have <5 grams carbohydrates per serving) I slice bread 1 cup skim milk 1 fruit exchange	1 cup cottage cheese, fat-free 1 fruit exchange
Mid-A.M. Snack	½ cup pretzels 1 fruit exchange	½ sandwich made with 2 oz fat-free lunch meat 1 fruit exchange	5 saltine crackers 1 fruit exchange
Lunch	½ sandwich made with 2 oz fat-free lunch meat 1 cup celery sticks 1 fruit exchange	Vegetable soup* (2 servings) 2 Tbsp Parmesan cheese	4 hard-boiled egg whites 1 cup spinach 1 tomato 1 cucumber Basic vinaigrette dressing* 1 fruit exchange
Mid-P.M. Snack	1 cup carrot sticks	¾ cup unsweetened breakfast cereal ½ cup skim milk 1 fruit exchange	1 cup sliced bell pepper
Supper	Green salad Basic vinaigrette dressing* 4–6 oz grilled lean meat or fish 2 cups cooked vegetables ½ cup brown rice 1 fruit exchange	Green salad Basic vinaigrette dressing* 4–6 oz grilled lean meat or fish 2 cups cooked vegetables 1 ear of corn 1 fruit exchange	Green salad Basic vinaigrette dressing* 4–6 oz grilled lean meat or fish 2 cups cooked vegetables 1 small potato 1 fruit exchange

Table 11.9 (continued)
THE BASIC MEAL PLAN

	Day 1	Day 2	Day 3
Bedtime Snack	1 cup fat-free yogurt 1 fruit exchange	1 cup fat-free yogurt 1 fruit exchange	1 cup fat-free yogurt 1 fruit exchange

Sandwich tips: Use lots of vegetables, sliced tomato, onion, lettuce, sprouts, and so on, to make the sandwich large and filling. Fat-free lunch meats include turkey, chicken, and ham. You may also substitute 2 oz grilled chicken, fish, or lean beef or canned tuna or salmon (in water). Use mustard and/or a very small amount of fat-free mayonnaise.

All fruit and vegetable exchanges listed are minimums. Additional fruits, vegetables, and egg whites can always be added if you are hungry.

* Recipe included

Make special effort to adhere to this diet as best you can. The quantities of fruits, vegetables, and egg whites on this diet are the *minimum* you should consume. You may always have more. If you are excessively hungry, eat only the "free foods" that you are allowed to have in unlimited quantities. These include "free food" exchanges, fresh fruits, vegetables, and egg whites. (Quantities for bananas, grapes, and watermelon are limited to a maximum of 5 exchanges per day.)

Many people, including myself, can follow this meal plan on a daily basis without getting bored of the simple meals. You do not have to follow such a simple eating style, however. After you become familiar with the basics of the diet, you can learn to become more creative with your meals, removing the monotony of this simplified approach.

Part of the fun of this eating style is that the choices are endless. The key is learning new ways to combine proteins, starches, fruits, and vegetables into delicious recipes that allow you to stay on the diet and not get bored. In the pages that follow the **Basic Meal Plan** is a 7-day version of the **Hormonal Health Diet**. The **7-Day Meal Plan** is designed to be a transition from the **Basic Meal Plan**. As you get used to this style of eating, you should be able to design your own diet, keeping the appropriate amount of protein, starches, and fats. And don't forget about fruits and vegetables—minimums always apply.

The key to long-term success is variety. Never let yourself get bored with the diet. The ingredients that you have to work with can be combined into an unlimited number of recipes. There are many outstanding cookbooks and Web sites devoted to healthy cooking. I also recommend the magazine *Cooking Light* as an ongoing resource. Experiment with at least two new recipes every week. Just keep cooking!

GET READY FOR SUCCESS!

The most basic element required for you to be successful in following this diet is something I've already talked about: preplanning. After all, you're going to have a lot of difficulty following the diet if you don't have the proper ingredients in your kitchen.

Think about it. You get home from work. It's late; you haven't exercised and you're tired and hungry. You look in the refrigerator and there is nothing to cook, so you order take-out Chinese, or a pizza, and pig out. There goes the day. Your diet may not be shot, but you've just taken a step backward.

On the other hand, if you have healthy food available, you will be much more likely to eat healthy. Make grocery-shopping part of your weekly diet routine. Plan on shopping on the same day every week, and plan on buying enough groceries to get you through the entire week. This may take some practice at first, but it can be done. The key is to buy enough vegetables and fruits, but not so much that you can't eat them all in a week's time. Use the shopping list on pages 355-356 as a guide for your shopping.

THE 7-DAY MEAL PLAN FOR HORMONAL BALANCE

The 7-Day Meal Plan is a more creative version of the Basic Meal Plan. This is a guideline to healthy eating. The portions of vegetables and fruits in this meal plan are the minimum amount you should eat. If you are hungry, you may include more free-food exchanges, vegetables, fruits, or egg whites. Remember, these items are unlimited. After you become accustomed to this style, you can start creating your own meals. Just use the exchanges in Table 11.9 as your guide. Be creative! Make healthy cooking and eating your passion. Following the 7-Day Meal Plan are recipes for selected meals.

DAY 1
Breakfast
1 slice whole-grain bread
1 oz low-fat cheese
1 cup yogurt plain/light sweetened low-fat or non-fat
1 cup mixed berries

Midmorning Snack
1 medium peach
¼ cup cottage cheese
3 (2½ inch square) Graham crackers

Lunch
Chicken with Broccoli*
½ cup whole-wheat pasta
2 small plums

Midafternoon Snack
Cut up carrots and celery sticks

Supper
Baked Salmon in Parchment with Lime and Cilantro*
1 small baked potato with skin
3 Tbsp low-fat sour cream
Zucchini with onions*
1 small pear

Bedtime Snack
¾ cup fresh pineapple
1 cup skim milk

*Recipe included.

DAY 2

½ cup bran cereal
1 cup skim milk
1 small banana
Egg White Omelet*

Midmorning Snack
One-Half Sandwich
    1 slice whole-grain bread
    1 oz lunch meat
    Lettuce and tomato
    1 Tbsp fat-free mayonnaise
1 small pear

Lunch
Large green salad
2 oz shrimp
1 cup croutons
Herb Vinaigrette*
1 medium peach

Midafternoon Snack
Cut up broccoli and cauliflower

Supper
Honey-Orange Chicken*
½ cup brown rice
Large green salad
Creamy Herb Dressing*
17 grapes

Bedtime Snack
1 cup cantaloupe
1 cup yogurt plain/light sweetened low-fat or non-fat

*Recipe included.

DAY 3

Breakfast
Cheese Grits
    ½ cup cooked grits
    1 oz low-fat cheese
½ grapefruit
1 cup skim milk

Midmorning Snack
One-Half Sandwich
    1 slice whole-grain bread
    ½ cup tuna
    Lettuce and tomato
    1 Tbsp fat-free mayonnaise
2 plums

Lunch
Middle Eastern Salad*
Add:
    ½ cup chickpeas
    1 oz crumbled low-fat feta cheese

Midafternoon Snack
Cut up green and red peppers

Supper
4 oz chicken breast, grilled
½ cup whole-wheat rice
Roasted Red Pepper Sauce*
2 servings Red Cabbage and Apples*

Bedtime Snack
1 small pear
1 cup yogurt plain/light sweetened low-fat or non-fat

*Recipe included.

DAY 4

Breakfast
Egg White Omelet*
½ cup orange juice
½ English muffin
1 tsp reduced-fat margarine
1 cup skim milk

Midmorning Snack
1 small pear
¼ cup low-fat cottage cheese
¾ oz pretzels

Lunch
Wild Rice and Chicken Salad with Broccoli Coleslaw*
¾ cup fresh pineapple

Midafternoon Snack
Cut up carrots and zucchini

Supper
4 oz lean ground beef or tofu
Vegetarian Pasta Sauce*
¾ cup whole-wheat pasta
Large green salad
Herb Vinaigrette*
1 small orange

Bedtime Snack
4 fresh apricots
1 cup yogurt plain/light sweetened low-fat or non-fat

*Recipe included.

DAY 5

Breakfast
1 slice whole-grain toast
1 oz Canadian bacon
½ cup apple juice
1 cup yogurt plain/light sweetened low-fat or non-fat

Midmorning Snack
Pita Pocket
>   1 small pita bread pocket
>   ½ cup vegetables
>   1 oz low-fat feta cheese
1 medium peach

Lunch
One-Half Sandwich
>   1 slice whole-grain bread
>   1 oz low-fat cheese
>   1 oz turkey
>   Lettuce and tomato
>   1 tbsp reduced-fat mayonnaise
17 grapes

Midafternoon Snack
Cucumber Rounds with Sour Cream and Chutney*

Supper
Charbroiled Tuna with Oregano Mango Sauce*
½ cup brown rice
Large green salad
Herb Vinaigrette*
1¼ cups strawberries

Bedtime
1 medium pear
1 cup skim milk

*Recipe included.

DAY 6

Breakfast
¾ cup unsweetened cereal
1 cup blueberries
1 cup skim milk
Egg White Omelet*

Midmorning Snack
1 medium pear
¼ cup cottage cheese
6 saltine crackers

Lunch
Green Beans with Dill*
½ cup steamed yellow squash
2 oz grilled chicken
Roasted Red Pepper Sauce*
½ cup whole-wheat pasta
2 small plums

Midafternoon Snack
Cut up broccoli and radishes

Supper
4 oz grilled chicken
½ cup brown rice
Sautéed Sugar Snap Peas*
½ cup sautéed green and red peppers
1 tsp olive oil
1 cup honeydew melon

Bedtime Snack
1 medium peach
1 cup yogurt plain/light sweetened low-fat or non-fat

*Recipe included.

DAY 7

Breakfast
½ cup oatmeal
1 small apple
2 hard-boiled egg whites
1 cup skim milk

Midmorning Snack
1 oz low-fat cheese
6 saltine crackers
1 kiwi

Lunch
½ cup whole-wheat pasta
2 oz grilled chicken
Sautéed mushrooms and broccoli
1 tsp olive oil
2 small tangerines

Midafternoon
Cut up celery and carrots

Supper
4 oz lean beef, grilled
Roasted Green Beans with Mushrooms and Onions*
½ cup garlic mashed potatoes
1 cup raspberries

Bedtime Snack
½ mango
1 cup yogurt plain/light sweetened low-fat or non-fat

*Recipe included.

RECIPES FOR THE HORMONAL HEALTH DIET

EGG WHITE OMELET

Makes 1 Serving

3	Egg whites
1	Egg yolk (optional)
1	slice Fat-free cheese (optional)
1 cup	Vegetables*
	Fat-free cooking spray
¼ teaspoon	Salt (optional)
¼ teaspoon	Pepper

*Onion, mushrooms, broccoli, peppers, asparagus, spinach, and/or squash

This recipe works best when an **8–10" nonstick omelet pan** is used.

1. Chop about 1 cup raw vegetables.
2. Cook vegetables in pan with fat-free cooking spray for 3–4 minutes until soft.
3. Remove vegetables from pan, place in small dish.
4. Clean vegetable residue from pan and place back on medium-high heat.
5. Combine egg whites, egg yolk, salt and pepper in a small bowl and whisk thoroughly.
6. After pan is hot (about 30–45 seconds), spray non-fat cooking spray, then add egg white mixture.
7. Place most (but not all) of the cooked vegetables over ½ of the egg white mixture as it is cooking.
8. Place 1 slice of fat-free cheese over the vegetables (optional).
9. Cover for 2–3 minutes. When egg mixture is completely solidified, gently fold the omelet together, keeping the half with vegetables on the bottom.
10. Gently slide the omelet onto a plate.
11. Garnish with remaining vegetables.

Nutritional Analysis
Per Serving: 273 Calories. 5.1g Fat (17.3% calories from fat), 49.7g Protein, 5.7g Carbohydrates. Exchanges: 4 Protein; 1 Fat.

BASIC VINAIGRETTE DRESSING

Makes 8 Servings

1½ cups	Vinegar (balsamic, red wine, rice)
⅛ cup	Olive oil
1 clove	Garlic, crushed
3 tablespoons	Sugar
½ teaspoon	Pepper
¼ teaspoon	Salt (optional)
2 tablespoons	Spices, fresh chopped*

* Chives, basil, oregano, cilantro, and/or tarragon

1. Combine all ingredients in a small jar or salad dressing container.
2. Shake well.
3. Serve over salad.

May be stored, without refrigeration, for 7–10 days.

Nutritional Analysis
Per Serving: 50 Calories. 3.4g Fat (59.7% calories from fat), 0.1g Protein, 5.1g Carbohydrates. Exchanges: ½ Fat.

VEGETABLE SOUP

Makes 10 Servings

1 cup	Chopped onions or leeks
2 cloves	Garlic, crushed
10–12 oz can	Diced or crushed tomatoes
2 cups	Yellow squash or zucchini, cut into small pieces
1 cup	Chopped celery
1 cup	Chopped carrots
8–10 oz can	Beans (pinto, navy, black, kidney)
1 box	Frozen cut corn
8 cups	Low-fat chicken broth or vegetable broth
1 Bay leaf	1 teaspoon Pepper
Optional	Salt

1. Heat a large pot with cooking spray and add onions or leaks and garlic. Cook for 4–5 minutes.
2. Add tomatoes, squash, carrots, celery, and corn; cook for 10 minutes, stirring occasionally.
3. Add beans, bay leaf, pepper, and broth.
4. Bring to a boil and simmer for 1½ hours.
5. Add salt if necessary.

Nutritional Analysis
Per Serving: 223 Calories. 3.6g Fat (13.9% calories from fat), 10.5g Protein, 39.8g Carbohydrates. Exchanges: 1 Starch; ½ Protein; 2½ Vegetable; ½ Fat.

BAKED SALMON IN PARCHMENT WITH LIME AND CILANTRO

Makes 4 Servings

1 teaspoon	Safflower oil, to grease parchment
1½ pounds	Salmon Filets, cut into 4 pieces
2 tablespoons	White wine
1 tablespoon	Lime juice
1 teaspoon	Lime zest
2 tablespoons	Fresh cilantro
1 teaspoon	Dark sesame oil
2 teaspoons	Garlic clove, minced

1. Preheat oven to 350° F. Lightly oil 4 sheets of parchment paper.
2. Place 1 salmon filet on the center of each sheet.
3. In a small bowl, combine garlic, white wine, lime juice, lime zest, cilantro, and sesame oil. Spoon equal amount over each salmon filet.
4. Roll edges of the parchment paper together to form a packet around the salmon. Bake for 12 minutes.
5. To serve, unroll parchment packets and gently slide the salmon on to plates. Spoon poaching liquid over the salmon and serve immediately.

NOTES: You can marinate the fish in the poaching liquid overnight before cooking. Fillets of red snapper, cod, flounder, or orange roughy also can be used with this recipe.

Nutritional Analysis
Per Serving: 105 Calories. 4.5g Fat (41.5% calories from fat), 12.9g Protein, 1.4g Carbohydrates. Exchanges: 2 Protein, ½ Fat.

CHICKEN WITH BROCCOLI

Makes 4 Servings

2	Whole chicken breasts, skinned and boned
2	Egg yolks
1½ cups	Chicken broth
1 tablespoon	Butter
1 clove	Garlic, minced (optional)
8 stalks	Broccoli
1 teaspoon	Sea salt
	Fresh ground black pepper
1 tablespoon	Lemon juice (optional)
2	Lemons, quartered
8 ounces	Chicken broth

1. Slice chicken breasts into 4 lengthwise strips.
2. Beat egg yolks in a non metal bowl with chicken broth. Stir together. Coat chicken with this egg mixture.
3. Heat butter and garlic (optional) to foaming in a sauté pan or skillet. Add chicken strips and cook over medium heat until golden brown on all sides. This will take about 4 minutes.
4. With a chef's knife, cut the tops off the broccoli (2-inch flowerettes). Chop coarsely.
5. Remove chicken from pan to a warm dish; put broccoli into pan over medium heat, stir in remaining chicken broth and lemon juice (optional). Catch all the cooked bits in the pan with your spoon. Cook broccoli for about 5 minutes. Season to taste.
6. Place chicken and broccoli together on plates. Pour sauce from pan over broccoli and garnish with quartered lemons.

Nutritional Analysis
Per Serving: 172 Calories. 6.8g Fat (31.4% calories from fat), 17.8g Protein, 15.6g Carbohydrates. Exchanges: 1½ Protein; 2 Vegetable; ½ Fruit; 1 Fat.

CREAMY HERB DRESSING

Makes 6 Servings

½ cup	Low-calorie mayonnaise
¼ cup	Plain nonfat yogurt
¼ cup	Parsley, minced
1 teaspoon	Chives, minced
2 tablespoons	Apple cider vinegar
1 dash	Sea salt
1 dash	Black pepper
½ tablespoon	Fresh basil, minced
1 clove	Garlic, minced

Blend all the ingredients until smooth. Makes about 1¼ cups.

NOTES: Snappy and low in calories. This dressing is also good on coleslaw or broccoli slaw.

Nutritional Analysis
Per Serving: 63 Calories. 5.5g Fat (75.4% calories from fat), 0.8g Protein, 3.2g Carbohydrates. Exchanges: 1 Fat.

HERB VINAIGRETTE

Makes 4 Servings

3 tablespoons	Balsamic vinegar
1 tablespoon	Rice vinegar
2 tablespoons	Lemon juice
3 tablespoons	Olive oil
2 tablespoons	Water
1 teaspoon	Dijon mustard
1 tablespoon	Cilantro, minced
1 tablespoon	Fresh basil, minced
1 tablespoon	Fresh oregano, minced
1	Garlic clove, minced
	Sea salt
	Fresh ground pepper

1. Pour vinegar, lemon juice, and water into a small bowl.
2. Stir in mustard, herbs, and seasonings. Adjust seasonings to taste.
3. Pour in olive oil and mix.
4. Refrigerate at least 1 day for best results.
5. Remove from refrigerator 1 hour before using.

Nutritional Analysis
Per Serving: 37 Calories. 3.5g Fat (75.8% calories from fat), .3g Protein, 2.2g Carbohydrates. Exchanges: ½ Fat.

HONEY-ORANGE CHICKEN

Makes 4 Servings

4	Chicken breasts, halves, boneless and skinless
1 tablespoon	Cornstarch
¼ teaspoon	Salt
¼ teaspoon	Pepper
1½ teaspoons	Butter
¼ cup	Chicken broth
1 teaspoon	Frozen orange juice concentrate
½ teaspoon	Dijon mustard
¼ teaspoon	Honey
1 tablespoon	resh parsley, minced
4	Orange slices

1. In a zip-lock bag or small paper bag, combine the cornstarch, salt, and pepper. Shake to mix. Add the chicken. Shake to coat evenly.
2. Remove the chicken from the bag. Save the excess cornstarch mixture.
3. In a large skillet, melt 1 tablespoon butter over medium heat. Add chicken breasts and brown on one side (about 5 minutes). If needed, add the remaining ½ tablespoon of butter.
4. Brown the second side. Transfer to a warm plate and set aside.
5. Dissolve the remaining cornstarch in the chicken. Whisk in orange juice concentrate, mustard, and honey. Pour in a large skillet. Bring to a boil over a medium stirring often
6. Add the chicken. Reduce the heat to low and cover the skillet. Cook until the chicken is tender.
7. Divide the chicken and sauce among 4 plates.
8. Divide chicken among the 4 dinner plates. Sprinkle with parsley and garnish with orange slices.

Nutritional Analysis
Per Serving: 205 Calories. 3.4g Fat (15.5% calories from fat), 35g Protein, 8.1g Carbohydrates. Exchanges: 4½ Protein; ½ Fruit; ½ Starch; ½ Fat.

CUCUMBER ROUNDS WITH SOUR CREAM AND CHUTNEY

Makes 4 Servings

2	Cucumbers
2 teaspoons	Light sour cream
1 teaspoon	Chutney
2 tablespoons	Lemon juice
	Sea salt

1. Slice cucumbers crosswise about ¼ inch thick.
2. Sprinkle with lemon juice. Lightly salt.
3. Top each slice with sour cream and purchased chutney.

NOTES: This is a simple recipe that will help lessen the burden of coming up with that perfect little something before dinner. Place on a bed of greens to serve as a salad

Nutritional Analysis
Per Serving: 44 Calories. 0.4g Fat (7% calories from fat), 2.1g Protein, 9.8g Carbohydrates. Exchanges: 2 Vegetable.

GREEN BEANS WITH DILL

Makes 16 Servings

2 pounds	Whole green beans
1 teaspoon	Cayenne pepper powder
4 cloves	Garlic
¼ teaspoon	Salt
4 sprigs	Fresh dill
2½ cups	Water
2 cups	Cider vinegar

1. Trim ends on the green beans.
2. Pack beans lengthwise into hot jars, leaving ¼ inch head space.
3. To each pint, add ¼ teaspoon Cayenne powder, 1 clove of garlic, and 1 sprig of dill.
4. Combine remaining ingredients and bring to boil. Pour, boiling hot, over beans, leaving ¼ inch head space.
5. Process 10 minutes in boiling-water bath. Let stand 2 weeks to allow flavor to develop.

Yields 4 pints.

NOTES: Makes a terrific appetizer, or garnish for Bloody Mary drinks. Also serve these as a vegetable side dish.

Nutritional Analysis
Per Serving: 23 Calories. 0.1g Fat (2.7% calories from fat), 1.1g Protein, 6.1g Carbohydrates. Exchanges: 1 Vegetable.

Middle Eastern Salad

Makes 4 Servings

Salad

2	Navel or Valencia oranges
1	Onion, sliced ¼" thick
1	Green bell pepper
16	Mediterranean black olives

Lemon-Garlic Dressing

1 clove	Garlic
1 teaspoon	Paprika
1 teaspoon	Hot pepper sauce
1 tablespoon	Lemon juice
3 tablespoons	Olive oil
¼ teaspoon	Ground cumin
¼ teaspoon	Salt

1. Grate zest from half an orange. Peel the oranges and cut them into approximately ¼-inch-thick slices.
2. Cut the onion into thin slices. Seed and cut the bell pepper into thin slices.
3. Pit the olives.
4. Combine the oranges, onion, bell pepper slices, and olives in a bowl and refrigerate until ½ hour before serving.

Lemon-Garlic Dressing Preparation

Lightly crush the garlic. In a bowl, whisk together crushed garlic, paprika, hot pepper sauce, salt, cumin, and lemon juice. Gradually add olive oil, whisking constantly. Recipe can be prepared to this point several hours ahead.

NOTES: Pour dressing over orange and vegetable mixture and stir gently. Let stand at room temperature for 30 minutes. Remove garlic.

TO SERVE:
Serve salad on lettuce and garnish with grated orange zest.

Nutritional Analysis (Salad)

Per Serving: 71 Calories. 2g Fat (23.3% calories from fat), 1.5g Protein, 13.6g Carbohydrates. Exchanges: 1 Vegetable; ½ Fruit; ½ Fat.

Nutritional Analysis (Dressing)

Per Serving: 93 Calories. 10.2g Fat (96.1% calories from fat), 0.1g Protein, 0.8g Carbohydrates. Exchanges: 2 Fat.

RED CABBAGE AND APPLES

Makes 4 Servings

½ tablespoon	Butter
2 cups	Chopped red cabbage
⅛ cup	Red wine
2	Unpeeled yellow apples

1. Melt butter over low heat in a sauté pan or skillet; slice apples into pan and add cabbage, stirring.
2. Cook 5 minutes over medium heat. Stir in wine.
3. Cover pan and cook 6–7 minutes.

Nutritional Analysis
Per Serving: 68 Calories. 1.8g Fat (22.8% calories from fat), 0.7g Protein, 12.8g Carbohydrates. Exchanges: ½ Vegetable; ½ Fruit; ½ Fat.

ROASTED GREEN BEANS WITH MUSHROOMS AND ONIONS

Makes 4 Servings

½ pound	Green beans
1 medium	White onion, sliced
½ pound	Shitake mushrooms, sliced
4 cloves	Garlic, sliced
½ tablespoon	Olive oil
¼ cup	Balsamic vinegar
	Salt
	Pepper

1. Preheat oven to 350°F.
2. Wash and dry green beans. Cut off tips.
3. Evenly distribute green beans and Shitake mushrooms in oblong roasting dish.
4. Top green beans with sliced onion and sliced garlic cloves. Season with salt and pepper.
5. Drizzle olive oil over the vegetables.
6. Bake for 30 minutes. Remove from oven when done.
7. Sprinkle with balsamic vinegar.

Nutritional Analysis
Per Serving: 110 Calories. 1.2g Fat (8.6% calories from fat), 3.5g Protein, 26.0g Carbohydrates. Exchanges: 4 Vegetable.

ROASTED RED PEPPER SAUCE

Makes 6 Servings

2 medium	Red bell peppers
1 tablespoon	Olive oil
1 medium	Onion, diced
1 tablespoon	White balsamic vinegar
2 tablespoons	Dry white wine
1 tablespoon	Fresh oregano, minced
1 cup	Chicken stock or canned chicken broth
1 clove	Garlic, minced
1 teaspoon	Salt
½ teaspoon	White pepper

1. Roast bell peppers over a gas flame, under the broiler, or on the grill, until skins blacken and blister. Cool, peel, seed, and chop bell peppers coarse; set aside.
2. Heat oil in a medium skillet. Add onions and bell peppers; sauté until onions soften, about 3 minutes. Add vinegar, simmer until vinegar evaporates, about 1 minutes. Add wine; simmer until liquid reduces to 1 tablespoon, about 2 minutes. Add stock; simmer until liquid reduces to ½ cup, about 10 minutes.
3. Cool slightly, then transfer to a food processor; add oregano, 1 teaspoon salt, and ½ teaspoon pepper; purée until smooth. Set sauce aside. (Can be cooled, covered, and refrigerated up to 3 days.)

TO SERVE: Warm over low heat. Spoon a portion of sauce onto each warm dinner plate. Arrange a portion of meat or roasted veal in each pool of sauce and serve immediately.

Nutritional Analysis
Per Serving: 48 Calories. 2.5g Fat (49.1% calories from fat), 0.8g Protein, 5.0g Carbohydrates. Exchanges: ½ Vegetable; ½ Fat.

Sautéed Sugar Snap Peas

Makes 4 Servings

2 teaspoons	Butter
2	Scallions, sliced
1 pound	Sugar snap peas
1 pinch	Sugar
	Salt, to taste
	Freshly ground pepper, to taste

1. In a large skillet over medium heat, melt butter; add sugar snap peas and scallions. Sauté, stirring frequently until tender, about 3 to 4 minutes.
2. Season to taste with sugar, salt, and pepper.

NOTES: Sugar snap peas remain succulent and colorful with this quick preparation.

Nutritional Analysis
Per Serving: 68 Calories. 2.1g Fat (27.4% calories from fat), 3.4g Protein, 9.4g Carbohydrates. Exchanges: 1½ Vegetable; ½ Fat.

VEGETARIAN PASTA SAUCE

Makes 8 Servings

1 tablespoon	Olive oil
1 medium	Onion, diced
1 cup	Mushrooms, sliced
¼ cup	Green bell pepper, diced
1 cup	Carrots, diced
½ cup	Celery, diced
¼ cup	Red wine
¾ cup	Tomato paste
3 cups	Tomatoes, chopped (fresh or canned)
3 cloves	Garlic, minced
2 tablespoons	Fresh basil (1 tablespoon dried)
1 tablespoon	Fresh oregano (½ tablespoon dried)
1 tablespoon	Fresh thyme (½ tablespoon dried)
1 teaspoon	Brown sugar
	Black pepper, to taste
	Salt, to taste

1. Melt butter in oil and swirl together.
2. Sauté onion until clear; add carrots, celery, and mushrooms. Sauté for about 5 more minutes, stirring frequently.
3. Add green bell pepper and the rest of the ingredients. Simmer for 30 minutes.
4. If sauce is too thick, add water. Cook 15 minutes more and salt and pepper to taste.

Yield: 4 cups

NOTES: Carrots, mushrooms and celery make this tomato sauce as hearty as a meat sauce. Best if prepared 1 day in advance.

Serve over pasta. Can also spoon sauce over boneless chicken breast and bake.

Nutritional Analysis
Per Serving: 95 Calories. 4.1g Fat (36.3% calories from fat), 2.4g Protein, 13.6g Carbohydrates. Exchanges: 2 Vegetable, ½ Fat.

WILD RICE AND CHICKEN SALAD WITH BROCCOLI COLESLAW

Makes 4 Servings

Chicken Salad

½ cup	Wild rice
½ pound	Chicken breast, no skin, boneless
1	Scallion, sliced
1 cup	Broccoli slaw
¾ cup	Granny smith apples, diced

Dressing

1 teaspoon	Olive oil
1½ tablespoon	Cider vinegar
1 clove	Garlic, minced
1 teaspoon	Dijon mustard
	Salt and pepper, to taste

Broccoli Slaw

¼ cup	Sour cream, light
¼ cup	2% buttermilk
2 tablespoons	Cider vinegar
1 cup	Broccoli slaw
1 large	Granny Smith apple, grated
½ teaspoon	Salt
¼ teaspoon	White pepper
1 tablespoon	Pine nuts, toasted and chopped

1. Combine broth and wild rice in a small sauce pan. Bring to a boil. Cover and simmer over medium-low heat until rice is tender and liquid is absorbed—about 50 minutes. Transfer to medium-size glass bowl. Cover and refrigerate until well chilled.
2. Add diced cooked chicken, broccoli coleslaw, apple, green onion, and garlic to the wild rice.
3. Whisk dressing ingredients together. Pour dressing over the wild rice mixture and toss well.
4. Season to taste with salt and pepper. Toss until coated. Sprinkle with pine nuts.

NOTES: Broccoli slaw mix, which consists of shredded broccoli stems, carrots, and red cabbage, is available packaged in many supermarkets. If you can't find it, you can make your own.

Nutritional Analysis

Per Serving: 204 Calories. 6.1g Fat (25.8% calories from fat), 15.4g Protein, 23.9g Carbohydrates. Exchanges: 1 Starch; ½ Fruit; 1 Fat, 1½ Protein, ½ Vegetable.

CHARBROILED TUNA WITH OREGANO MANGO SAUCE

Makes 4 Servings

1½ pounds	Tuna steaks
2 cloves	Garlic, minced
1	Lime, juiced
1 cup	2% milk
¼ cup	Sherry
1 tablespoon	Fresh oregano, minced
1	Mango, peeled

1. Preheat broiler.
2. Season tuna with a little salt and fresh crushed garlic. Sprinkle with lime juice. Broil for about 2 minutes on each side.
3. Blend mango into a puree. In a saucepan, reduce milk to about half. Add mango, sherry, lemon juice, and oregano. Boil for 2 minutes. Store in plastic container.
4. Pour mango sauce over tuna. Broil 3 minutes. Serve immediately.

Nutritional Analysis
Per Serving: 320 Calories. 10g Fat (29.3% calories from fat), 42.7g Protein, 11.5g Carbohydrates. Exchanges: 5½ Protein; ½ Fruit; ½ Fat.

Shopping List

VEGETABLES

Minimum of 35 servings

__ Artichokes
__ Asparagus
__ Beans
__ Beets
__ Broccoli
__ Brussels sprouts
__ Cabbage
__ Cauliflower
__ Celery
__ Cucumbers
__ Eggplant
__ Greens
__ Leeks
__ Lettuce
__ Mushrooms
__ Okra
__ Onions
__ Pea pods
__ Peppers
__ Pumpkin

__ Radishes
__ Spinach
__ Sprouts
__ Squash
__ Tomatoes
__ Turnips
__ Zucchini

FRUITS

Minimum of 35 servings

__ Apples
__ Apricots
__ Bananas
__ Blackberries
__ Blueberries
__ Cantaloupe
__ Cherries
__ Grapefruit
__ Grapes
__ Honeydew melon
__ Kiwi

FRUITS (CONTINUED)
__ Lemons
__ Limes
__ Mangos
__ Nectarines
__ Oranges
__ Peaches
__ Pears
__ Pineapple
__ Plums
__ Raspberries
__ Strawberries
__ Tangerines
__ Watermelon

DAIRY

__ Cheese, fat-free
__ Cheese, Parmesan
__ Cottage cheese
__ Egg substitute
__ Eggs
__ Skim milk
__ Soy milk, low-fat
__ Yogurt, fat-free

STARCHES

__ Breakfast cereal
__ Pasta
__ Potatoes
__ Pretzels
__ Rice, brown
__ Saltine crackers
__ Whole-wheat bread

JUICE

__ Apple
__ Grapefruit
__ Orange

PROTEIN

__ Beef
__ Chicken
__ Fish
__ Pork
__ Soy burger
__ Soy links

LUNCH MEAT

__ Chicken
__ Ham
__ Turkey breast
__ Turkey, smoked

CANNED FISH

__ Salmon, in water
__ Tuna, in water

OTHER

__ Gelatin, sugar-free
__ Mustard
__ Olive oil
__ Pickles
__ Salsa
__ Spices
__ Vinegar

HORMONE DISORDERS:
A GUIDE TO SYMPTOMS

THIS CHART IS DESIGNED to help you determine if your symptoms are associated with a particular hormone problem. A single symptom can be nonspecific and may be associated with a variety of possible problems.

DM   =   Type 2 diabetes (Chapter 3)
IR   =   Insulin resistance (Chapter 3)
RH   =   Reactive hypoglycemia (Chapter 2)
IN   =   Insulinoma (Chapter 2)
MH   =   Male hypogonadism (Chapter 4)
FLAS   =   Female low-androgen syndrome (Chapter 5)
PCOS =   Polycystic ovary syndrome (Chapter 5)
MP   =   Menopausal or perimenopausal (Chapter 6)
HT   =   Hypothyroidism (Chapter 7)
CS   =   Cushing's syndrome (Chapter 8)
PC   =   Pseudo-Cushing's (Chapter 8)
GHD   =   Growth hormone deficiency (Chapter 9)
VIR   =   Virilism (Chapter 5)

	DM	IR	RH	IN	MH	FLAS	PCOS	VIR	MP	HT	CS	PC	GHD
Acanthosis nigricans	X	X					X	X			X	X	
Aches and pains									X	X		X	X
Acne	X	X					X	X	X		X	X	
Aggressiveness								X		X	X		
Allergies/Hives										X			
Anemia					X	X				X			X
Anxiety			X	X	X	X	X		X	X	X	X	X
Bloating							X		X	X	X	X	
Blurred vision	X			X									
Body odor, excessive								X					
Bruising											X	X	
Buffalo hump											X	X	
Carbohydrate cravings	X	X	X				X				X	X	
Carpal tunnel syndrome	X									X			
Cheeks red											X		
Cheeks round	X	X									X	X	
Circulation problems	X	X							X				
Concentration problems	X	X	X	X					X		X		X
Confusion				X									
Constipation										X			
Decreased endurance					X	X			X	X	X	X	X
Depression					X	X	X	X	X	X	X	X	X
Deterioration in work performance				X	X	X			X	X	X	X	X
Difficulty concentrating				X	X	X			X	X	X	X	X
Difficulty relating to others					X	X			X	X	X	X	X

	DM	IR	RH	IN	MH	FLAS	PCOS	VIR	MP	HT	CS	PC	GHD
Dry skin					X	X			X	X			X
Edema										X	X	X	
Eyebrows thinner										X			
Face, round (moon face)	X	X								X	X	X	
Facial puffiness										X	X	X	
Family history of diabetes	X	X					X						
Family history of heart disease		X					X						
Family history of high blood pressure		X					X						
Family history of thyroid problems										X			
Fat over the collarbones											X	X	
Fatigue	X	X	X	X	X	X	X	X	X	X	X	X	X
Feeling cold										X			
Fingernails brittle						X				X			
Fluid retention						X				X	X	X	
Fractures					X	X			X		X		X
Goiter										X			
Hair falling out									X	X	X	X	
Hair thin					X	X			X				
Headaches			X	X	X			X			X	X	X
Heart disease	X	X					X		X		X	X	X
Heart palpitations			X	X							X		
Heartburn											X		
High blood pressure	X	X					X		X	X	X	X	
High cholesterol	X	X					X	X	X	X	X	X	
High-fat food preference	X	X					X				X	X	

	DM	IR	RH	IN	MH	FLAS	PCOS	VIR	MP	HT	CS	PC	GHD
High-carb food preference	X	X	X				X					X	
High triglycerides	X	X					X				X	X	
Hot flashes					X	X					X		
Hunger, excessive	X	X	X	X			X				X	X	
Inability to lose weight	X	X	X	X	X	X	X	X	X	X	X	X	X
Increased body fat	X	X		X	X	X	X		X	X	X	X	X
Increased fat in the belly	X	X			X	X	X		X		X	X	X
Infections, frequent	X										X		
Insomnia									X		X		
Irritability				X					X	X			X
Joint aches									X	X			X
Kidney stones											X		
Libido, decreased					X	X		X	X		X		X
Loss of consciousness				X									
Loss of zest for life					X	X			X	X	X	X	X
Memory loss				X					X	X	X	X	X
Mood swings					X	X	X	X	X	X	X	X	
Muscle wasting					X	X					X		X
Muscle weakness					X	X				X	X		X
Nausea			X										
Numbness or tingling	X			X						X	X		
Osteoporosis or osteopenia					X	X							X
Peripheral vascular disease	X	X							X				
Personality changes				X				X	X		X		
Poor general health	X	X			X	X	X	X	X	X	X	X	X

	DM	IR	RH	IN	MH	FLAS	PCOS	VIR	MP	HT	CS	PC	GHD
Sedentary lifestyle	X	X										X	
Seizure				X									
Sense of well-being, decreased					X	X			X				X
Skin tags	X	X			X	X					X	X	
Skin, darker	X	X			X	X					X	X	
Skin, pale					X	X				X			X
Skin, thin									X		X		X
Skin, yellow										X			
Sleep apnea										X	X	X	
Sleeping too much					X	X			X	X			X
Slow reflexes										X			
Smoke cigarettes		X							X				
Snoring					X	X				X	X	X	
Social isolation							X				X		X
Stomach ulcers											X		
Stretch marks, pink or white											X	X	
Stretch marks, red or purple											X		
Stretch marks, wider than ½ inch											X		
Strokes	X	X							X				
Stuffy nose										X			
Sweating, decreased										X			
Sweating, increased									X		X	X	
Thin arms and legs											X	X	
Thirst, excessive	X										X		
Urination, frequent	X										X		

	DM	IR	RH	IN	MH	FLAS	PCOS	VIR	MP	HT	CS	PC	GHD
Urinary incontinence						X			X				
Voice, deeper									X	X			
Weight gain	X	X	X	X	X	X	X	X	X	X	X	X	X
Weight loss					X	X		X					X
Female only													
Balding							X	X			X		
Birth to child over 10 pounds	X	X				X							
Breast shrinkage						X		X			X		
Enlargement of the clitoris								X			X		
Extensive muscle growth								X			X		
Hirsutism	X	X					X	X	X		X	X	
Infections, urinary	X										X		
Infections, yeast	X										X		
Infertility	X	X				X	X	X	X	X	X		
Menstrual problems	X	X				X	X	X	X	X	X	X	
Pain with intercourse						X		X	X				
PMS						X	X	X	X	X	X		
Waistline greater than 35 "	X	X					X	X			X	X	
Pregnancy, weight gain (excessive)	X	X					X					X	
Vaginal dryness									X				

	DM	IR	RH	IN	MH	FLAS	PCOS	VIR	MP	HT	CS	PC	GHD
Male only													
Breast growth					X						X	X	X
Erectile dysfunction					X						X	X	
Infertility					X						X		
Less body hair					X								
Shaving less					X								
Softening of the voice					X								
Softening of the testicles					X								
Waistline greater than 40 inches	X	X									X	X	

BIBLIOGRAPHY

CHAPTER 1

Albu JB, Bray GA, Despres MJP, Pi-Sunyer FX. Obesity: Is It a Disease? If So, How Should It Be Treated? *Medical Crossfire*. 1999;Oct:35–43.

The Bantam Medical Dictionary. 1981. Bantam Medical Books, Inc.

Bender R, Jockel KH, Truatner C, Spraul M, Berger M. Effect of Age on Excess Mortality in Obesity. *Journal of the American Medical Association*. 1999;281:1498–1504.

Bjorntorp P. The Regulation of Adipose Tissue Distribution in Humans. *International Journal of Obesity and Related Metabolic Disorders*. 1996;20:291–302.

Borzo G. Fat of the Land. *American Medical News*. 1999;Nov:27.

Kushner R. The Treatment of Obesity: A Call for Prudence and Professionalism. *Archives of Internal Medicine*. 1997;157:602–604.

Leach HM. Popular Diets and Anthropological Myths. *New Zealand Medical Journal*. 1989;102:474–477.

Perusse L, et al. The Human Obesity Gene Map: The 2000 Update. *Obesity Research*. 2001;9:135–170.

Ross R, Dagnone D, Jones PJH, et al. Reduction in Obesity and Related Comorbid Conditions after Diet-Induced Weight Loss or Exercise-Induced Weight Loss in Men: A Randomized, Controlled Trial. *Annals of Internal Medicine*. 2000;133:92–103.

Ruderman N, Chisholm D, Pi-Sunyer X, Schneider S. The Metabolically Obese, Normal-Weight Individual Revisited. *Diabetes*. 1998;47:35–48.

Willett WC, Dietz WH, Colditz GA. Guidelines for Healthy Weight. *New England Journal of Medicine*. 1999;341:427–434.

CHAPTER 2

Astrup A, Vrist E, Quaade F. Dietary Fibre Added to Very Low Calorie Diet Reduces Hunger and Alleviates Constipation. *International Journal of Obesity*. 1990;14:105–112.

Avenell A, Richmond PR, Lean MEJ, Reid DM. Bone Loss Associated with a High Fibre Weight Reduction Diet in Postmenopausal Women. *European Journal of Clinical Nutrition*. 1994;48:561–566.

Baron JA, Schori A, Crow B, et al. A Randomized Controlled Trial of Low Carbohydrate and Low Fat/High Fiber Diets for Weight Loss. *American Journal of Public Health*. 1986;76:1293–1296.

Calle-Pascual AL, Gomez V, Leon E, Bordiu E. Foods with a Low Glycemic Index Do Not Improve Glycemic Control of Both Type 1 and Type 2 Diabetic Patients After One Month of Therapy. *Diabetes and Metabolisme*. 1988;14:629–633.

Cham BE, Roeser HP, Linton I, Gaffney T. Effect of a High Energy, Low Carbohydrate Diet on Serum Levels of Lipids and Lipoproteins. *Medical Journal of Australia*. 1981;1:237–240.

Chandalia M, et al. Beneficial Effect of High Dietary Fiber Intake in Patients with Type 2 Diabetes Mellitus. *New England Journal of Medicine*. 2000;342:1392–1398.

Davidson MH, Hauptman J, DiGirolamo M, et al. Weight Control and Rsk Factor Reduction in Obese Subjects Treated for Two Years with Orlistat. *Journal of the American Medical Association*. 1999;281:235–279.

Epstein LH, et al. Increasing Fruit and Vegetable Intake and Decreasing Fat and Sugar Intake in Families at Risk for Childhood Obesity. *Obesity Research*. 2001;9:171–178.

Forster H. Is the Atkins Diet Safe in Respect to Health? *Fortschr Med*. 1978;96:1697–1702.

Guerciolini R, et al. Comparative Evaluation of Fecal Fat Excretion Induced by Orlistat and Chitosan. *Obesity Research*. 2001;6:364–367.

Hollenbeck CB, Coulston AM. The Clinical Utility of the Glycemic Index and Its Application to Mixed Metals. *Canadian Journal of Physiology & Pharmacology*. 1991;69:100–107.

Hu FB, Stampfer MJ, Rimm EB, et al. A Prospective Study of Egg Consumption and Risk of Cardiovascular Disease in Men and Women. *Journal of the American Medical Association*. 1999;281:1387–1394.

Kaumudi J, et al. The Effect of Fruit and Vegetable Intake on Risk for Coronary Heart Disease. *Annals of Internal Medicine*. 2001;134:1106–1114.

Jenkins DJA, Jenkins AL. Nutrition Principles and Diabetes: A Role for "Lente Carbohydrate"? *Diabetes Care*. 1995;18:1491–1498.

Jenkins DJ, Wolever TM, Kalmusky J, et al. Low-Glycemic Index Diet in Hyperlipidemia: Use of Traditional Starchy Foods. *American Journal of Clinical Nutrition*. 1987;46:66–71.

Joshipura KJ, et al. Fruit and Vegetable Intake in Relation to Risk of Ischemic Stroke. *Journal of the American Medical Association*. 1999;282:1233–1239.

Lichenstein AH, Ausman LM, Jalbert SM, Schaefer EJ. Effects of Different Forms of Dietary Hydrogenated Fats on Serum Lipoprotein Cholesterol Levels. *New England Journal of Medicine*. 1999;340:1933–1998.

Ludwig DS, Perieira MA, Kroenke CH, et al. Dietary Fiber, Weight Gain and Cardiovascular Disease Risk Factor in Young Adults. *Journal of the American Medical Association*. 1999;282:1539–1546.

Mickelsen O, Makdani DD, Cotton RH, et al. Effects of a High Fiber Bread Diet on Weight Loss in College-Age Males. *American Journal of Clinical Nutrition*. 1979;32:1703–1709.

Natt N, Service FJ. The Highway to Insulinoma: Road Signs and Hazards. *The Endocrinologist*. 1997;7:89–96.

Pasman WJ, Westerterp-Plantega MS, Saris WHM. The Effectiveness of Long-Term Supplementation of Carbohydrate, Chromium, Fibre and Caffeine on Weight Management. *International Journal of Obesity*. 1997;21:1143–1151.

Phinney SD, Bistrian BR, Wolfe RR, Blackburn GL. The Human Metabolic Response to Chronic Ketosis Without Caloric Restriction: Physical and Biochemical Adaptation. *Metabolism*. 1983;32:757–768.

Raben A, Jensen ND, Marckmann P, et al. Spontaneous Weight Loss During 11 Weeks' *ad libitum* Intake of a Low Fat/High Fibre Diet in Young, Normal Weight Subjects. *International Journal of Obesity*. 1995;19:916–923.

Rendell M. Dietary Treatment of Diabetes Mellitus. *New England Journal of Medicine*. 2000;342:1440–1441.

Rigaud D, Ryttig KR, Angel LA, Apfelbaum M. Overweight Treated with Energy Restriction and a Dietary Fibre Supplement: A 6-Month Randomized, Double-Blind, Placebo-Controlled Trial. *International Journal of Obesity*. 1990;14:763–769.

Rolls BJ. Carbohydrates, Fats, and Satiety. *American Journal of Clinical Nutrition*. 1995;61(Suppl 4):960S–967S.

Rolls BJ. Is the Low-Fat Message Giving People a License to Eat More? *Journal of the American College of Nutrition*. 1997;16:535–543.

Service FJ. Hypoglycemic Disorders. *New England Journal of Medicine*. 1995;332:1114–1150.

Slabber M, Barnard HC, Kuyl JM, et al. Effects of a Low-Insulin-Response, Energy-Restricted Diet on Weight Loss and Plasma Insulin Concentrations in Hyperinsulinemic Obese Females. *American Journal of Clinical Nutrition*. 1994;60:48–53.

Stevens, J. Does Dietary Fiber Affect Food Intake and Body Weight? *Journal of the American Dietetic Association.* 1988;88:939–945.

St. Jeor, et al. Dietary Protein and Weight Reduction: A Statement for Healthcare Professionals from the Nutrition Committee of the Council on Nutrition, Physical Activity, and Metabolism of the American Heart Association. *Circulation.* 2001;104:1869–1874.

Vogel RA. The Mediterranean Diet and Endothelial Function: Why Some Dietary Fats May Be Healthy. *Cleveland Clinic Journal of Medicine.* 2000;67:232–236.

Wolever TM, Jenkins DJA, Vuksan V, et al. Beneficial Effect of Low-Glycemic Index Diet in Overweight NIDDM Subjects. *Diabetes Care.* 1992;15:562–564.

Yang MU, Van Itallie TB. Composition of Weight Lost During Short-Term Weight Reduction. Metabolic Responses of Obese Subjects to Starvation and Low-Calorie Ketogenic and Nonketogenic Diets. *Journal of Clinical Investigation.* 1976;58:722–730.

Zambon D, Sabate J, Munoz S, et al. Substituting Walnuts for Monounsaturated Fat Improves the Serum Lipid Profile of Hypercholesterolemic Men and Women. *Annals of Internal Medicine.* 2000;132:538–546.

CHAPTER 3

Anderson RA. Nutritional Role of Chromium. *Sci Total Environ.* 1981;17:13–29.

Andreu AL, Hanna MG, Reichman H, et al. Exercise Intolerance Due to Mutations in the Cytochrome *b* Gene of Mitochondrial DNA. *New England Journal of Medicine.* 1999;341:1037–1044.

Arioglu E, Duncan-Morin J, Sebring N, et al. Efficacy and Safety of Troglitazone in the Treatment of Lipodystrophy Syndromes. *Annals of Internal Medicine.* 2000;133:263–274.

Badmaev V, Prakash S, Majeed M. Vanadium: A Review of Its Potential Role in the Fight Against Diabetes. *Journal of Alternative and Complementary Medicine.* 1999;5:273–291.

Battilana P, et al. Effects of Free Fatty Acids on Insulin Sensitivity and Hemodynamics During Mental Stress. *Journal of Clinical Endocrinology and Metabolism.* 2001;86:124–128.

Bell DSH. Inflammation, Insulin Resistance, Infection, Diabetes, and Atherosclerosis. *Endocrine Practice.* 2000;6:272–276.

Ben-Noun L, et al. Neck Circumference as a Simple Screening Measure for Identifying Overweight and Obese Patients. *Obesity Research.* 2001;8:470–477.

Bjorntorp P, Fahlen M, Grimby G, et al. Carbohydrate and Lipid Metabolism in Middle-Aged, Physically Well-Trained Men. *Metabolism.* 1972;21:1037–1044.

Cam MC, Li WM, McNeill JH. Partial Preservation of Pancreatic Beta-Cells by Vanadium: Evidence for Long-Term Amelioration of Diabetes. *Metabolism.* 1997;46:769–778.

Cam MC, Rodrigues B, McNeill JH. Distinct Glucose Lowering and Beta Cell Protective Effects of Vanadium and Food Restriction in Streptozotocin Diabetes. *European Journal of Endocrinology.* 1999;141:546–554.

Capes SE, Hunt D, Malmberg K, Gerstein HC. Stress Hyperglycaemia and Increased Risk of Death After Myocardial Infarction in Patients With and Without Diabetes: A Systematic Overview. *Lancet.* 2000;355:773–778.

Cunningham JJ. Micronutrients as Nutraceutical Interventions in Diabetes Mellitus. *J Am Coll Nutr.* 1998;17:7–10.

DeFronzo RA, Ferrannini E. Insulin Resistance: A Multifaceted Syndrome Responsible for NIDDM, Obesity, Hypertension, Dyslipidemia, and Atherosclerotic Cardiovascular Disease. *Diabetes Care.* 1991;14:173–194.

Elias AN, Grossman MK, Valenta LJ. Use of the Artificial Beta Cell (ABC) in the Assessment of Peripheral Insulin Sensitivity: Effect of Chromium Supplementation in Diabetic Patients. *Gen Pharmacol.* 1984;15:535–539.

Eriksson J, Taimela S, Koivisto VA. Exercise and the Metabolic Syndrome. *Diabetologia.* 1997;40:125–135.

Fantus IG, Tsiani E. Multifunctional Actions of Vanadium Compounds on Insulin Signaling Pathways: Evidence for Preferential Enhancement of Metabolic Versus Mitogenic Effects. *Molecular and Cellular Biochemistry.* 1998;182:109–119.

Faure P, Roussel A, Coudray C, et al. Zinc and Insulin Sensitivity. *Biol Trace Elem Res.* 1992;Jan–Mar:305–310.

Ganda OP. Lipoatrophy, Lipodystrophy, and Insulin Resistance. *Annals of Internal Medicine.* 2000;133:304–306.

Ginsberg H, Olefsky JM, Kimmerling G, et al. Induction of Hypertriglyceridemia by a Low-Fat Diet. *Journal of Clinical Endocrinol Metab.* 1976;45:729–735.

Groop L, Lehto M. Molecular and Physiological Basis for Maturity Onset Diabetes of Youth. *Current Opinion in Endocrinology and Diabetes.* 1999;6:157–162.

Halberstam M, Cohen N, Shlimovich P, et al. Oral Vandyl Sulfate Improves Insulin Sensitivity in NIDDM but Not in Obese Nondiabetic Subjects. *Diabetes.* 1996;45:659–666.

Hooper PL. Hot-Tub Therapy for Type II Diabetes Mellitus. *New England Journal of Medicine.* 1999;341:924–925.

Hu F. Diet, Lifestyle, and the Risk of Type 2 Diabetes Mellitus in Women. *New England Journal of Medicine.* 2001;345:790–797.

Jancin B. High-Protein Diet May Boost Insulin Sensitivity. *Internal Medicine News.* 2000;Jan:15.

Jeejeebhoy KN. The Role of Chromium in Nutrition and Therapeutics and as a Potential Toxin. *Nutr Rev.* 1999;57:329–335.

Jeppesen J, Schaaf P, Jones C, et al. Effect of Low-Fat, High-Carbohydrate Diets on Risk Factors for Ischemic Heart Disease in Postmenopausal Women. *American Journal of Clinical Nutrition.* 1997;65:1027–1033.

Jovanovic L. Rationale for Prevention and Treatment of Postprandial Glucose-Mediated Toxicity. *The Endocrinologist.* 1999;9:87–92.

Karam JH. Reversible Insulin Resistance in Non-Insulin-Dependent Diabetes Mellitus. *Hormone and Metabolism Research.* 1996;28:440–444.

Koivisto VA, Yki-Jarvinen H, DeFronzo RA. Physical Training and Insulin Sensitivity. *Diabetes/Metabolism Reviews.* 1986;1:445–481.

Kumar D. One-Hour Meal Tolerance Test to Assess Withdrawl of Insulin Therapy in Overweight Patients with Type 2 Diabetes. *Endocrine Practice.* 2001;7:256–261.

Kuroki R, Sadamoto Y, Imamura M, et al. *Acanthosis nigricans* with Severe Obesity, Insulin Resistance and Hypothyroidism: Improvement by Diet Control. *Dermatology.* 1999;198:164–166.

Levine JA, Eberhardt NL, Jensen MD. Role of Nonexercise Activity Thermogenesis in Resistance to Fat Gain in Humans. *Science.* 1999;283:212–185.

McCarty MF. Homologous Physiological Effects of Phenformin and Chromium Picolinate. *Medical Hypotheses.* 1993;41:316–324.

McCarty MF. Chromium and Other Insulin Sensitizers May Enhance Glucagon Secretion: Implications for Hypoglycemia and Weight Control. *Medical Hypotheses.* 1996;46:77–80.

McCarty MF. Complementary Measures for Promoting Insulin Sensitivity in Skeletal Muscle. *Medical Hypotheses.* 1998;51:451–464.

McCarty MF. High-Dose Biotin, an Inducer of Glucokinase Expression, May Synergize with Chromium Picolinate to Enable a Definitive Nutritional Therapy for Type II Diabetes. *Medical Hypotheses.* 1999;52:401–406.

Mertz W. Chromium in Human Nutrition: A Review. *Journal of Nutrition.* 1993;123:117–119.

Mogul, H. Syndrome W. *Internal Medicine News.* July 1, 1999.

Mori TA, Bao DQ, Burke V, et al. Dietary Fish as a Major Component of a Weight-Loss Diet: Effect on Serum Lipids, Glucose, and Insulin Metabolism in Overweight Hypertensive Subjects. *American Journal of Clinical Nutrition.* 1999;70:817–825.

Morris BW, MacNeil S, Hardist CA, et al. Chromium Homeostasis in Patients with Type II (NIDDM) Diabetes. *Journal of Trace Elem Med Biol.* 1999;13:57–61.

Nakanishi N, Nakamura K, Matsuo Y, et al. Cigarette Smoking and Risk for Impaired Fasting Glucose and Type 2 Diabetes in Middle-Aged Japanese Men. *Annals of Internal Medicine.* 2000;133:183–191.

National Institute of Diabetes and Digestive and Kidney Diseases. *The Pima Indians: Pathfinders for Health.* NIH Publication No. 95-3821.

Offenbacher EG, Pi-Sunyer FX. Beneficial Effect of Chromium-Rich Yeast on Glucose Tolerance and Blood Lipids in Elderly Subjects. *Diabetes.* 1980;29:919–925.

O'Keffe JH, Harris WS. From Inuit to Implementation: Omega-3 Fatty Acids Come of Age. *Mayo Clinic Proceedings.* 2000;75:607–614.

Olatunbosun ST, Bella AF. Relationship Between Height, Glucose Intolerance, and Hypertension in an Urban African Black Adult Population: A Case for the "Thrifty Phenotype" Hypothesis? *Journal of the National Medical Association.* 2000;92:265–268.

Pohl JH, Greer JA, Hasan KS. Type 2 Diabetes Mellitus in Children. *Endocrine Practice.* 1998;4:413–416.

Poucheret P, Verma S, Grynpas MD, McNeill JH. Vanadium and Diabetes. *Molecular and Cellular Biochemistry.* 1998;188:73–80.

Preuss HG. Effects of Glucose/Insulin Perturbations on Aging and Chronic Disorders of Aging: The Evidence. *Journal of the American College of Nutrition.* 1997;16:397–403.

Pruthi S, et al. Vitamin E Supplementation in the Prevention of Coronary Artery Disease. *Mayo Clinic Proceedings.* 2001;76:1131–1136.

Rabinowitz D, Maffezzoli R, Merimer TJ, Burgess JA. Patterns of Hormonal Release After Glucose, Protein, and Glucose Plus Protein. *The Lancet.* 1966; 2(7461):454–456.

Reaven GM. Role of Insulin Resistance in Human Disease. *Diabetes.* 1988;37:1595–1607.

Reddi A, DeAngelis B, Frank O, et al. Biotin Supplementation Improves Glucose and Insulin Tolerances in Genetically Diabetic KK Mice. *Life Sciences.* 1988;42:1323–1330.

Rexrode KM, Carey VJ, Hennekens CH, et al. Abdominal Adiposity and Coronary Heart Disease in Women. *Journal of the American Medical Association.* 1998;280:1843–1848.

Riales R, Albrink MJ. Effect of Chromium Chloride Supplementation on Glucose Tolerance and Serum Lipids Including High-Density Lipoprotein of Adult Men. *American Journal of Clinical Nutrition.* 1981;34:2670–2678.

Ristow M, Moller-Wieland D, Pfeiffer A, et al. Obesity Associated with a Mutation in a Genetic Regulator of Adipocyte Differentiation. *New England Journal of Medicine*. 1998;339:953–959.

Rosen ED, Spiegelman BM. Tumor Necrosis Factor-a as a Mediator of the Insulin Resistanace of Obesity. *Current Opinion in Endocrinology and Diabetes*. 1999;6:170–176.

Rupp H. Insulin Resistance, Hyperinsulinemia, and Cardiovascular Disease. The Need for Novel Dietary Prevention Strategies. *Basic Research in Cardiology*. 1992;87:99–105.

Ryan AS, Pratley RE, Goldberg AP, Elahi D. Resistive Training Increases Insulin Action in Postmenopausal Women. *Journal Gerontol A Biol Sci Med Sci*. 1996;51:M199–205.

Samaras K, Kelly PJ, Chiano MN, et al. Genes Versus Environment. *Diabetes Care*. 1998;21:2069–2076.

Saris WHM. Fit, Fat and Fat Free: The Metabolic Aspects of Weight Control. *International Journal of Obesity*. 1998;22(Supp 2):S515–S521.

Shecter Y and Shisheva A. Vanadium Salts and the Future Treatment of Diabetes. *Endeavour*. 1993;17:27–31.

Shepherd, PR, Kahn BB. Glucose Transporters and Insulin Action: Implications for Insulin Resistance and Diabetes Mellitus. *New England Journal of Medicine*. 1999;341:248–246.

Shim ML, Geffner ME. Insulin Resistance in Children. *The Endocrinologist*. 1999;9:270–276.

Singh RB, Niaz MA, Rastogi SS, et al. Current Zinc Intake and Risk of Diabetes and Coronary Artery Disease and Factors Associated with Insulin Resistance in Rural and Urban Populations of North India. *Journal of American College of Nutrition*. 1998;17:564–570.

Striffler JS, Law JS, Polansky MM, et al. Chromium Improves Insulin Response to Glucose in Rats. *Metabolism*. 1995;44:1314–1320.

Striffler JS, Polansky MM, Anderson RA. Dietary Chromium Decreases Insulin Resistance in Rats Fed a High-Fat, Mineral-Imbalanced Diet. *Metabolism*. 1998;47:396–400.

Striffler JS, Polansky MM, Anderson RA. Overproduction of Insulin in the Chromium-deficient Rat. *Metabolism*. 1999;48:1063–1068.

Tessedre PL, Krosniak M, Portet K, et al. Vanadium Levels in French and Californian Wines: Influence on Vanadium Dietary Intake. *Food Addit Contam*. 1998;15:585–591.

Thompson WG. Early Recognition and Treatment of Glucose Abnormalities to Prevent Type 2 Diabetes Mellitus and Coronary Heart Disease. *Mayo Clinic Proceedings*. 2001;76:1137–1143.

Tuomilehto J, et al. Prevention of Type 2 Diabetes Mellitus by Changes in Lifestyle Among Subjects with Impaired Glucose Tolerance. *New England Journal of Medicine*. 2001;344:1343–1350.

Turley ML, Skeaff CM, Mann JI, Cox B. The Effect of a Low-Fat, High-Carbohydrate Diet on Serum High Density Lipoprotein Cholesterol and Triglyceride. *European Journal of Clinical Nutrition.* 1998;52:728–732.

Verma S, Cam MC, McNeill JH. Nutritional Factors That Can Favorably Influence the Glucose/Insulin System: Vanadium. *Journal of the American College of Nutrition.* 1998;17:11–18.

Vinik AI, Wing RR. The Good, the Bad, and the Ugly in Diabetic Diets. *Endocrinology and Metabolism Clinics of North America.* 1992;21:237–279.

Wallach S. Clinical and Biochemical Aspects of Chromium Deficiency. *Journal of the American College of Nutrition.* 1985;4:107–120.

Wei M, Gibbons LW, Kampert JB, et al. Low Cardiorespiratory Fitness and Physical Inactivity as Predictors of Mortality in Men with Type 2 Diabetes. *Annals of Internal Medicine.* 2000;132:605–670.

Wilmore JH. Variations in Physical Activity Habits and Body Composition. *International Journal of Obesity.* 1995;19(Suppl 4):S107–S112.

Wojtaszewski JFP, Goodyear LJ. Cellular Effects of Exercise to Promote Muscle Insulin Sensitivity. *Current Opinion in Endocrinology and Diabetes.* 1999;6:129–134.

Zamboni M, Armellini F, Turcato E, et al. Relationship Between Visceral Fat, Steroid Hormones and Insulin Sensitivity in Premenopausal Obese Women. *Journal of Internal Medicine.* 1994;236:521–527.

Zhang H, Osada K, Maebashi M, et al. A High Biotin Diet Improves the Impaired Glucose Tolerance of Long-Term Spontaneously Hyperglycemic Rates with Non-Insulin-Dependent Diabetes Mellitus. *Journal of Nutr Sci Vitaminol.* 1996;42:517–526.

Zhang H, Osada K, Sone H, and Furukawa Y. Biotin Administration Improves the Impaired Glucose Tolerance of Streptozotocin-Induced Diabetic Wistar Rats. *Journal of Nutr Sci Vitaminol.* 1997;43:271–280.

CHAPTER 4

AACE Clinical Practice Guidelines for the Evaluation and Treatment of Hypogonadism in Adult Male Patients. 1996.

Bagatell CJ, Bremner WJ. Androgens in Men—Uses and Abuses. *Drug Therapy.* 1996;334:707–713.

Bhasin S, Storer TW, Berman N, et al. The Effects of Supraphysiologic Doses of Testosterone on Muscle Size and Strengths in Normal Men. *New England Journal of Medicine.* 1996;335:1–7.

Corcoran C, Grinspoon S. Treatments for Wasting in Patients with the Acquired Immunodeficiency Syndrome. *New England Journal of Medicine.* 1999;340:1740–1750.

Dobs AS. Is There a Role for Androgenic Anabolic Steroids in Medical Practice? *Journal of the American Medical Association.* 1999;281:1326–1327.

Ghusn HF, Cunningham GR. Evaluation and Treatment of Androgen Deficiency in Males. *The Endocrinologist.* 1991;1:399–408.

Goodman NF. Hyperandrogenism: Defining the Reference Range for "Normal" Androgens. *Endocrine Practice.* ; :357–376.

Griffin JE. Androgen Resistance—The Clinical and Molecular Spectrum. *New England Journal of Medicine.* 1992;326:611–618.

Isidori AM, et al. Leptin and Androgen Levels in Male Obesity. *Journal of Clinical Endocrinology and Metabolism.* 1999;84:3673–3680.

Jensen MD. Androgen Effect on Body Composition and Fat Metabolism. *Mayo Clinic Proceedings.* 2000;75:S65–S69.

Katznelson L. Neuroendocrine Aspects of Testosterone Insufficiency with Aging. *The Endocrinologist.* 1999;9:190–196.

King DS, Sharp RL, Vukovich MD, et al. Effet of Oral Androstenedione on Serum Testosterone and Adaptations to Resistance Training in Young Men. *Journal of the American Medical Association.* 1999;281:2020–2044.

Leder BZ, Longcope C, Catlin DH, et al. Oral Androstenedione Administration and Serum Testosterone Concentrations in Young Men. *Journal of the American Medical Association.* 2000;283:779–782.

Ly LP, et al. Effects of Dihydrotestosterone Gel in Older Men. *Journal of Endocrinology and Metabolism.* 2001;86:4078–4088.

Madden CC. Are Creatine Supplements Safe and Effective? What to Tell Active Patients. *Your Patient and Fitness.* 2000;14:17–20.

Marin P, Holmang S, Jonsson L, et al. Androgen treatment of Abdominally Obese Men. *Obesity Research.* 1993;1:245–251.

McPhaul MJ, Marcelli M, Zoppi S, et al. Genetic Basis of Endocrine Disease 4: The Spectrum of Mutations in the Androgen Receptor Gene That Causes Androgen Resistance. *Journal of Clinical Endocrinology and Metabolism.* 1993;76:17–23.

Morley JE. Testosterone Replacement and the Physiologic Aspects of Aging in Men. *Mayo Clinic Proceedings.* 2000;75:S83–S87.

Report of the National Institute on Aging Advisory Panel on Testosterone Replacement in Men. *Journal of Clinical Endocrinology and Metabolism.* 2001;86:4611–4614.

Sattler FR, Jaque SV, Schroeder ET, et al. Effects of Pharmacological Doses of Nandrolone Decanoate and Progressive Resistance Training in Immunodeficient Patients Infected with Human Immunodeficiency Virus. *Journal of Clincial Endocrinology and Metabolism.* 1999;84:1268–1275.

Sheffield-Moore M, Urban RJ, Wolf SE, et al. Short-Term Oxandrolone Administration Stimulates Net Muscle Protein Synthesis in Young Men. *Journal of Clinical Endocrinology and Metabolism.* 1999;84:2705–2711.

Snyder PJ. Effects of Age on Testicular Function and Consequences of Testosterone Treatment. *Journal of Clinical Endocrinology and Metabolism.* 2001;86:2369–2372.

Snyder PJ, Peachey H, Hannoush P, et al. Effect of Testosterone Treatment on Body Composition and Muscle Strength in Men Over 65 Years of Age. *Journal of Clinical Endocrinology and Metabolism.* 1999;84:2467–53.

Strawford A, Barbieri T, Van Loan M, et al. Resistance Exercise and Supraphysiologic Androgen Therapy in Eugonadal Men with HIV-Related Weight Loss: A Randomized Controlled Trial. *Journal of the American Medical Association.* 1999;281:1282–1290.

Wang C, et al. Transdermal Testosterone Gel Improves Sexual Function, Mood, Muscle Strength and Body Composition Parameters in Hypogonadal Men. *Journal of Clinical Endocrinology and Metabolism.* 2000;85:2839–2853.

CHAPTER 5

AACE Medical Guidelines for Clinical Practice for the Diagnosis and Treatment of Hyperandrogenic Disorders. *Endocrine Practice.* 2001;2:120–134.

Arlt W, Callies FC, Van Viljmen JC, et al. Dehydroepiandrosterone Replacement in Women with Adrenal Insufficiency. *New England Journal of Medicine.* 1999;341:1013–1020.

Ayala C, Steinberger E, Smith KD, et al. Serum Testosterone Levels and Reference Ranges in Reproductive-Age Women. *Endocrine Practice.* 1999;5:322–329.

Azziz R. Adrenal Androgen Excess in the Polycystic Ovary Syndrome. *The Endocrinologist.* 2000;10:245–254.

Azziz R, Hincapie LA, Knochenhauer ES, et al. Screening for 21-Hydroxylase Deficient Non-Classic Adrenal Hyperplasia Among Hyperandrogenic Women: A Prospective Study. *Fertil Steril.* 1999;72:915–925.

Birdsall MA, Farquhar CM, White HD. Association Between Polycystic Ovaries and Extent of Coronary Artery Disease in Women Having Cardiac Catheterization. *Annals of Internal Medicine.* 1997;126:32–35.

Bloomgarden ZT, et al. Use of Insulin Sensitizing Agents in Polycystic Ovary Syndrome. *Endocrine Practice.* 2001;4:279–286.

Branhardt KT, Freeman E, Grisso JA, et al. The Effect of Dehydroepiandrosterone Supplementation to Symptomatic Perimenopausal Women on Serum Endocrine Profiles, Lipid Parameters, and Health Related Quality of Life. *Journal of Clinical Endocrinology and Metabolism.* 1999;84:3896–3901.

Callies F, et al. Dehydroepiandrosterone Replacement in Women with Adrenal Insufficiency: Effects on Body Composition, Serum Leptin, Bone Turnover, and Exercise Capacity. *Journal of Clinical Endocrinology and Metabolism.* 2001;86:1968–1972.

Casson PR, Buster JE. DHEA Replacement After Menopause: HRT 2000 or Nostrum of the 90s? *Contemporary Ob/Gyn.* 1997;April:119–133.

Franks S. Polycystic Ovary Syndrome. *The New England Journal of Medicine.* 1995;333:853–860.

Gallagher JC, et al. Prevention of Bone Loss with Tibolone in Postmenopausal Women: Results of Two Randomized, Double-Blind, Placebo-Controlled, Dose-Finding Studies. *Journal of Clinical Endocrinology and Metabolism.* 2001;86:4717–4726.

Geisthovel F, Olbrich M, Frorath B, et al. Obesity and Hypertestosteronaemia Are Independently and Synergistically Associated with Elevated Insulin Concentrations and Dyslipidaemia in Pre-menopausal Women. *Human Reproduction.* 1994;9:610–616.

Lobo RA, Carmina E. The Importance of Diagnosing the Polycystic Ovary Syndrome. *Annals of Internal Medicine.* 2000;132:989–993.

Lucas KJ. Finasteride Cream in Hirsutism. *Endocrine Practice.* 2001;1:5–10.

Miller KK. Androgen Deficiency in Women with Hypopituitarism. *Journal of Clinical Endocrinology and Metabolism.* 2001;86:561–567.

Miller KK. Androgen Deficiency in Women. *Journal of Clinical Endocrinology and Metabolism.* 2001;86:2395–2401.

Nestler JE, Jakubowicz DJ. Decreases in Ovarian Cytochrome P450c17a Activity and Serum Free Testosterone After Reduction of Insulin Secretion in Polycystic Ovary Syndrome. *New England Journal of Medicine.* 1996;335:617–623.

Nestler JE, Jakubowicz DJ, Evans WS, Pasquali R. Effects of Metformin on Spontaneous and Clomiphene-Induced Ovulation in the Polycystic Ovary Syndrome. *New England Journal of Medicine.* 1998;338:1876–1880.

Shrifen JL. Transdermal Testosterone Treatment in Women with Impaired Sexual Function After Oophorectomy. *New England Journal of Medicine.* 2000;343:682–688.

Snyder PJ. Role of Androgens in Women. *Journal of Clinical Endocrinology and Metabolism.* 2001;86:1006–1007.

Verma S, Mather K, Dumont AS, Anderson TJ. Pharmacological Modulation of Insulin Resistance and Hyperinsulinemia in Polycystic Ovary Syndrome: The Emerging Role. *The Endocrinologist.* 1998;8:418–424.

CHAPTER 6

AACE Medical Guidelines for Clinical Practice for Management of Menopause. *Endocrine Practice.* 1999;5:355–366.

Abramowicz M, ed. A Progestin-Releasing Intrauterine Device for Long-Term Contraception. *The Medical Letter.* 2001;43:7–8.

Adlercreutz H. Diet, Breast Cancer and Sex Hormone Metabolism. *Annals of New York Academy of Sciences.*

Andersson B, Mattsson LA, Hahn L, et al. Estrogen Replacement Therapy Decreases Hyperandrogenicity and Improves Glucose Homeostasis and Plasma Lipids in Postmenopausal Women with Noninsulin-Dependent Diabetes Mellitus. *Journal of Clinical Endocrinology and Metabolism.* 1997;82:638–643.

Berger PB, Herrmann RR, Dumesic DA. The Effect of Estrogen Replacement Therapy on Total Plasma Homocysteine in Healthy Postmenopausal Women. *Mayo Clinic Proceedings.* 2000;75:18–23.

Binder EF, et al. Effects of Hormone Replacement Therapy on Serum Lipids in Elderly Women. *Annals of Internal Medicine.* 2001;134:754–760.

Brussard HE, Gevers LJA, Frolich M, et al. Short-Term Estrogen Replacement Therapy Improves Insulin Resistance, Lipids and Fibrinolysis in Postmenopausal Women with NIDDM. *Diabetologia.* 1997;40:843–849.

Chlebowski, RT. Reducing the Risk of Breast Cancer. *New England Journal of Medicine.* 2000;343:191–198.

Clarkson, MA, et al. Inhibition of Postmenopausal Atherosclerosis Progression: A Comparison of the Effects of Conjugated Equine Estrogens and Soy Phytoestrogens. *Journal of Clinical Endocrinology and Metabolism.* 2001;86:41–47.

Colacurci N, Zarcone R, Mollo A, et al. Effects of Hormone Replacement Therapy on Glucose Metabolism. *Panminerva Med.* 1998;40:18–21.

Dimmock PW, et al. Efficacy of Selective Serotonin-Reuptake Inhibitors in Premenstrual Syndrome: A Systematic Review. *Lancet.* 2000;356:1131–1136.

Fitzpatrick LA. Selective Estorgen Receptor Modulators and Phytoestrogens: New Therapies for the Postmenopausal Woman. *Mayo Clinic Proceedings.* 1999;74:601–607.

Frost G, Leeds A, Trew G, et al. Insulin Sensitivity in Women at Risk of Coronary Heart Disease and the Effect of a Low Glycemic Diet. *Metabolism.* 1998;47:1245–1251.

Gebhart SSP, Watts NB, Clark RV, et al. Reversible Impairment of Gonadotropin Secretion in Critical Illness: Observations in Postmenopausal Women. *Archives of Internal Medicine.* 1989;149:1637–1641.

Godsland IF, Gangar K, Walton C, et al. Insulin Resistance, Secretion, and Elimination in Postmenopausal Women Receiving Oral or Transdermal Hormone Replacement Therapy. *Metabolism.* 1993;42:846–853.

Herrington DM, Reboussin DM, Brosnihan KB, et al. Effects of Estrogen Replacement on the Progression of Coronary-Artery Atherosclerosis. *New England Journal of Medicine.* 2000;343:522–528.

Herrington DM. The HERS Trial Results: Paradigms Lost? *Annals of Internal Medicine.* 1999;131:463–466.

Huerta R, Mena A, Malacara JM, de Leon JD. Symptoms at the Menopausal and Premenopausal Years: Their Relationship with Insulin, Glucose, Cortisol, FSH, Prolactin, Obesity and Attitudes Toward Sexuality. *Psychoneuroendocrinology.* 1995;20:851–864.

Hurskainen R, et al. Quality of Life and Cost-Effectiveness of Levonorgestrel-Releasing Intrauterine System Versus Hysterectomy for Treatment of Menorrhagia. *Lancet.* 2001;357:273–277.

Keating NL, Cleary PD, Rossi AS, et al. Use of Hormone Replacement Therapy by Postmenopausal Women in the United States. *Annals of Internal Medicine.* 1999;130:545–553.

LeBlanc ES, et al. Hormone Replacement Therapy and Cognition. *Journal of the American Medical Association.* 2001;285:1489–1499.

Lindeheim SR, Buchanan TA, Duffy DM, et al. Comparison of Estimates of Insulin Sensitivity in Pre- and Postmenopausal Women Using the Insulin Tolerance Test and the Frequently Sampled Intravenous Glucose Tolerance Test. *Journal of Soc Gynecol Investig.* 1994;1:150–154.

Lindeheim SR, Duffy DM, Kojima T, et al. The Route of Administration Influences the Effect of Estrogen on Insulin Sensitivity in Postmenopausal Women. *Fertil Steril.* 1994;62:1176–1180.

Lindeheim SR, Presser SC, Ditkoff EC, et al. A Possible Bimodal Effect of Estrogen on Insulin Sensitivity in Postmenopausal Women and the Attenuating Effect of Added Progestin. *Fertil Steril.* 1993;60:664–667.

McMillan PJ, Dorsa DM. Estrogen Actions in the Central Nervous System. *Neuroendocrinology.* 1999;6:33–37.

McNagny SE. Prescribing Hormone Replacement Therapy for Menopausal Symptoms. *Annals of Internal Medicine.* 1999;131:605–616.

Medelsohn ME, Karas RH. The Protective Effects of Estrogen on the Cardiovascular System. *New England Journal of Medicine.* 1999;340:1801–1811.

Scully RE, ed. Case Records of the Massachusetts General Hospital: Case 12-2000. *New England Journal of Medicine.* 2000;342:1196–1204.

Scuteri A, et al. Hormone Replacement Therapy and Longitudinal Changes in Blood Pressure in Postmenopausal Women. *Annals of Internal Medicine.* 2001;135:229–238.

Shlipak MG, Simon JA, Vittinghoff E, et al. Estrogen and Progestin, Lipoprotein(a), and the Risk of Recurrent Coronary Heart Disease Events After Menopause. *Journal of the American Medical Association.* 2000;283:1845–1852.

Sorensen MB, et al. Obesity and Sarcopenia After Menopause Are Reversed by Sex Hormone Replacement Therapy. *Obesity Research.* 2001;9:622–626.

Spencer CP, Godsland IF, Stevenson JC. Is There a Menopausal Metabolic Syndrome? *Gynecol Endocrinol.* 1997;11:341–355.

Stampfer MJ, Hu FB, Manson JE, et al. Primary Prevention of Coronary Heart Disease in Women Through Diet and Lifestyle. *New England Journal of Medicine.* 2000:343:16–22.

Steinmetz R, Brown NG, Allen DL, et al. The Environmental Estrogen Bisphenol A Stimulates Prolactin Release *in Vitro* and *in Vivo. Endocrinology.* 1997;138:1780–1786.

Stevenson JC. Metabolic Effects of the Menopause and Estrogen Replacement. *Baillieres Clin Obstet Gynaecol.* 1996;10:449–467.

Stevenson JC, Proudler AJ, Walton C, Godsland IF. HRT Mechanisms of Action: Carbohydrates. *International Journal of Fertility and Menopausal Studies.* 1994;39:50–55.

Tehernof A, Calles-Escandon J, Sites CK and Poehlman ET. Menopause, Central Body Fatness, and Insulin Resistance: Effects of Hormone-Replacement Therapy. *Coron Artery Dis.* 1998;9:503–511.

Tham DM, Gardner CD, Haskell WL. Potential Health Benefits of Dietary Phytoestrogens: A Review of the Clinical, Epidemiological, and Mechanistic Evidence. *Journal of Clinical Endocrinology and Metabolism.* 1998;83:2223–2235.

Vanderbroucke JP, et al. Oral Contraceptives and the Risk of Venous Thrombosis. *New England Journal of Medicine.* 2001;344:1527–1535.

Vincent A, Fitzpatrick LA. Soy Isoflavones: Are They Useful in Menopause? *Mayo Clinic Proceedings.* 2000;75:1174–1184.

Viscoli, CM, et al. A Clinical Trial of Estrogen-Replacement Therapy After Ischemic Stroke. *New England Journal of Medicine.* 2001;345:1243–1249.

Walsh B, Paul S, Wild R, et al. The Effects of Hormone Replacement Therapy and Raloxifene on C-Reactive Protein and Homocysteine in Healthy Postmenopausal Women: A Randomized, Controlled Trial. *Journal of Clinical Endocrinology and Metabolism.* 2000;85:214–218.

Whitaker MD. Selective Estrogen Receptor Modulators: From Bench to Bedside and Back. *Endocrine Practice.* 2001;7:113–119.

Wise PM, Hyde JF. Changes in the Neuroendocrine Control of the Female Reproductive Axis with Aging. *Neuroendocrinology.* 1999;6:50–54.

CHAPTER 7

AACE Clinical Practice Guidelines for the Evaluation and Treatment of Hyperthyroidism and Hypothyroidism. Endocrine Practice. 1995;1(1).

Abramowicz M, ed. Generic Drugs. *The Medical Letter on Drugs and Therapeutics.* 1999;41:47–50.

Adler GK. Hormonal Changes and Fibromyalgas. *Current Opinions in Endocrinology and Diabetes.* 1999;6:55–60.

Anselmo J, Cesar R. Resistance to Thyroid Hormone: Report of Two Kindreds with 35 Patients. *Endocrine Practice.* 1998;4:368–374.

Arafa BM. Increased Need for Thyroxine in Women with Hypothyroidism During Estrogen Therapy. *New England Journal of Medicine.* 2001;344:1743–1749.

Bauer DC, et al. Risk for Fracture in Women with Low Serum Levels of Thyroid-Stimulating Hormone. *Annals of Internal Medicine.* 2001;134:561–568.

Bell DS, Ovalle F. Use of Soy Protein Supplement and Resultant Need for Increased Dosage of Levothyroxine. *Endocrine Practice.* 2001;7:134–194.

Brennan MD, Bahn RS. Thyroid Hormones and Illness. *Endocrine Practice.* 1998;4:396–402.

Bunevicius R, Kazanavicius G, Zalinkevicius R, Prange AJ. Effects of Thyroxine as Compared with Thyroxine Plus Triiodothyronine in Patients with Hypothyroidism. *New England Journal of Medicine.* 1999;340:424–429.

Canaris GJ, Manowitz NR, Mayor G, Ridgway EC. The Colorado Thyroid Disease Prevalence Study. *Archives of Internal Medicine.* 2000;160:526–534.

Clinical Guidelines, American College of Physicians. Screening for Thyroid Disease. *Annals of Internal Medicine.* 1998;129:141–158.

Cushing GW. Subclinical Hypothyroidism: Understanding Is the Key to Decision Making. *Postgraduate Medicine.* 1993;94:1–7.

Ferretti E, Persani L, Jaffrain-Rea ML, et al. Evaluation of the Adequacy of Levothyroxine Replacement Therapy in Patients with Central Hypothyroidism. *Journal of Clinical Endocrinology and Metabolism.* 1999;84:924–929.

Gordon MB, Gordon MS. Variations in Adequate Levothyroxine Replacement Therapy in Patients with Different Causes of Hypothyroidism. *Endocrine Practice.* 1999;5:233–301.

Hak E, Huibert APP, Visser TJ, et al. Subclinical Hypothyroidism Is an Independent Risk Factor for Atherosclerosis and Myocardial Infarction in Elderly Women: The Rotterdam Study. *Annals of Internal Medicine.* 2000;132:270–278.

Helfand M, Redfern CC, Sox HC. Screening for Thyroid Disease. *Annals of Internal Medicine.* 1998;129:141–158.

Hollowell JG Jr, Garbe PL, Miller DT. Maternal Thyroid Deficiency during Pregnancy and Subsequent Neuropsychological Development of the Child. *New England Journal of Medicine.* 1999;341(26):2016–2017.

Hussein WI, Green R, Jacobsen DW, Faiman C. Normalization of Hyperhomocysteinemia with L-Thyroxine in Hypothyroidism. *Annals of Internal Medicine.* 1999;131:348–351.

Jackson IMD, Asamoah EO. Thyroid Function in Clinical Depression: Insights and Uncertainties. *Thyroid Today*. 1999;22:1–11.

Klein I, Ojamaa K. Thyroid Hormone and the Cardiovascular System. *New England Journal of Medicine*. 2001;344:501–509.

Ladenson PW, Singer PA, Ain KB, et al. American Thyroid Association Guidelines for Detection of Thyroid Dysfunction. *Archives of Internal Medicine*. 2000;160:1573–1575.

Liang BA, ed. A Case-Based Review of the AACE Clinical Practice Guidelines for the Management of Thyroid Disease. *Hospital Physician*. 1996;Oct:26–48.

McDermott MT, Ridgway EC. Subclinical Hypothyroidism Is Mild Thyroid Failure and Should Be Treated. *Journal of Clinical Endocrinology and Metabolism*. 2001;86:4585–4590.

Mohammed IA, Aldasouqi S, Schnute R, et al. The Syndrome of Resistance to Thyroid Hormone Misdiagnosed and Treated as Thyrotoxicosis. *Endocrine Practice*. 1998;4:391–394.

Monzani F, Del Guerra P, Caraccio N, et al. Subclinical Hypothyroidism: Neurobehavioral Features and Beneficial Effect of L-Thyroxine Treatment. *The Clinical Investigator*. 1993;71:367–371.

Polikar R, Burger AG, Scherrer U, Nicod P. The Thyroid and the Heart. *Circulation*. 1993;87:1435–1441.

Pollock MA, et al. Thyroxine Treatment in Patients with Symptoms of Hypothyroidism but Thyroid Function Tests Within the Reference Range: Randomised Double Blind Placebo Controlled Crossover Trial. *British Medical Journal*. 2001;323:891–895.

Singer PA, Cooper DS, Levy EG, et al. Treatment Guidelines for Patients with Hyperthyroidism and Hypothyroidism. *Journal of the American Medical Association*. 1995;273:808–812.

St. Germain DL. Selenodeiodinases: Preceptor Regulators of Thyroid Action. *Thyroid Today*. 1999;22:1–11.

Tagliaferri M, et al. Subclinical Hypothyroidism in Obese Patients, Relation to Resting Energy Expenditure, Serum Leptin, Body Composition, and Lipid Profile. *Obesity Research*. 2001;9:196–201.

Teegardin C. State Drug Agents Looking for Link Between Thyroid Capsules, Ailments. *The Atlanta Journal-Constitution*. March, 29, 2001.

Toft AD. Thyroxine Therapy. *New England Journal of Medicine*. 1994;331:174–180.

Vaisman M, Soares DV, Buesca A. Chronic Inappropriate TSH Elevation in a Hypothyroid Patient During Replacement Therapy with Levothyroxine. *Endocrinologist*. 2000;10:125–126.

Woeber KA. Subclinical Thyroid Dysfunction. *Archives of Internal Medicine*. 1997;157:1065–1068.

Chapter 8

Annane D, Sébille V, Troche G, et al. A 3-Level Prognostic Classification in Septic Shock Based on Cortisol Levels and Cortisol Response to Corticotropin. *Journal of the American Medical Association.* 2000;283:1038–1045.

Castro M, Elias PC, Quidute AR, et al. Outpatient Screening for Cushing's Syndrome: The Sensitivity of the Combination of Circadian Rhythm and Overnight Dexamethasone Suppression Salivary Cortisol Tests. *Journal of Clinical Metabolics.* 1999;84:878–882.

Graham KE, Samuels MH. Recent Advances in the Evaluation of Cushing's Syndrome. *The Endocrinologist.* 1998;8:425–435.

Herman JP. Neurocircuit Control of the Hypothalamo-Pituitary-Adrenocortical Axis During Stress. *Current Opinion in Endocrinology and Diabetes.* 1999;6:3–9.

Jessop DS, et al. Resistance to Glucocorticoid Feedback in Obesity. *Journal of Clinical Endocrinology and Metabolism.* 2001;86:4109–4114.

Kung AWC. Cytokines and Hormonal Regulations. *Current Opinion in Endocrinology and Diabetes.* 1999;6:77–83.

Magiakou MA, Mastorakos G, Oldfield EH, et al. Cushing's Syndrome in Children and Adolescents: Presentation, Diagnosis, and Therapy. *New England Journal of Medicine.* 1994;331:629–636.

McCarty MF. Enhancing Central and Peripheral Insulin Activity as a Strategy for the Treatment of Endogenous Depression—an Adjuvant Role for Chromium Picolinate? *Medical Hypotheses.* 1994;43:247–252.

Newell-Price J, Trainer P, Besser M, et al. The Diagnosis and Differential Diagnosis of Cushing's Syndrome and Pseudo-Cushing's States. *Endocrine Reviews.* 1998;19:647–672.

Orth DN. Cushing's Syndrome. *New England Journal of Medicine.* 1995;332:791–802.

Papanicolaou DA, Yanovski JA, Cutler GB, et al. A Single Midnight Serum Cortisol Measurement Distinguishes Cushing's Syndrome from Pseudo-Cushing States. *Journal of Clinicial Endocrinolgy and Metabolism.* 1998;83:1163–1167.

Pittler MH and Ernst E. Efficacy of Kava Extract for Treating Anxiety: Systematic Review and Meta-analysis. *Journal of Clinical Psychopharmacology.* 2000;20:84–89.

Richard D. The Role of Corticotropin-Releasing Hormone in the Regulation of Energy Balance. *Current Opinion in Endocrinology and Diabetes.* 199;6:10–18.

Ridker PM, Hennekens CH, Buring JE, Rifai N. C-Reactive Protein and Other Markers of Inflammation in the Prediction of Cardiovascular Disease in Women. *New England Journal of Medicine.* 2000;342:836–843.

Rossi R, et al. Subclinical Cushing's Syndrome in Patients with Adrenal Incidentaloma: Clinical and Biochemical Features. *Journal of Clinical Endocrinology and Metabolism.* 2000;85:1440–1448.

Visser M, Bouter LM, McQuillan GM, et al. Elevated C-Reactive Protein Levels in Overweight and Obese Adults. *Journal of the American Society of Medicine.* 1999;282:2131–2135.

Wand GS. Alcohol and the Hypothalamic-Pituitary-Adrenal Axis. *The Endocrinologist.* 1999;9:333–341.

Weinstein JA, Isaacs SD, Shore DA, Blevins LS. Diagnosis and Management of Pituitary Tumors. *Comprehensive Therapy.* 1997;23:594–604.

Williams JE, et al. Anger Proneness Predicts Coronary Heart Disease Risk: Prospective Analysis from the Atherosclerosis Risk in Communities Study. *Circulation.* 2000;101:2034–2039.

Wing RR, Jeffrey RW. Benefits of Recruiting Participants with Friends and Increasing Social Support for Weight Loss and Maintenance. *Journal of Consulting and Clinical Psychology.* 1999;67:132–138.

Yanovski JA. The Dexamethasone-Suppressed Corticotropin-Releasing Hormone Test in the Differential Diagnosis of Hypercortisolism. *The Endocrinologist.* 1995;5:169–175.

CHAPTER 9

AACE Clinical Practice Guidelines for Growth Hormone Use in Adults and Children. *Endocrine Practice.* 1998;4:165–173.

Bach MA, Cambira M. Growth Hormone Releasing Peptides: Growth Studies. *Current Opinion in Endocrinology and Diabetes.* 1999;6:100–105.

Baker B. Growth Hormone Not Tied to Increased Mortality. *Internal Medicine Review.* 1999;Sept:40.

Bengtsson BA, et al. Therapeutic Controversy: Treatment of Growth Hormone Deficiency in Adults. *Journal of Clinical Endocrinology and Metabolism.* 2000:86:933–942.

Beuschlein F, Strasburger CJ, Siegerstetter V, et al. Acromegaly Caused by Secretion of Growth Hormone by a Non-Hodgkin's Lymphoma. *New England Journal of Medicine.* 2000;342:1871–1876.

Buckway CK, et al. The IGF-1 Generation Test Revisited: A Marker of GH Sensitivity. *Journal of Clinical Endocrinology and Metabolism.* 2001;86:5176–5183.

Cook DM. A Cardiovascular Pespective: The Impact of Long-Term Recombinant Human Growth Hormone Replacement Therapy (GHRT) in Adult GH-Deficient Patients. *Consults in Endocrinology.* 2000;1:1–9.

DeBoer H, Blok GJ, Voerman B, et al. Changes in Subcutaneous and Visceral Fat Mass During Growth Hormone Replacement Therapy in Adult Men. *International Journal of Obesity.* 1996;20:580–587.

Ferry RJ, Liu B, Cohen P. New Roles for IGF Binding Proteins. *The Endocrinologist.* 1999;9:438–450.

Frasier DS. The Diagnosis and Treatment of Childhood and Adolescent Growth Hormone Deficiency—Consensus or Confusion? *Journal of Clinical Endocrinology and Metabolism.* 2000;11:3988–3989.

Freda PU. Advances in the Diagnosis of Acromegaly. *The Endocrinologist.* 2000;10:237–244.

Gasperi M, Aimaretti G, Scarcello G, et al. Low Dose Hexarelin and Growth Hormone (GH)-Releasing Hormone as a Diagnostic Tool for the Diagnosis of GH Deficiency in Adults: Comparison with Insulin-Induced Hypoglycemia Test. *Journal of Clinical Endocrinology and Metabolism.* 1999;84:2633–2637.

Gibney J, Wallace JD, Spinks T, et al. The Effects of 10 Years of Recombinant Human Growth Hormone (GH) in Adult GH-Deficient Patients. *Journal of Clinical Endocrinology and Metabolism.* 1999;84:2596–2602.

Gotherstrom G, et al. A Prospective Study of 5 Years of GH Replacement Therapy in GH-Deficient Adults: Sustained Effects on Body Composition, Bone Mass and Metabolic Indices. *Journal of Clinical Endocrinology and Metabolism.* 2001;86:4657–4665.

Johannson G, et al. Growth Hormone Treatment of Abdominally Obese Men Reduces Abdominal Fat Mass, Improves Glucose and Lipoprotein Metabolism and Reduces Diastolic Blood Pressure. *Journal of Clinical Endocrinology and Metabolism.* 1997;82:727–734.

Kamel A, et al. Growth Hormone Treatment for Childhood Obesity. *Journal of Clinical Endocrinology and Metabolism.* 2000;85:1412–1419.

Klibanski A, Clemmons DR, Christiansen J, Underwood L. Growth Hormone Replacement Therapy for Growth Hormone Deficiency in Adults: The Changing Role of Growth Hormone Therapy. *Endocrine Practice.* 1999;5:88–96.

Laron Z, Klinger B. Comparison of the Growth-Promoting Effects of Insulin-like Growth Factor 1 and Growth Hormone in the Early Years of Life. *Acta Paediatr.* 2000;89:38–41.

Lo JC, et al. The Effects of Recombinant Human Growth Hormone on Body Composition and Glucose Metabolism in HIV-Infected Patients with Fat Accumulation. *Journal of Clinical Endocrinology and Metabolism.* 2001;86:3480–3487.

Mahajan T, Lightman SL. A Simple Test for Growth Hormone Deficiency in Adults. *Journal of Clinical Endocrinology and Metabolism.* 2000;85:1473–1476.

Roemmich JN, Rogol AD. Evidence Supporting an Adipo-Leptin-Growth Hormone Axis in Obesity-Related Hyposomatotropism. *The Endocrinologist.* 1999;9:424–430.

Shalet SM, Toogood A, Rahim A, Brennan BM. The Diagnosis of Growth Hormone Deficiency in Children and Adults. *Endocr Rev.* 1998;19(2):203–223.

Slonim AE, Bulone L, Damore M, et al. A Preliminary Study of Growth Hormone Therapy for Crohn's Disease. *New England Journal of Medicine.* 2000;342:1633–1637.

Takala J, Ruokonen E, Webster NR, et al. Increased Mortality Associated with Growth Hormone Treatment on Critically Ill Adults. *New England Journal of Medicine.* 1999;341:785–792.

Trainer PJ, Drake WM, Katznelson L, et al. Treatment of Acromegaly with the Growth Hormone-Receptor Antagonist Pegvisomant. *New England Journal of Medicine.* 2000;342:1171–1209.

Twigg SM, Baxter RC. Regulation of Serum Insulin-like Growth Factor Bioavailability. *Current Opinion in Endocrinology and Metabolism..* 1999;6:84–90.

Van Cauter E, Leproulot R, Plat L. Age-Related Changes in Slow Wave Sleep and REM Sleep and Relationship with Growth Hormone and Cortisol Levels in Healthy Men. *Journal of the American Medical Association.* 2000;284:861–868.

Vance ML, Mauras N. Growth Hormone Therapy in Adults and Children. *New England Journal of Medicine.* 1999;341:1206–1215.

Wallace JD, Cuneo RC. Growth Hormone Abuse in Athletes: A Review. *The Endocrinologist.* 2000;10:175–184.

Weinstein JA, Isaacs SD, Shore DA, Blevins LS. Diagnosis and Management of Pituitary Tumors. *Comprehensive Therapy* 1997;23:594–604.

Chapter 10

Apfelbaum M, Vague P, Ziegler O, et al. Long-term Maintenance of Weight Loss After a Very-Low-Calorie Diet: A Randomized Blinded Trial of the Efficacy and Tolerability of Sibutramine. *American Journal of Medicine.* 1999;106:179–184.

Bray GA, Blackburn GL, Ferguson JM, et al. Sibutramine Produces Dose-Related Weight Loss. *Obesity Research.* 1999;7:189–198.

Cangiano C, Ceci F, Cascino A, et al. Eating Behavior and Adherence to Dietary Prescriptions in Obese Adult Subjects Treated with 5-Hydroxytryptophan. *American Journal of Clinical Nutrition.* 1992;56:863–867.

Ceci F, Cangiano C, Cairella M, et al. The Effects of Oral 5-Hydroxytryptophan Administration on Feeding Behavior in Obese Adult Female Subjects. *Journal of Neural Transm.* 1989;76:109–117.

Considine RV, Caro JF. Pleiotropic Cellular Effects of Leptin. *Journal of Clinical Endocrinology and Diabetes.* 1999;6:163–169.

Farooqi IS, Jebb SA, Langmack G, et al. Effects of Recombinant Leptin Therapy in a Child with Congenital Leptin Deficiency. *New England Journal of Medicine.* 1999;341:879–884.

Finer N, Bloom SR, Frost GS, et al. Sibutramine Is Effective for Weight Loss and Diabetic Control in Obesity with Type 2 Diabetes: A Randomized, Double-Blind, Placebo-Controlled Study. *Diabetes, Obesity and Metabolism.* 2000;2:105–112.

Flier JS. The Adipocyte: Storage Depot or Node on the Energy Information Superhighway? *Cell.* 1995;80:15–18.

Gadde KM, et al. Bupropion for Weight Loss: An Investigation of Efficacy and Tolerability in Overweight and Obese Women. *Obesity Research.* 2001;9:544–550.

Hall JE, Shek EWM, Brands MW. Does Leptin Contribute to Obesity Hypertension? *Current Opinion in Endocrinology and Diabetes.* 1999;6:225–229.

Heymsfield SB, Greenberg AS, Fujioka K, et al. Recombinant Leptin for Weight Loss in Obese and Lean Adults: A Randomized, Controlled, Dose-Escalation Trial. *Journal of the American Medical Association.* 1999;282:1568–1575.

Kamal A, et al. Central Exendin-4 Infusion Reduces Body Weight Without Altering Plasma Leptin in (*fa/fa*) Zucker Rats. *Obesity Research.* 200;8:317–323.

Leibowitz SF. Brain Peptides and Obesity: Pharmacologic Treatment. *Obesity Research.* 1995;3(Suppl 4):S573–S589.

Lin L, Okada S, York DA, Bray GA. Structural Requirements for the Biological Activity of Enterstatin. *Peptides.* 1994;15(Suppl 5):S849–S854.

Lunetta M, DiMauro M, LeMoli R, Burrafato S. Long-term Octreotide Treatment Reduced Hyperinsulinema, Excess Body Weight and Skin Lesions in Severe Obesity with *Acanthosis nigricans. Journal of Endocrinol Invest.* 1996;19:699–703.

Mantzoros CS. The Role of Leptin in Human Obesity and Disease: A Review of Current Evidence. *Annals of Internal Medicine.* 1999;130:671–680.

McCarty MF. Vegan Proteins May Reduce Risk of Cancer, Obesity, and Cardiovascular Disease by Promoting Increased Glucagon Activity. *Medical Hypotheses.* 1999;53:459–485.

Mertens IL, Van Gaal LF. Promising New Approaches to the Management of Obesity. *Drugs.* 2000;60:1–9.

Moran TH, Sawyer TK, Seeb DH, et al. Potent and Sustained Satiety Actions of a Cholecystokinin Octapeptide Analogue. *American Journal of Clinical Nutrition.* 1992;55:S286–S290.

National Task Force on the Prevention and Treatment of Obesity. Long-Term Pharmacotherapy in the Management of Obesity. *Journal of the American Medical Association.* 1996;276:1907–1915.

Pellymounter MA, Cullen MJ, Baker MB, et al. Effects of the *obese* Gene Product on Body Weight Regulation in *ob/ob* Mice. *Science.* 1995;269:540–543.

Picard F, et al. Topiramate Reduces Energy and Fat Gains in Lean and Obese Zucker Rats. *Obesity Research.* 2000;9:656–663.

Ranganath L, Schaper F, Gama R, et al. Effect of Glucagon on Carbohydrate-Mediated Secretion of Glucose-Dependent Insulinotropic Polypeptide (GIP) and Glucagon-like Peptide-1 (7-36 amide) (GLP-1). *Diabetes and Metabolism Research Review.* 1999;15:390–394.

Rodriquez de Fonesca F, Navarro M, Alvarez E, et al. Peripheral Versus Central Effects of Glucagon-like Peptide-1 Receptor Agonists on Satiety and Body Weight Loss in Zucker Obese Rats. *Metabolism.* 2000;49:709–717.

Roemmich JN, Rogol AD. Evidence Supporting an Adipo-Leptin-Growth Hormone Axis in Obesity-Related Hyposomatotropism. *The Endocrinologist.* 1999;9:424–430.

Schwartz MW, Seeley RJ. Neuroendocrine Responses to Starvation and Weight Loss. *New England Journal of Medicine.* 1997;336:1802-1811.

Shuldiner AR, et al. Resistin, Obesity and Insulin Resistance—The Emerging Role of the Adipocyte as an Endocrine Organ. *New England Journal of Medicine.* 2001;345:1345–1345.

Steppan CM, et al. The Hormone Resistin Links Diabetes to Obesity. *Nature.* 2001;409:307–312.

Szayna M, Doyle ME, Betkey JA, et al. Exendin-4 Decelerates Food Intake, Weight Gain, and Fat Deposition in Zucker Rats. *Endocrinology.* 2000;141:1936–1941.

Weyer C, et al. Hypoadiponectinemia in Obesity and Type 2 Diabetes: Close Association with Insulin Resistance. *Journal of Clinical Endocrinology and Metabolism.* 2001;86:1930–1935.

Williamson DF. Pharmacotherapy for Obesity. *Journal of the American Medical Association.* 1999;281:278–280.

Yanovski JA, Yanovski SZ. Recent Advance in Obesity Research. *Journal of the American Medical Association.* 1999;228:1504–1506.

INDEX